Fundamentals of Frontline Surgery

Fundamentals of Frontline Surgery

Edited by
Professor Mansoor Khan
Consultant Oesophagogastric, General and Trauma Surgeon, Honorary
Clinical Professor of Trauma Surgery, Brighton and Sussex University
Hospital, Brighton, UK
Surgeon Commander Royal Navy (Retired)

and

Professor David Nott
Professor of Humanitarian Surgery, Imperial College London
Consultant Vascular, General and Trauma Surgeon. St Mary's Hospital,
Paddington, London, UK

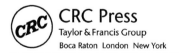

CRC Press
Taylor & Francis Group
Boca Raton London New York

CRC Press is an imprint of the
Taylor & Francis Group, an **informa** business

First edition published 2021
by CRC Press
6000 Broken Sound Parkway NW, Suite 300, Boca Raton, FL 33487-2742

and by CRC Press
2 Park Square, Milton Park, Abingdon, Oxon, OX14 4RN

CRC Press is an imprint of Taylor & Francis Group, LLC

This book contains information obtained from authentic and highly regarded sources. While all reasonable efforts have been made to publish reliable data and information, neither the author[s] nor the publisher can accept any legal responsibility or liability for any errors or omissions that may be made. The publishers wish to make clear that any views or opinions expressed in this book by individual editors, authors, or contributors are personal to them and do not necessarily reflect the views/opinions of the publishers. The information or guidance contained in this book is intended for use by medical, scientific, or health-care professionals and is provided strictly as a supplement to the medical or other professional's own judgement, their knowledge of the patient's medical history, relevant manufacturer's instructions, and the appropriate best practice guidelines. Because of the rapid advances in medical science, any information or advice on dosages, procedures, or diagnoses should be independently verified. The reader is strongly urged to consult the relevant national drug formulary and the drug companies' device or material manufacturers' printed instructions and their websites, before administering or utilising any of the drugs, devices, or materials mentioned in this book. This book does not indicate whether a particular treatment is appropriate or suitable for a particular individual. Ultimately, it is the sole responsibility of the medical professional to make his or her own judgments, so as to advise and treat patients appropriately. The authors and publishers have also attempted to trace the copyright holders of all material reproduced in this publication and apologize to copyright holders if permission to publish in this form has not been obtained. If any copyright material has not been acknowledged, please write and let us know so we may rectify in any future reprint.

Library of Congress Cataloging-in-Publication Data
Names: Khan, Mansoor, 1977- editor. | Nott, David (David M.), editor.
Title: Fundamentals of frontline surgery / edited by Professor Mansoor Khan and David Nott.
Description: First edition. | Boca Raton : CRC Press, 2021. | Includes bibliographical references and index. |
Summary: "Fundamentals of Frontline Surgery is an easy to read text, written by world class faculty, that provides clinicians with succinct and didactic information about what to do in high intensity, resource limited situations. With global conflicts and humanitarian emergencies on the rise, there has been a dramatic uptake in the number of volunteers for both military and humanitarian operations. This manual aids best practice and fast decision making in the field"-- Provided by publisher.
Identifiers: LCCN 2020035126 (print) | LCCN 2020035127 (ebook) | ISBN 9780367435592 (paperback) | ISBN 9780367437497 (hardback) | ISBN 9781003005469 (ebook)
Subjects: MESH: Surgical Procedures, Operative | Wounds and Injuries--surgery | Armed Conflicts | Disasters | Developing Countries | Health Resources
Classification: LCC RD31 (print) | LCC RD31 (ebook) | NLM WO 500 | DDC 617.--dc23

LC record available at https://lccn.loc.gov/2020035126
LC ebook record available at https://lccn.loc.gov/2020035127

ISBN: 978-0-367-43749-7 (hbk)
ISBN: 978-0-367-43559-2 (pbk)
ISBN: 978-1-003-00546-9 (ebk)

Typeset in Sabon
by MPS Limited, Dehradun

'Ut alii vivant'

(So others may live)

Contents

Forewords to Fundamentals of Frontline Surgery

Victims of armed conflict deserve the best trauma care possible. They already endure too much misery. Traditionally, humanitarian assistance has not excelled in the quality of care delivered. Good intentions are not good enough. Austere environments do not justify assistance with limited resources or poor skills. If a deployment for assistance is undertaken, there should be a well-prepared team, with the necessary skills, and the equipment as required.

Currently, there is a clear picture of the minimum requirements for emergency medical teams in disasters and conflicts. The (regrettable) experience of our military medical colleagues in recent conflicts has changed the concept of trauma care. Over the past 10 years, there have been good examples of sharing this military medical experience with humanitarian actors. The WHO Emergency Medical Team project, with professional input from humanitarian, military, and academic colleagues, has now defined these minimum requirements, and is in the process of verifying that emergency medical teams meet these standards. Patients with injuries from armed conflict and natural disasters do require a different approach as compared to trauma management 'at home'.

Additional training of the surgical teams is required. The book in front of you, Fundamentals of Frontline Surgery, will be an important tool for colleagues who would embark on humanitarian assistance or on military deployments. Extensive field experience of the international faculty is shared in this book, and thus, you will be able to identify your skill gaps, and act on it, before going on a mission.

On behalf of your future patients, I hereby thank you for your efforts in making good preparations for a mission, and optimising the assistance you will deliver. The victims deserve it!

Harald Veen, FRCSEd
Humanitarian and Conflict Surgeon

The end of the combat operations in Iraq and Afghanistan provided a sense of relief to all who bore the burden of those wars. However, the return to a period of relative peace can have the insidious effect of eroding the knowledge base and operational skills needed to manage the first casualties of the next war. This has been referred to as the *peacetime effect*.[1] In addition to maintaining surgical currency for future casualty care, there is an abundant need for proficiency in managing those who are ill or injured around the world as a result of political unrest, cross-border conflicts, natural disasters, poverty or a combination of these situations.

In this context, the editors of *Fundamentals of Frontline Surgery* have assembled a comprehensive set of exceptionally informative chapters that represents a weighty contribution to mitigating the peacetime effect. Professors Khan and Nott have combined decades of their own patient care experiences in resource-limited settings with their international prominence to provide a timely resource that is practical and straightforward to read, and that is addressed to all levels of training and experience. The range of topics explored in the textbook stretches from managing common injury patterns, to treatment of non-traumatic life-threatening conditions, to tips on the use of basic diagnostic tools and simple lifesaving maneuvers.

The opening chapter, entitled 'The Resource Limited Environment', is written by the editors and provides a strong foundation for the remainder of the book's content. In their opening, Professors Khan and Nott ready the reader with an overview of the utility of various echelons of care, the categories of humanitarian response and the laws of conflict. The subsequent chapters, written by seasoned, international experts, build upon the book's opening to provide a resource that is a "must read" for those learning about or going into harm's way to provide care. Although there are other resources dedicated to wartime and humanitarian surgery, *Fundamentals of Frontline Surgery* is a new approach with an aperture that captures just the right amount of practical content and detail. The textbook is an appropriate resource for the teacher, the learner and the practitioner.

No one academic initiative or group of authors can mitigate the dangers of the peacetime effect on surgical readiness. However, professionally created and timely projects like this textbook can help keep us, our students, our trainees focused and prepared. I congratulate the authors of *Fundamentals of Frontline Surgery* on their impressive accomplishments and recommend that we use the book's publication as an opportunity to shore up our knowledge base, our

professional partnerships and to maximize our readiness for the next mission.

Todd E. Rasmussen, MD
Professor of Surgery and Attending Vascular Surgeon,
The F. Edward Hébert School of Medicine at the
Uniformed Services University and Walter Reed
National Military Medical Center, Bethesda, MD

REFERENCE

1. Cannon JW, Gross KR, Rasmussen TE. *Combating the Peacetime Effect in Military Medicine. JAMA Surg.* 2020 Sep 16. doi: 10.1001/jamasurg.2020.1930. Online ahead of print.

Preface

Conflicts, war, and disasters. There is nothing new to describe these words when used; they are as old as history itself. What has changed, though, is the belief and acceptance that we must now provide the best possible medical care given the resources we have. Many may state that this is not possible or achievable. However, we will counter by saying that only with aspiration and the best possible care can we, given the resources available to us, stride to achieve frontline medical care.

This book is written for those who either voluntarily undertake risk or have no choice, those who are caught up in the web of humanitarian disasters and conflict. The expertise, experience, compassion, and dedication of the contributors to this text is immeasurable. Every author has dedicated a significant portion of their life and career to care for those who are in need, often putting their safety as a secondary concern.

Why did we choose to write, collate, and edit this text? There are now multiple textbooks and online resources available that can show how to undertake the practical aspects of conflict and humanitarian surgery. There is the International Committee of the Red Cross War Surgery text, present in two volumes, as well as the Surgical Training for Austere Environments course, held under the auspices of the Royal College of Surgeons of England. What this book provides is an invaluable, slim, and easy-to-access resource which highlights the fundamentals of frontline surgery and provides an excellent, easy-to-access text when deployed.

MAK
DMN

The Editors

Mansoor Khan is a Consultant Oesophagogastric, Trauma and General Surgeon as well as Honorary Clinical Professor of Trauma Surgery at Brighton and Sussex University Hospitals. He has recently retired from the Royal Navy, with the rank of Surgeon Commander after completing over two decades of military service with distinction. After graduation from King's College London in 2000, he undertook his House Officer training in Plymouth and Portsmouth, followed by three years of military posts. In November 2001 he graduated from Britannia Royal Naval College in Dartmouth and was deployed in the Northern Arabian Gulf on military operations upon completion. The remainder of his General Duties saw deployments in the Baltic and North Sea on NATO's Immediate Reaction Force of Minehunters, the 2003 Gulf War, and Counternarcotics deployment in the Caribbean.

Upon completion of three years of Military General Duties, he commenced surgical training, completing his rotations in Peterborough, Birmingham, and South Yorkshire. Having successfully obtained his FRCS in General Surgery in 2010, he subsequently got deployed on a busy tour at Camp Bastion in Afghanistan, followed directly by a one-year Trauma Critical Care Fellowship at the world-renowned R Adams Cowley Shock Trauma Center in Baltimore, Maryland, USA. He was appointed as a Consultant General Surgeon in the Defence Medical Services of the UK and subsequently was awarded a Fellowship of the European Board of Surgery and Fellowship of the American College of Surgeons. Since appointment as a Consultant Trauma Surgeon, he has undertaken multiple operational tours and was the Lead Clinician for the Military Team that was awarded the Military-Civilian Health Partnership Award in 2014 for Team of the Year, for his work in Afghanistan. He completed his military career with a four-month tour of South Sudan on a United Nations deployment. His military positions include the Consultant Advisor in General Surgery (Head of General Surgery) to Medical Director-General Royal Navy, and the Senior Lecturer in Military Surgery at the Royal Centre for Defence Medicine. Current positions include Visiting Professor of Physics at Imperial College London and a number of international Adjunct Professor of Surgery (USUHS, Bethesda and Shock Trauma, Baltimore), NIHR positions, overseas academic positions, Editor/Associate Editor and Reviewer for multiple journals, undergraduate and postgraduate examiner, Co-Director of the Definitive Surgical Trauma Skills course at the Royal College of Surgeons of England, and memberships in multiple international surgical organisations as well as being faculty on multiple international surgical training courses. He is keen on research and has published more than 200 publications, including book chapters, and conference papers and secured more than £3 million in research grants. His interests include research in primary injury prevention, blast mitigation strategies, haemorrhage control, trauma education, physiological monitoring, gut microbiome studies in relation to trauma and hypoperfusion, and oesophagogastric and general surgical techniques/advances.

David Nott trained to be a doctor at St Andrews and Manchester University, became a Fellow of the Royal College of Surgeons in 1985, and was subsequently awarded an MD for a thesis on Liver Surgery in 1989 from Manchester. He is a full-time NHS surgeon specialising in General, Vascular, Sarcoma, and Trauma Surgery at St Mary's Hospital and the Royal Marsden Hospital in London. Alongside a very busy civilian job, working in crowded major teaching hospitals, he has – for the past 25 years taken – took unpaid leave from the NHS to volunteer to work for the major aid agencies and has worked in

27 areas of conflict, most notably and recently, in Syria. He has also worked in areas of natural disasters, as in the earthquakes that affected Haiti and Nepal.

He has reservist military experience working as a surgeon in Basrah, Iraq, and Camp Bastion, Afghanistan, during the worst of the fighting in 2010. Over the years, he has gained enormous experience operating on every region and every speciality that is required to save lives from the effects of fragmentation and bullets. He has operated on thousands of patients, saving countless number of lives—sometimes in extreme circumstances both to the patient and himself. He was able to document most of these cases and use this knowledge to set up the David Nott Foundation in 2015 with his wife, Elly. This offers scholarships to surgeons from all over the world to come to get trained by him and his faculty on the Surgical Training for the Austere Environment course at the Royal College of Surgeons of England. This training is a distillation of all the most important procedures, including training in all the aspects of surgical and obstetric practice.

His foundation also takes the training to the frontline and recently ran the Hostile Environment Surgical Training course in Hajjah, Northern Yemen, in January 2020, using bespoke surgical simulations that accompany this course. In the last five years, over 800 surgeons have received training both in the UK and abroad, with an estimated 2.2 million patients benefitting from the training. His other love is flying, and he adapts human factors from flying into his work. A relatively little-known fact is that he holds an airline transport pilot licence and a helicopter licence, as well as being a fully accredited flying instructor. His humanitarian work has been recognised by the Queen of England, who awarded him an OBE in 2012; he also holds the prestigious Roberts Burns Humanitarian award, as well as doctorates and awards from both Welsh and UK universities.

List of Contributors

Nicholas Alexander FRCS, Consultant Paediatric Surgeon, St Mary's Hospital, Imperial College Hospitals NHS Trust, Praed Street, London, UK

Daniel Christopher Allison, MD, MBA, FACS, Assistant Professor of Surgery, Cedars-Sinai Medical Center, Los Angeles, California, USA

John H. Armstrong, MD, FACS, Former Florida Surgeon General and Secretary of Health, Tallahassee, Florida, USA

Mohammed Mar'ae Asieri, MD, MBBS, SB-Surg, Consultant Trauma/Critical Care Surgeon, Director of Trauma Center, Dammam Medical Complex, Dammam, Saudi Arabia

Avi Benov, MD, Israel Defense Forces, Medical Corps, Tel Hashomer, Ramat Gan, Israel; The Azrieli Faculty of Medicine, Bar-Ilan University, Safed, Israel

Richard J. Blanch, FRCS, Consultant Ophthalmologist, Academic Department of Military Surgery and Trauma, Royal Centre for Defence Medicine, Birmingham, UK

Johno Breeze, PhD, FRCS, Consultant Maxillofacial Surgeon, Royal Centre for Defence Medicine, University Hospitals Birmingham, Birmingham, UK

Katherine A. Brown, Institute of Shock Physics, Blackett Laboratory, Imperial College London, London, UK

Andrew P. Cap, MD, Department of Medicine, Division of Hematology/Oncology, San Antonio Military Medical, San Antonio, Texas, USA; Acute Combat Casualty Care Research Division, U.S. Army Institute of Surgical Research (USAISR), Ft. Sam Houston, Texas, USA, Department of Medicine, The Uniformed Services University of the Health Sciences Bethesda, Maryland, USA

Christopher Coulson, PhD, FRCS(ORL-HNS), Consultant Otologist & Skull Base Surgeon, Queen Elizabeth Hospital, Birmingham, UK

Paul J.H. Drake, MBChB, BSc, FRCS(Plast), MFCI, Consultant Plastic, Reconstructive & Aesthetic Surgeon, Queen Victoria Hospital Foundation Trust, East Grinstead & Brighton and Sussex University Hospitals Trust, East Grinstead, UK

Charles Anton Fries, MB, BChir, MA, MSc, FRCS (Plast), Consultant Plastic Surgeon, Oxford University Hospitals, Forward Surgical Team, Commando Forward Support Group, Oxford, UK

William G. Gensheimer, MD, Warfighter Eye Center, Malcolm Grow Medical Clinics and Surgery Center, Joint Base Andrews, Maryland, USA; Department of Surgery, Division of Ophthalmology, Uniformed Services University, Bethesda, Maryland, USA

Elon Glassberg, MD, Israel Defense Forces, Medical Corps, Tel Hashomer, Ramat Gan, Israel; The Azrieli Faculty of Medicine, Bar-Ilan University, Safed, Israel; Department of Medicine, The Uniformed Services University of the Health Sciences, Bethesda, Maryland, USA

Lorraine Harry, PhD, FRCS (Plast), MA (Cantab), MB, BChir, Plastic Surgery Consultant, Queen Victoria Hospital Foundation Trust, East Grinstead & Brighton and Sussex University Hospitals Trust, East Grinstead, UK

Kristin Hummel, DO, FACS, Major USAF (Retired), General Surgeon/Surgical Critical Care, SIM Galmi Hospital, Madaoua, Niger

Johann A. Jeevaratnam, FRCS, Plastic Surgery Registrar, Oxford University Hospitals, Oxford, UK

Dimitrios Kanakopoulos, MD, MSc, Trauma and Reconstructive Fellow, Plastic Surgery, Queen Victoria Hospital Foundation Trust, East Grinstead & Brighton and Sussex University Hospitals Trust, East Grinstead, UK

David S. Kauvar, MD, MPH, Lieutenant Colonel, United States Army Medical Corps, Vascular Surgery Service, San Antonio Military Medical Center, Department of Surgery, Uniformed Services University, Houston, Texas, USA

Boris Kessel, MD, Associated Professor of Surgery, Chief of Surgical Division, Hillel Yaffe Medical Center, Rappoport Medical School, Technion, Hadera, Israel

Mansoor Khan, MBBS, PhD, PGDip, FRCS, FEBS, FACS, CMgr, FCMI, Consultant Oesophagogastric, General and Trauma Surgeon, Honorary Clinical Professor of Trauma Surgery, Brighton and Sussex University Hospital, Brighton, UK

David R. King, MD, FACS, DABS, COL, US Army, Associate Professor of Surgery, Harvard Medical School, Division of Trauma, Acute Care Surgery, and Surgical Critical Care, Massachusetts General Hospital, Boston, Massachusetts, USA

Jonathan D.E. Lee, M.B., ChB, University Hospitals Birmingham NHS Foundation Trust, Birmingham, UK

Danyal Magnus, Institute of Shock Physics, Blackett Laboratory, Imperial College London, London, UK

Carlos Augusto M. Menegozzo, MD, Attending Surgeon, Division of General Surgery and Trauma, Hospital das Clínicas, University of Sao Paulo, Brazil; Head of the Surgical Point of Care Ultrasound Group, Sao Paulo, Brazil

Carlos Pilasi Menichetti, MD, MSc, Consultant General and Trauma surgeon, Consultant Obstetrician & Gynaecologist, Chief of Trauma and Emergency Surgery, Hospital San Juan de Dios, Santiago, Chile

Mark Midwinter, BMedSci (Hons), MB, BS, MD (Res), FRCS, CBE, Chair Clinical Anatomy, School of Biomedical Sciences, The University of Queensland, Brisbane, Australia

Jameel Muzaffar, MSc, FRCS(ORL-HNS), Research Fellow of University Hospitals Birmingham NHS Foundation Trust, Birmingham, UK

Roy Nadler, MD, Israel Defense Forces, Medical Corps, Tel Hashomer, Ramat Gan, Israel; Department of General Surgery and Transplantation-Surgery B, Chaim Sheba Medical Center, Tel Hashomer, Affiliated to Sackler School of Medicine, Tel Aviv, Israel

David Nott, DSc, MD, FRCS, Professor of Humanitarian Surgery, Imperial College London, London, UK; Consultant Vascular, General and Trauma Surgeon. St Mary's Hospital, London, UK

James V. O'Connor, MD, FACS, FCCP, Professor of Surgery, University of Maryland School of Medicine; Chief Thoracic and Vascular Trauma, Chief, Critical Care, R Adams Cowley Shock Trauma Center, Baltimore, Maryland, USA

Linda E. Orr, DM FRCS(ORL-HNS) OBE, Consultant ENT Surgeon, Queen Elizabeth Hospital, Birmingham, UK

Jowan Penn-Barwell, Consultant Orthopaedic Surgeon, John Radcliffe Hospital, Oxford University Hospitals, Oxford, UK

Bruno M. Pereira, MD, MSc, PhD, FACS, FCCM, Full Professor of Surgery – Post Graduation and Research Division, Masters Program in Health Applied Sciences, University of Vassouras, Rio de Janeiro, Brazil, CEO, Grupo Surgical, Campinas, Sao Paulo, Brazil; Director, General Surgery Residency Program – Campinas Holly House Hospital, Campinas, Sao Paulo, Brazil

William G. Proud, Institute of Shock Physics, Blackett Laboratory, Imperial College London, London, UK

Viktor Reva, MD, PhD, Assistant Professor, Department of War Surgery, Kirov Military Medical Academy, Saint-Petersburg, Russian Federation, Russia

Marcelo A. F. Ribeiro Jr., MD, MSc, PhD, FACS, Professor of General and Trauma Surgery, Chief of Acute Care and Trauma Surgery, Hospital Moriah, São Paulo, Brazil

Rebekka Troller, MD, General, Trauma and Humanitarian Surgeon, Addenbrookes Hospital, Cambridge, UK

Kevin Tsang, FRCS, Consultant Neurosurgeon, St Mary's Hospital, Imperial College Healthcare NHS Trust, Praed Street, London, UK

Avishai M. Tsur, MD, Israel Defense Forces, Medical Corps, Tel Hashomer, Ramat Gan, Israel

Carrie Valdez, MD, Spectrum Health Grand Rapids Level 1 Trauma Center, Michigan, USA; Acute Care Surgeon – Trauma, Emergency General Surgery, Trauma Surgery, Surgeon and Mission Co-leader: International Surgical Health Initiatives, Peru

Ori Yaslowitz, MD, Department of Surgery "A" Meir Medical Center, Kfar Saba and the Sackler Faculty of Medicine, Tel-Aviv University, Israel

Mark H. Yazer, MD, Department of Pathology, University of Pittsburgh, Pittsburgh, Pennsylvania, USA; Department of Pathology, Tel Aviv University, Tel Aviv, Israel

The Resource-Limited Environment 1

Mansoor Khan and David Nott

INTRODUCTION

There has been significant change in injury patterns of conflict over the last 100 years. In the initial Great War (World War I), there was a high burden of penetrating trauma from ballistic weaponry. Subsequently, the Second World War saw a rise in both blast and ballistic injury, the former occurring in maritime forces and the latter predominately in combat infantry units.

With the evolution of weaponry, defensive strategies also improved, especially in the advent of modern armour. There were significant number of torso injuries in the Korean and Vietnam conflicts, whereas, with the evolution of body armour, the injury pattern changed in the Iraq and Afghanistan conflicts to target junctional regions – neck, axillae, and groins.

The most recent conflicts in Iraq and Afghanistan have led to the widespread adoption of Improvised Explosive Devices (IEDs). These low-cost, easy-to-produce-and-distribute explosives have established themselves as 'territory depriver' and 'fear' weapons of choice by those who utilise them.

It is important to note that frontline surgery does not just refer to conflicts, but also surgical responses to humanitarian disasters. These, invariably by the time surgical facilities have been established, are not for the management of acute waves of injuries but rather for managing humanitarian and second waves of debridement and corrective surgeries. In these environments, particularly outside military evacuation chains, individuals with a high burden of injury invariably fail to survive in definitive care. The application point of wounding limb tourniquets has undisputedly led to substantial gains in casualty survival. Patients who survive require a spectrum of surgical care seldom in the skill set of a single surgeon. Humanitarian disaster relief, particularly from a surgical perspective, has a high burden of obstetric care.

WHAT MAKES CONFLICT OR DISASTER SURGERY DIFFERENT?

There are multiple, noticeable differences between conflict/military/humanitarian surgery when compared with normal civilian practice. Even within the conflict and disaster setting, there are different levels of care available compounded by hostilities, availability of resources, location of the conflict, manpower, and skill set availability. All of these factors greatly influence the capability of care available and, in some circumstances, rationalisation of healthcare with organisational and governmental matrices. The phrases 'austere' and 'resource-limited' are not interchangeable and, although sometimes interdependent, carry significantly different meanings.

Hostilities play a factor in terms of not only personal safety but also logistical supply lines. One of the greatest reasons for the survival of casualties is the evacuation chain and timeline. The vast majority of casualties during the conflicts in Iraq and Afghanistan reached definitive care in under one hour from time of injury. The greatest reason for this was air superiority; if the airspace isn't controlled, then this would not be a viable option. Humanitarian disasters, such as volcanic eruptions and severe weather, would invariably prevent an air evacuation chain and, needless to say, would compound the problems experienced by ground evacuation. Therefore, without air evacuation and air replenishment, a relatively well-stocked facility has the potential to become resource-limited.

An austere medical facility is not necessarily resource-limited. For example, Camp Bastion, although present in an austere environment, had all of the facilities – including the manpower of a fully functioning Westernised hospital. On the other hand, there are also many locations in the world where a Forward Surgical Team or a Non-Governmental Organisation Hospital facility is located in an austere setting with limited resources.

The level of facility and care available also plays a significant role in casualty management. The principles of damage control are often applied to allow transfer of patients between 'roles' or 'echelons' of care.

ECHELONS AND ROLES OF MEDICAL SUPPORT

The term 'role' or 'echelon' is used to describe the different levels of medical support in deployed operations. Different nations and armed forces will have differing notations to describe these roles/echelons, but they universally have the same definitions (Figure 1.1):

- Role 1 – Combat Medical Support provides medical care for routine primary care ailments and point of injury care for injured personnel, dealing with the CABC paradigm (Catastrophic bleed, Airway, Breathing, and Circulation). This is usually a key component in all forward-deploying military units, allowing for control of most compressible haemorrhage sites.
- Role 2 – Forward surgical team provides a significantly higher level of care than Role 1 and is able to manage non-compressible torso haemorrhage (NCTH). It has the ability to provide damage control resuscitation and damage control

surgery, allowing casualties to have immediate, life-threatening haemorrhage control before onward transfer. In certain circumstances, it may also offer a holding facility for casualties.
- Role 3 – Combat Support Hospital provides a significantly resourced facility in terms of specialities (determined by medical intelligence prior to deployment), diagnostics, and overall resources. In the last two decades, these have evolved into hardstanding facilities established for medium- to long-term missions.
- Role 4 – Repatriated Definitive Care Facility is usually located in the home country, or outside the conflict zone, of an allied nation. It provides the complete range of facilities and care that are unsuitable to deploy in conflict zones.

There are no defined echelons or roles of care in a humanitarian environment; the two broad categories that can be applied are immediate stabilisation and onward surgical care – in effect similar to Role 2 and Role 3 or Role 4 in the military setting.

EVACUATION CHAIN BETWEEN ROLES OR ECHELONS OF CARE

The injured has to transfer from one role to another to receive subsequent levels of care. They are usually managed in Role 1 by a Combat Medic and then transported either by vehicle or foot to the First Aid Post. From this point, they are transferred to a Role 2 facility by vehicle or an aeromedical asset. This usually occurs within the first hour of injury.

Once the patient has been stabilised and life-threatening injuries have been contained, he or she is transferred by aeromedical assets to Role 3; this can occur on the first 72 hours, depending on the operational environment. Subsequent transfer from Role 3 to Role 4 is taken as required but can be anywhere over 72 hours post-arrival.

For the patient to be transferred, a number of conditions need to be met:

- The patient must be physiologically stable for transfer;
- The patient's airway must be patent without danger of compromise;

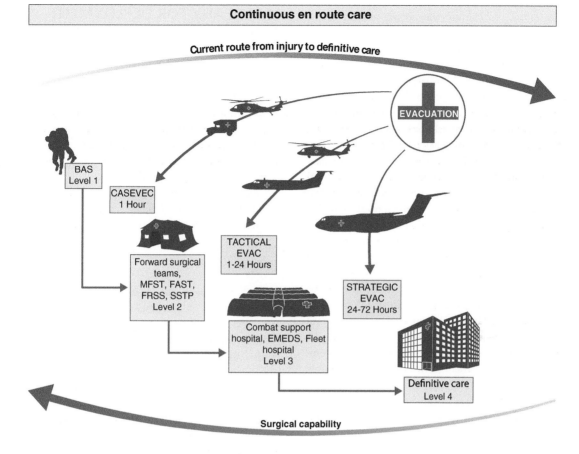

Figure 1.1 Roles of care.

- All access and tubing must be secured;
- A thorough CABC assessment should be made to identify any life-threatening injuries and treated prior to transfer (i.e. thoracotomies); and
- Patient should have protective measures against hypothermia implemented.

HUMANITARIAN OR CONFLICT RESPONSE CATEGORIES

The following classifications are based on the authors' experience and, to their knowledge, there are no similar references in literature. These classifications are borne of necessity, and arbitrarily, but they will help understand the different scenarios conflict and humanitarian surgeons may find themselves in.

In general, the situations faced in humanitarian work can be broadly divided into five categories:

1. High public financing
2. Developed country
3. Lesser developed country
4. Non-state actors, guerrilla groups
5. Natural disaster, earthquake, and tsunami

The first category, involving high public financing, is exemplified by the Defence Medical Services response within Afghanistan. This was a highly funded multi-national campaign which had arguably the best trauma hospital and prehospital facilities in the world.

An example of a developed country conflict would be that of the Libyan conflict in 2011. The environment is tagged as a warzone with unsafe infrastructure – difficult to enter and exit. The amenities are not reliable; there is depletion in manpower and an unreliable logistics chain.

The third category is still in a warzone but involves a lesser developed country, Yemen being a prime example. Much like Libya, entry and exit from the country is extremely difficult. There are comparable problems to that of Libya in 2011, but the general infrastructure and development of resources within the country are substantially less than those displayed by countries in Category 2.

Non-state actors and guerilla groups make up Category 4. Again, a warzone, but with several factions fighting for power. Invariably, there is an absence of a supply chain and logistical support, with depleted manpower and no facilities for transfer. This is without a doubt a resource-limited environment, usually in an extremely austere setting.

Category 5 can occur in a relatively well-developed country but, due to the nature of the event, can leave the region devastated. Initial entry may have to be via rotary-wing platforms, as runways and ports may be made inaccessible. Invariably, there will be a complete loss of infrastructure with no electricity supply or running water. The supply chains will take at least 7–10 days to establish. The major cause of morbidity after the first 24–48 hours is the lack of sanitation and potable water supply.

LAWS OF CONFLICT

All conflicts must abide by the International Humanitarian Law regulations. Modern laws have been generated over the last 100 years from the Geneva Conventions, charters set about by the United Nations and The Hague. They not only provide medical personnel with rights in times of armed war but also assign duties encompassing these rights. What is paramount is that healthcare professionals are bound by ethics to treat patients and prioritise care based on illness/injury and not according to their nationality, race, religion, gender, or political beliefs.

All healthcare professionals and facilities in times of conflict are protected by law and should not be immune from attack. However, this may not be feasible due to location constraints and identifying military healthcare facilities as modern conflict is unconventional.

AM I READY FOR DEPLOYMENT WITHIN A RESOURCE-LIMITED ENVIRONMENT?

The management strategies will invariably depend on the resources available, whether it be consumables, diagnostic/therapeutic equipment, or skill set of staff to name a few. The principles of Damage Control Resuscitation will invariable apply, as it involves sticking to the basics of combat casualty care. Decision-making of this nature is invariably complex and difficult and requires practice in the context of exposure, simulation, exercises, and courses.

Again, the question is: how do I prepare to be deployed in a resource-limited environment? There is an old military saying:

The more you sweat in Peace, the less you bleed in War.

To undertake such an arduous task, it is necessary to assume all planned procedures in an elective, non-resource limited setting. This is not just attending lectures and courses to brush up and learn new skills. Healthcare professionals must go and get regular exposure, not only to the operative skill set but also the high-level decision-making involved in these scenarios. Also, resilience must be augmented; not only will you have the operative stress but also the potential threat of risk to life.

When all is said and done, treat the casualty in front of you as your prime responsibility, and this is summed up well by the International Committee of the Red Cross Code of Conduct:

1. The humanitarian imperative comes first.
2. Aid is given regardless of the race, creed, or nationality of the recipients and without adverse distinction of any kind. Aid priorities are calculated on the basis of need alone.
3. Aid will not be used to further a particular political or religious standpoint.
4. We shall endeavour not to act as instruments of government foreign policy.
5. We shall respect culture and custom.
6. We shall attempt to build disaster response on local capacities.
7. Ways shall be found to involve programme beneficiaries in the management of relief aid.

8. Relief aid must strive to reduce future vulnerabilities to disaster as well as meeting basic needs.

9. We hold ourselves accountable to both those we seek to assist and those from whom we accept resources.

10. In our information, publicity, and advertising activities, we shall recognise disaster victims as dignified human beings, not hopeless objects.

Patterns of Injury 2

Danyal Magnus, Katherine A. Brown, Mansoor Khan,
and William G. Proud

CONTENTS

ENERGY RELEASE PROCESSES

How different are the effects of explosion from a large anti-tank mine and a knife wound? There are several ways: a range of effect, mortality rate, the number affected. The main parameter used in this chapter is the energy delivered to the human body and its effect. When an anti-personnel system operates, there is a combination of blast effect, projectile impact, fragments, and shrapnel cutting and burns – this can be described as simultaneously blown up, shot, and stabbed.

Bombs

Explosives are a particular example of a range of substances called 'energetic materials' (EMs). The term describes a variety of materials that can be divided into three broad categories: explosives, propellants, and pyrotechnics. Explosives are defined as materials which react to produce a violent expansion of hot gas – an explosion which rapidly delivers energy to its surroundings. The rate of transformation from solid to hot gas takes place in microseconds. Propellants are less violent in reaction and, as the name implies, are used to accelerate objects such as missiles and bullets. The time taken to go from solid to gas is in milliseconds. Some materials such as gunpowder can be used either as an explosive charge or as a propellant. The difference in behaviour is dependent on the amount of containment/confinement around the gunpowder – the more confined, the more violent the reaction. The last class is pyrotechnics, which are a myriad of chemical mixtures which react to produce intense heat, smoke, light, or noise with reaction times from milliseconds to several minutes. While the effect of a white-light flare can be easily appreciated, the blinding light and accompanying heat in pyrotechnics can present significant, hidden hazards. Magnesium Teflon, Viton (MTV) is a classic composition used in infrared-emitting flares, the flame is invisible to the naked eye, but the megawatt of energy released can cause deep, thorough skin burns. Several components of pyrotechnics can be toxic (or can release toxic materials), which can add a longer-term toxic effect on top of any acute effect.

A general way of thinking about an overall energetic system is the 'explosive train'. The train is a series of steps going from a low energy stimulus (e.g., standing on a pressure pad through a series of increasingly higher-energy intermediate states, finally detonating the main explosive charge. Amongst a range of activities, bomb disposal officers try to break the explosive train by separating the sensitive low-energy trigger from the main charge or de-activating the main charge directly.

The output of an explosive can be defined in terms of two factors: brisance and heave. The shock wave associated with a detonating explosive can be transmitted into materials causing them to shatter – brisance. In general, this only happens when the explosive and target material are in physical contact (e.g., the metal casing of a shell will produce a range of fragments).

The second effect is produced by the expansion of the hot, gaseous products which lift, separate, and throw materials – this is called heave. For example, 1 cm^3 of solid, room-temperature explosive can produce approximately 10 L of hot gas at temperatures well over 3,500 °C – a change in less than 1 ms, resulting in an expansion of volume by 10,000 times. The initial pressure of the product gases is in the range of 240,000 atmospheres. Hence, the violent expansion.

Most explosive devices produce both brisance and heave; the ultimate application determines the desired balance. Mining explosives tend to be of low brisance, high heave; military explosives tend to have more brisance and less heave. In this case, the aim is to shatter the target directly or to fragment a shell casing, afterwards accelerating the fragments outwards.

The expansion of product gases from explosives produces the blast wave. A blast is a supersonic wave

(velocity > 330 m s^{-1}) of compressed high-pressure air pushed by hot explosive products.

Figure 2.1 shows the pressure-time profile of a classic blast wave. This particular form is sometimes called a 'Friedlander' wave, an initial rapid rise of pressure expanding outwards from the explosion. The speed of the gas moving behind the blast front, the 'blast wind', can be as high as 2,000 km/h^{-1}. This is followed by a drop which can take the pressure below atmospheric pressure. This release occurs as both air and product gases rapidly expand away from detonating explosive.

This leaves a partial vacuum in the region of the initial explosion and this lower pressure causes air and gas to flow backwards. This push–pull movement can be especially damaging to structures and humans.

From an efficiency viewpoint, using an explosive against a vehicle or a human is a very energy-inefficient way of producing damage and injury but – the vital factor – is that the human body is not extraordinarily strong compared to the available energy in the explosive charge. A 10 kg charge of TNT will release approximately 40,000,000 J of energy, while only a fraction of a joule of appropriately placed energy will kill or maim a human.

Often, explosive charges are placed in the ground and the movement of a vehicle or an observer triggers the device. There are many factors that influence the behaviour of the floor during an under-vehicle explosion including vehicle design, explosive size, burial

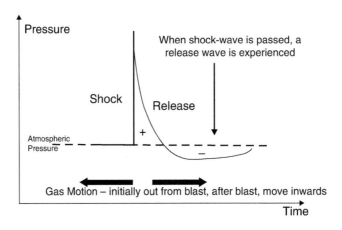

Figure 2.1 The classic Friedlander form of a blast wave.

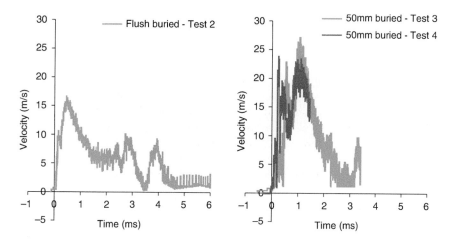

Figure 2.2 A comparison of the velocity–time graphs measured at the centre of the plate for the flush-buried and 50 mm deep-buried experiments with a 1 kg charge.

depth, and soil properties. Figure 2.2 shows a comparison of velocity-time data recording a sensor located at the centre of a rectangular flat armoured steel plate (Weldox 700 E, SSAB, Stockholm, Sweden), $20 \times 2500 \times 2000$ mm was used as a vehicle-floor surrogate. The experiment was on a charge flush-buried and a 50 mm deep-buried. The peak velocity in the 50 mm buried tests was higher than that in the flush-buried test and the time to peak was shorter.

The peak velocity measured in the buried tests was higher (by approximately 35%) than the flush tests. It is possible that this is because of a plug of soil being thrown against the plate in the buried tests, flush burying the explosive – the absence of a soil plug means that most of the impulse is transmitted through the expanding gas alone.

Projectile Injury

In principle, the penetrative process is quite simple: the strength of the skin is overcome and the projectile pushes through the bulk of the body, delivering kinetic energy to the surrounding flesh. If a sufficiently high velocity is used, the projectile will fully penetrate the body and an exit wound will be formed.

To put the levels of energy and pressure in perspective, a standard NATO round (7.62 mm diameter) has a muzzle velocity of $\sim$830 m s^{-1} and a kinetic energy of $\sim$1000 J. The impact pressure of such a projectile will be up to 320 kbars if a steel-on-steel impact occurs. If impacting water, gel, or the human body, the pressure is much lower – $\sim$15 kbars due to the lower density and strength of the flesh. As a result of the difference in impact pressure, projectiles striking armour steel are often severely deformed, while those penetrating flesh are not.

In the initial stages of impact, the projectiles send out a compressive pulse into the material, as seen in the experiments reported in part 1 of this review. For a small projectile, the release waves originate from the sides of the impact zone. When these waves overlap, a tensile region is formed where tears and cavities can be nucleated. In the body, this cavitation occurs in front of the projectile, tearing and weakening the structure. This is coupled with two more effects. First, the projectile pushes the target both forward and outwards. This results in a radial expansion of the hole carved out by the projectile, widening the overall cavity. It is this momentum transfer that opens the cavity, not the popular misconception that the cavity 'inflates' with gas rushing in. This would only be the case if the gun were at a remarkably close range (e.g., significantly below 1 m). A second effect occurs if the projectile is moving faster than the speed of sound in the air ($\sim$330 m s^{-1}), where

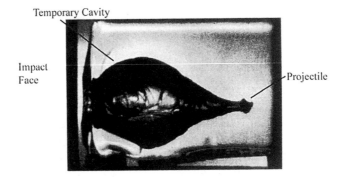

Figure 2.3 Cavities in gelatine caused by projectile penetration.

a sub-atmospheric pressure region with turbulent flow is found immediately behind the projectile. The effect of this is that air and other debris can be sucked into the expanding wound cavity.

This initial cavity is not permanent, as the flesh will spring back, forcing the air out of the cavity and reducing its volume. The maximum volume is referred to as the temporary cavity volume; it can easily be more than 200 cm^3 for a small arm (around 5.56 mm diameter), travelling at 800 m s^{-1}. Figure 2.3 shows the substantial extent of cavitation seen in simple gel targets.

Drapela et al. suggested for a 50% probability of skin penetration with an energy level of 25 J cm^{-2}. This is based on statistical averages of hit locations on the body taken from a wide database of injuries. However, they suggest the use of a lower value of 10 J cm^{-2} for practical purposes – to allow for the probability of impact on less robust areas of the body, such as the face and hands.

In broadest terms, the damage produced is dependent on the amount of energy transferred to the target. In many cases, a low-velocity projectile which penetrates but stops inside the body will produce more overall damage and probably push the target to the ground than a higher velocity projectile which penetrates fully, with a small reduction in velocity.

The penetration depth and energy loss of a 7.75 mm pistol around 300 m s^{-1} into gelatine showed the following penetration depth: 65 cm for 10% gelatine, 36 cm for 20% gelatine; energy loss rates averaged 3.48 and 5.93 J cm^{-1}, respectively. Pig flesh, regarded as a good human stimulant, showed a loss rate of 6.90 J cm^{-1}.

The path of the projectile can vary markedly even in homogeneous materials like soap. Assumptions of straight-line motion can be wildly inaccurate. The initial angle of impact, organ structure, presence of bones, lungs, etc. can all cause the bullet to change direction by 90° or more in a relatively short distance.

Bones do not tend to stop bullets, except if they enter at a very low speed (<100 m s^{-1} or much lower). Bones tend to shatter while deflecting the bullet, causing bone splinters which can lead to extensive secondary damage.

Sometimes, the projectile itself will shatter and cause multiple injury tracks. A 1995 Danish study examined fragmentation of 7.62 mm NATO systems. Rounds from one manufacturer were found to be unusually susceptible to shattering and would fragment after travelling ~100 m in free flight, when the projectile had been significantly slowed by the air. While fragmenting, explosive bullets are subject to legislation even in the 1899 Hague convention. However, in practice, a projectile may fragment in an unexpected fashion due to manufacturing processes, by ricochet, or by penetrating an armour system.

Body armour itself can sometimes modify the injury process in less predictable ways. Police reports show incidents where victims wearing Kevlar and other protective clothing have been injured or killed by gunfire, but that the protective clothing was not penetrated – a process called 'pencilling'. The physics of the injury is straightforward. The protective garments in these cases were worn as loose fitting or not backed by a solid support. The impacting bullet pushes both itself and part of the garment into the body. The garment captures the kinetic energy of the projectile and spreads the wound over a wider part of the body, as the projectile drives the garment into the body. Afterwards, the garment can be pulled from a relatively wide wound cavity, leaving a mildly distorted projectile in its folds.

Knives (and Fragments)

Knife crime amongst juveniles is of increasing concern. It is the simplest weapon, widely available, and requires little formal training. On average, it takes about 10 J of energy to push a sharp pointed knife into the human body if no bones are encountered. Data from knife injuries are of use in blast situations if one considers tertiary blast effects – the carrying of fragments and debris in the blast wind, shattered glass being driven by the blast wave, or falling from a height.

BLAST EFFECTS ON THE HUMAN BODY

When a blast wave reaches the human body, two effects dominate the interaction. First, the blast wave is directional. The wave strikes one part of the body first, compressing it into the so-far unaffected part of the body. This is the result of the higher sound speeds seen in the body compared to that of the blast wave. The softer biological organs

compress against the harder ones. The second effect, occurring milliseconds later when the body is completely enveloped in the blast wave, is a less directional, general compression of the soft tissues. The precise compression of a particular body part during the blast is difficult to precisely determine without the use of advanced diagnostics and computational models.

The two organs most affected by blast waves are those with the greatest air content: the lungs and ears. Figure 2.4 shows a compilation of data on the blast loading of the human body over a range of pressure and time. Shorter pulses have higher survival as there is less time, resulting in lower compression, so lung damage is limited. However, as the lungs have a fixed volume, there is a point when the lungs become non-functional, so little more damage can happen, and the survivability curves tend to flatten off.

It is important to note that survival rates are significantly lowered if the subject is close to a wall or other large, immobile, structure. In this case, the blast wave reflects from the wall and subjects the body to a second higher pressure pulse. As a general approximation, the pressure seen from waves reflected from walls and the earth tends to be twice than from the blast wave moving, unimpeded, through the air.

These data were produced over several experimental studies using a variety of animals (performed in a period when animal testing was not strongly regulated). This showed that creatures with small lung volumes per unit body mass were more susceptible to blast; also, those animals with denser lung

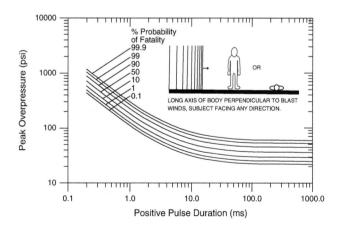

Figure 2.4 Data on survival rates against blast loading for the human body.

material were more vulnerable, probably due to increased stress transmission into the lung.

Blast Effects in Vehicles

These are most likely to occur for occupants of armoured vehicles, passing over a land mine or being stuck by non-penetrating projectile Lightweight vehicles (18 tons or less) are more susceptible than heavier ones; landmines of 12 kg TNT, equivalent content, or higher are estimated to incapacitate the whole crew. Large land mines may contain over 23 kg of explosive. Many papers exist on explosive loading of the vehicles and there is ongoing attention to isolating the crew from the violent vehicle motion.

Civilian medical knowledge of these injury types is well known due to sports such as boxing, traffic, and pedestrian-car accidents seen each year. Crash test and aerospace studies also provide good data. Some values of the acceleration required to incapacitate a subject are shown in Table 2.1.

Blunt Impact

These are impacts which do not penetrate the skin but cause pain and internal injury. Many of the studies relevant to this are found in non-lethal weapon systems – the flexing of helmets and body armour. Here, the energy is transmitted into the body by stress waves. These move across the interfaces from the impactor, through any intervening layers of armour or clothing, into the target. Most of the studies from the US Army land warfare laboratory use energy per unit area to allow comparison between slower-moving large projectiles and smaller high-velocity systems. The levels of energy are quite

small; non-penetrating projectiles with striking energy between 40 and 120 J can cause dangerous injuries (contusions, broken ribs, concussions, blindness, and damage in organs near the surface). With more than 120 J, considerable damage is expected (cranial breaks, renal and heart wounds, strong bleeding).

Other effects have been seen in blunt impact, the so-called two-strike phenomenon, and the effect of wave focusing.

The two-strike process is seen when a hard projectile strikes a target of finite thickness but does not penetrate. The target material initially moves with the projectile, but as waves reflect from the rear of the impacted material, the target loses contact with the impactor for a period (up to 1 s may be seen in some experiments) but is then restruck by the impactor. This effect is illustrated in the high-speed photograph in Figure 2.5.

In Figure 2.5, a steel ball is fired against a rubber band at several hundred metres per second. The rubber band is 2 mm thick. In frame one, the ball has started to push into the band, the time difference between each frame is 2.5 μs; the entire process is quite quick. The net effect is that the second contact can transfer a significant level of energy into the target as the first contact.

The second effect which may be seen in non-penetrative impact is that of shock-focusing based on the shape of the target. Figure 2.6 shows this effect in a disc of gelatine hit by a falling hammer. The timescale is short, a microsecond between each image. In the first frames, a wave is seen moving through this disc. This wave is compressive in nature. However, in frame 7 onwards, the wave has reached the sides of the gelatine disc and has now reflected as a release wave (taking the material from the high-stress state back to normal pressures).

Table 2.1 Accelerative forces and durations required for complete incapacitation		
Body part	**Impulse (nm)**	**Duration (ms)**
Head	>22	>2
Pelvis (vertical motion)	>111	>7
Spine (instantaneous)	>400	0
Spine (longer loading pulse)	>275	>30

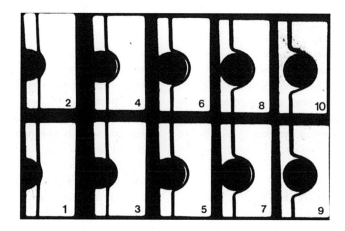

Figure 2.5 High velocity impact between a steel ball and a rubber band. Interframe time 2.5 μs, field of view 25 × 45 mm.

However, when the release wave focuses into a small region in frames 9 and 10, the net result is that the material in that region is put into tension. If the material is weak, then a cavity will be opened in the material. If, instead of gelatine, the material was brain tissue and the shape more like the cross-section of the human skull, the focusing of the wave will occur in a region towards the rear skull, near the spinal column – a particularly vulnerable region of the human body.

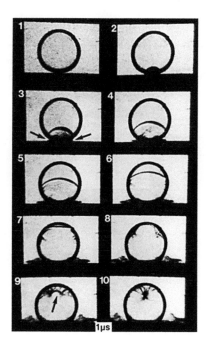

Figure 2.6 Gelatine disc struck from below by a metal plate.

Burns

A further effect of the shock is heating of the air and combustion of metal fragments – the pyrophoric effect. Depleted uranium is a known pyrophore and this is one of its many operational 'advantages'. This has increased the incidence of 'behind armour' burns. While some of the energy producing the burn is from direct contact with hot gasses (convective burning) and hot fragments, it is estimated that up to 50% of the energy can come from radiative sources (light) and bright flashes.

Numerous studies on the level of heat that can be supported by the skin have been conducted. Skin is thinnest on the eyelids (~0.5 mm) and thickest on the back (5 mm); an average value of 2.00 mm is used in many cases, when the skin reaches a temperature of 58 °C, pain is triggered.

Energy absorption in the skin is not a simple process; reflectivity and light absorption vary with wavelength. For high-temperature sources (4000 K), white skin will reflect 40% of the incident visible light incident upon it. The 60% energy absorbed can penetrate deeply and is absorbed through a thickness of 2.0 mm. Black skin reflects less and absorbs strongly in the outer melanin-containing layer, concentrating energy in a relatively small volume. This means that white skin is less susceptible to thermal heat flashes. It must also be added that white skin rates poorly compared to black skin in relation to ultraviolet-induced skin cancer for precisely the same reason – the depth of light penetration.

THE GLOBAL OVERVIEW: META-ANALYSIS OF BLAST INJURY

Fear of terrorism is common and understandable; it must be placed within the wider context of human activity. In this section, a meta-analysis of terrorist bombings is presented, but this is prefaced by a discussion of domestic and industrial explosions, where accident or negligence, as opposed to malice aforethought, was the cause.

Deliberate Acts

An upsurge of terrorist activity has occurred in the past two decades (Figures 2.7 and 2.8). As part of this, explosive devices continue to be extensively deployed against civilians in wide-ranging environments. Bombings remain the leading cause of civilian

fatalities worldwide due to terrorism. This demands an understanding of modern terrorist bombing trends to devise mitigation strategy. The objective of the study cited here is to identify the occurrence and severity of bombings against civilian targets in diverse attack settings and to establish corresponding blast injury profiles. Data were obtained from analysis of the Global Terrorism Database (GTD) and a meta-analysis of blast injury data is derived from the PubMed database.

Closed environment explosions were associated with significantly greater ($p < 0.05$) mortality than open spaces. The injury profiles were found to be influenced by attack setting, with higher rates of primary injury on trains and buses, and secondary injury in open space.

To link the casualties to injury mechanism and scenario, the following tables give a summary of types of injury seen and the scenarios. Further details on the types and causes of injury form the second section of this chapter. In medical literature, the types of blast injury are classified into four groups: primary are injuries associated with the blast wave alone, secondary are due to fragments or projectiles thrown by the blast, tertiary are due to the human body being thrown against other objects, and quaternary include burns, toxic shock, and acts as a catch-all class for injury types which are not mechanical in nature (Tables 2.2 and 2.3).

Table 2.4 compiles the range of injuries encountered. It is clear that tympanic membrane

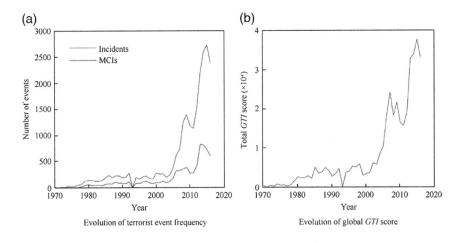

(a) Evolution of terrorist event frequency

(b) Evolution of global *GTI* score

Figure 2.7 Terrorist activity during the period 1970–2016.

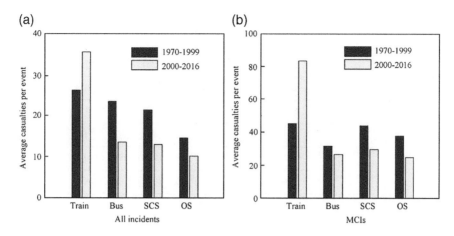

Figure 2.8 Distribution of terrorist events across attack settings.

Table 2.2 Blast injury classifications for review of epidemiological data

Blast injury mechanism	Classification
Blast lung injury (BLI)	Primary
Tympanic membrane perforation (TMP)	Primary
Intra-abdominal rupture	Primary
Penetrating torso	Secondary
Penetrating head, neck, and face	Secondary
Penetrating extremity	Secondary
Skull fracture	Tertiary
Other fracture	Tertiary
Traumatic amputation	Tertiary
Burns	Quaternary

Table 2.3 Key to attack setting

Attack setting	Example environments
Train	Train, trolley, subway
Bus	Bus, van, vehicle, taxi
Semi-confined space (SCS)	Restaurant, bank, hotel
Open space (OS)	City, village, road

perforation (TMP) is the most prevalent blast injury because it has been found to occur at a low peak pressure threshold of approximately 100 kPa for loading durations longer than 10 ms. The highest contrast comparison was observed between most enclosed environments (trains and buses) and open space. Open-space targets are less likely to suffer PBI or fireball injuries, with significantly fewer casualties presenting BLI, TMP, and intra-abdominal rupture. However, such targets are more susceptible to penetrating trauma due to the uninhibited trajectory of fragments. Tertiary injuries do not present a clear dependence on setting, though it is

Table 2.4 Injury rates across attack settings

Injury	Proportion Presenting Injury (± 95% CI)			
	Train	Bus	SCS	OS
BLI	8.40 (1.22)	17.69 (2.65)	6.87 (1.43)	2.96 (1.09)
TMP	46.29 (4.62)	29.70 (3.30)	40.96 (1.86)	11.53 (3.53)
Intra-abdominal Rupture	5.47 (1.00)	6.88 (3.47)	6.91 (2.77)	1.00 (1.07)
Penetrating Torso	7.81 (1.18)	26.39 (7.87)	22.35 (3.67)	28.25 (7.42)
Penetrating Head, Neck and Face	18.36 (1.71)	68.06 (8.33)	26.48 (2.75)	38.33 (7.40)
Penetrating Extremity	15.04 (1.57)	36.11 (8.58)	40.97 (5.81)	40.02 (9.68)
Skull Fracture	1.76 (0.58)	11.11 (5.61)	6.85 (1.75)	5.87 (3.33)
Other Fracture	33.40 (2.08)	6.75 (1.85)	23.38 (2.35)	16.28 (4.20)
Traumatic Amputation	7.34 (3.07)	0.77 (0.41)	2.55 (2.2)	0.00 (0.00)
Burns	17.38 (1.67)	16.49 (2.77)	28.9 (3.63)	7.08 (3.60)

noted that the mobile nature of trains and buses may be a key factor due to the potential for rapid deceleration of the vehicle. In terms of quaternary injury, burns are suffered to a greater extent in enclosed environments due to transient confinement of the fireball.

Addressing the threat of terrorism has been a long-standing priority of international agenda, particularly following the events of 9/11. Terrorism remains the subject of intense analysis by a broad range of research disciplines – studying changes in terrorist tactics, recruitment, operational scope, ideology, and weaponry. Though attacks may vary in their execution – from lone wolves to coordinated incidents – a hallmark of modern terrorism has been psychological warfare achieved through indiscriminate and ostensibly random attacks on the public, to inflict maximum morbidity and mortality. For this purpose, Improvised Explosive Devices (IEDs) have been utilised globally by terrorists with devastating effect. A wide range of epidemiological studies report blast injuries sustained by military populations, with less focus on civilians. For blast mitigation research, the civilian setting may be of special interest due to victims being unequipped with Personal Protective Equipment (PPE), allowing the unmitigated impact to be assessed. The civilian case raises challenges in the nature of the available data. Patients will often experience varied medical response and transit to trauma centres. In terms of clinical blast injury data, different trauma registries or

investigators provide wide-ranging degrees of medical record detail. The objective of the present study is to establish the incidence of blast attacks on civilian targets, and how this has changed in recent years. The effect of the blast environment was examined by determining the severity of these events based on the attack setting. Finally, epidemiological data for blast injuries sustained in these events were analysed with respect to attack setting.

The large casualty population over the studies included in the meta-analysis enable conclusions that may assist with devising blast mitigation strategy. Enclosed spaces are associated with enhanced primary blast injury, placing greater emphasis on the need to mitigate the blast wave. In open space, protection from fragment impact must be prioritised. Mitigation material design is fundamentally different in both cases. Blast-wave mitigants may incorporate deformable component for impulse energy absorption.

In the case of secondary injury, armour is conventionally designed to defeat ballistic or penetrating threats, typically utilising combinations of hard ceramic plates and aramid fibres. For civilians, structural rather than personal solutions must be sought. The greatest potential for structural design to provide mitigation is in the enclosed environment. There is a need for effective primary blast injury mitigation. Though terrorist activity has increased across all attack settings, a key finding of the GTD study was the upsurge of bus and train attack frequency and severity. This is supported by the blast injury meta-analysis, with train incidents resulting in greatest morbidity. In response to this, O'Neill et al. identified the structural components of trains and rail systems that must be addressed to mitigate the effects of the blast wave. Areas such as the walls, doors, and roof are of interest in introducing mitigation layers. An analogous need also exists in buildings where retrofitted cladding may be preferred. Such applications demand cost-effective, practical, and lightweight solutions.

In such scenarios, it should be remembered that the widespread use of various gases as a portable form of energy also entails some risk of explosion.

Domestic Explosions

Looking at the safety record of the UK with respect to gas supply and distribution, from 2010/2011 to 2014/2015, there was an average of 25 explosions/fires, resulting in an average of two deaths and 32 injuries each year (Table 2.5). Most of these deaths are likely due to the resulting fires rather than explosions. There was a significantly higher incident of carbon monoxide poisoning each year in the same period, resulting in seven deaths on average a year and an average of 290 incidents of non-fatal carbon monoxide poisoning in the same period. Overall, the fatality rate from methane is exceptionally low, as each year there may be up to 500,000 gas leakages. Technology to prevent gas being released, without being ignited, on heating and cooking appliances plus cut out systems to switch off the gas if CO is produced, have had a major effect.

Industrial Activity and Explosive Storage

Industrial explosions can be more devastating in both industrial plants destroyed or lives lost. In some cases, this may be due to fires during transport of flammable, volatile, or explosive materials. Three examples show the variety and scale of the effects seen.

Bhopal in India is globally remembered due to pressure developing in a storage vessel, leading to an explosive gas release followed by further gas venting, in December 1984. The release of methyl isocyanate led to the immediate death of between 3,787 and 16,000. A few 500,000 are said to have suffered ill effects.

The Ryongchon Station disaster, April 22, 2004, occurred when a flammable cargo exploded in North Korea, near the border of People's Republic of China. According to the Red Cross, 160 people were killed and 1,300 were injured in the disaster. A wide area was reported to have been affected, with some airborne debris reportedly falling across the border in China. The Red Cross reported that 1,850 houses and buildings had been destroyed and another 6,350 had been damaged.

Lethal fires in explosive storage facilities or factories occur worldwide, on average, once every two years, with other fires not causing immediate harm. This relative safety is due to the strength, remoteness, and security of explosive factories and storage facilities, the use of safety-distance rules, lightning

Table 2.5 UK gas leak incidents injuries and deaths between 2010 and 2015					
Incident type	**2010/11**	**2011/12**	**2012/13**	**2013/14**	**2014/15**
CO poisoning incidents	229	142	193	188	138
Explosion/fire incidents	36	24	25	20	20
CO poisoning fatalities	13	3	9	3	6
Explosions/fires fatalities	3	1	1	3	-
CO poisoning non-fatal	368	226	313	39	214
Explosions/fires non-fatal	48	32	34	22	23

protection, and specialist handling capabilities. However, on July 11, 2011, a large amount of ammunition and military explosives that had been stored outdoors for over two years at the Evangelos Florakis Naval Base, Cyprus, self-detonated. This killed 13 people, including the commander of the navy, the base commander, and six firefighters. Sixty-two people were injured. The ammunition had been seized in 2009 from a cargo ship bound for Syria. The explosion severely damaged hundreds of buildings and the nearby Vasilikos power station, causing widespread disruption in power supply to the island.

Quarrying and mining account for approximately 99% of all explosive use in the world. The petrochemical industry uses explosive charges in exploration, in perforating oil and water-bearing rock, and in general blasting. This is not without hazard and incidents related to explosion regularly occur, though the main dangers occur due to the collapse and flooding of tunnels, accidents with vehicles and machinery, plus long-term effects of dust and exposure to toxic materials.

The Natural World

There are two general scenarios of true explosions involving the rapid release of energy and gas expansion. These are volcanic eruptions, where the sudden release of pressure can produce blast waves and pyroclastic flows. Pyroclastic flows are fast-moving mixtures of hot gas and fragments. Volcanic activity is a well-documented phenomenon, and humans have tended to settle near active or dormant volcanoes due to the fertility of the soil. The second natural phenomena that are dramatically explosive is the impact of asteroids, meteorites, and comets. With impact velocities of up to 70 km/s^{-1}, the contact between the incoming body and the planet results in dramatic localised heating, vaporisation, and explosion with fragmentation. Such impacts are associated with the death of the dinosaurs and the explosion in Tunguska, Siberia, the early twentieth century.

If the effects of the natural world are classified by effects and not cause, then explosive-like effects are produced by tornados, whirlwinds, and hurricane conditions. The extreme winds produce strong loading on structures, and objects are entrained into the flow. Secondary injuries are produced by being thrown or violently carried by the wind, while tertiary injuries from projectile impact are common. Unlike explosive loading which is generally a millisecond to a second long, the loading from these extreme weathers can last minutes to hours leading building responses from sudden demolition to slow progressive collapse. For buildings in tornado areas, any added protection in terms of shielding, construction regulation, and the removal of objects and external features which can be moved by the wind along with the presence of internal safe spaces will assist in producing more blast-resistant structures.

THE EFFECT OF HIGH-STRAIN RATE ON BIOLOGICAL MATERIALS

Materials behave differently depending on the rate at which they are deformed. A simple example is a polymer sheet, which can be pulled slowly and will extend with little effort. If the same sheet is given a violent tug, the material behaves as if it was very rigid and may snap as opposed to deforming. Biological tissues are a form of complex polymeric composite often with collagen being a key material (e.g., in skin). In this section, we describe the effects of high loading rare on selected materials, skin, bone, and trachea, in each case indicating how the mechanical properties have changed the physical effect. The effects of strain rate and mechanical response influence the severity and areas of the injury.

Strain rates and the speed of deformation of the sample are a measure of the violence of the loading. The strain rates must be combined with the length of time, over which the loading takes place. Violent loading for short periods only produce superficial injury, colloquially we might call these a 'hard slap'. A low-rate, quasi-steady but severe load maintained over an extended period will result in crushing injuries throughout the body. Blast injuries tend to be produced by loading between these extremes. Alternatively, an extremity can be violently accelerated while the rest of the body, due to inertia, hardly moves – this will again lead to remarkably high localised strain rates and severe localised injury.

Bone

In most impact situations, one of the most common injuries is to the bones. A typical blast loading produces strain rates of 100 s^{-1} maintained over 10 ms can produce a localised strain of 0.1 or 10%. Effectively, a 30 cm bone will be crushed by 3 cm in a hundredth of a second. A result of the short time scales involves most of the damage occurring at the end. Medical evidence shows that injury caused by jumping from a building in the lower limb is less severe and more widely distributed over the length of the limb compared to the much more localised, more severe effects from an explosion.

Figure 2.9 shows the effect of strain rate on the strength of bone. The precise details of the loading can be found in the work of Cloete (2014). The main result is that bone behaves as a stronger material for strain rates around 10 s^{-1}. The strain rates associated with falling or jumping indicate the mechanical behaviour of the bone changes at these rates. The data in Figure 2.9 come from bovine specimens; however, the results are general across a range of mammalian species. The specimen goes to strain rates in the region of 100 s^{-1} and above the strength levels with no further increase. This means that bones subject to strong but sub-injury loads will behave as a stronger material. However, if this loading rate is increased, bones in the

region will break. This combination of increased strength at sub-injury levels combined with rapid failure leads to the strong localisation of bone injury seen in blast.

Skin

Soft tissues associated with skin and respiratory system are often damaged by blast. Characterising the material properties of these tissues over a range of loading rates representative of injury conditions is a crucial step towards developing biofidelic models for mitigation and biomedical applications. Comparative studies of the heterogeneous properties of fresh porcine skin are harvested from different anatomical regions (rump, upper back, and thigh). Compression experiments were performed at different strain rates using an Instron (low rate) and a SHPB system to mimic blast loading. Data obtained at a low strain rate of 1.0 s^{-1} using the Instron are shown in Figure 2.10. These data illustrate the variation in the relative stiffness of the skin samples over the body, reflecting differences in their underlying structure and compositions.

Other skin samples were subject to either low loading rate or high rate. Figure 2.11 shows optical images of histological sections stained with

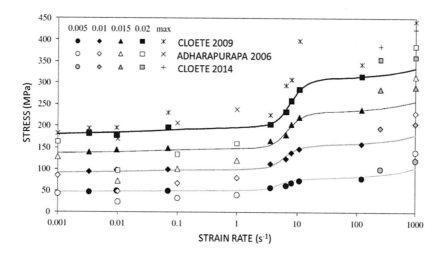

Figure 2.9 The bovine bone stress as a function of strain rate at strains of 0.005, 0.01, 0.015, and 0.02. Also shown is the maximum stress attained at each strain rate.

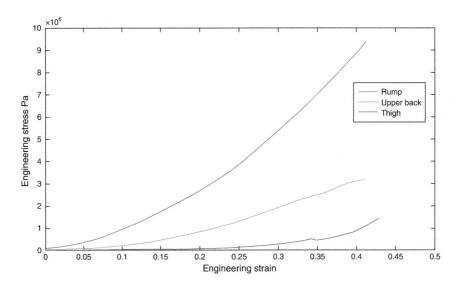

Figure 2.10 Comparison of the engineering stress-strain curves for skin taken from different anatomical regions. These were obtained on an Instron testing rig at a strain rate of 1 s^{-1}.

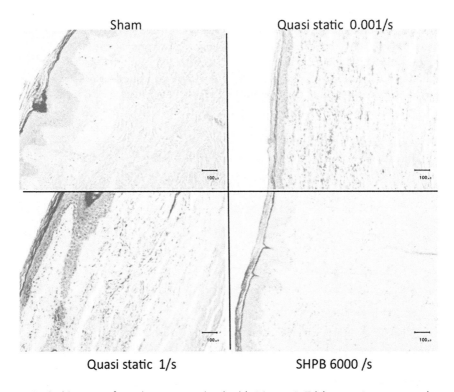

Figure 2.11 Optical images of porcine rump stained with Masson's Trichrome. Instron samples are labelled 'Quasi-static' and a Split Hopkinson Pressure Bar sample is labelled 'SHPB'. The dye infiltration pattern is greater in the samples subjected to compression compared to sham.

Masson's trichrome to investigate skin histology. These images show increased infiltration of dye in the samples subjected to compression, compared to a sample which was not loaded ('sham'). The level of dye infiltration decreases as the applied strain rate of loading increases. The increased presence of dye in slowly compressed samples indicates disruption of tissue organisation, most likely due to damage of collagen structures. At the higher loading rates, the severe localised disruption gives a clear region where infection can start, toxic materials intrude, and drive the severe disruption of the biochemical systems and provoke extreme histamine response.

The significant localised damage with increased strain rates associated with a blast seen in the both the bones and soft tissues indicates that the distribution and severity of the injury will increase markedly in a fashion not simply an extrapolation of that in 'normal' medical experience.

CONCLUSION

Overall, we can conclude with the following points:

1. Explosions produce high-rate loading both on people and the environment.
2. Injury processes are varied because of different physical mechanisms resulting in blast lung, heterotopic ossification, burns, and a range of localised bone and soft tissue damage. Many body areas are affected at once.
3. Blast injuries from terrorist activity will be increasingly seen from train and other easily accessible transport systems.
4. The severity and localisation of blast injuries within a limb or body part is, in part, caused by the marked changes in the mechanical behaviour of the human body tissues when loaded.
5. Blast injury severity and treatment are not a simple extension of 'normal' impact injuries.

ACKNOWLEDGEMENTS

The authors acknowledge the support of Imperial College London, AWE Aldermaston, EPSRC and the Royal British Legion Centre for Blast Injury Studies. Assistance and critical discussion were provided by Prof Sara Rankin, Dr David Sory, Dr Gareth Tear, Dr Thuy-Tien Nyugen Ngoc, and Dr Spyros Masouros.

FURTHER READING

1. Kinney GF, Graham KJ. *Explosive shocks in air.* Berlin: Springer-Verlag, 1985.
2. Cullis IG. Blast wave and how they interact with structures. *J R Army Med Corps* 2001;**147**:16–26.
3. Ngo TD, Mendis P, Gupta A, et al. *Blast loading and blast effects on structures.* EJSE 2007;**7**:76–91.
4. Magnus D, Khan MA, and Proud WG. Epidemiology of civilian blast injuries inflicted by terrorist bombings from 1970-2016. Defence Technol 2018.
5. Born CT. Blast trauma: the fourth weapon of mass destruction. *Scand J Surg* 2005;**94**:279–285.
6. Proud WG. The physical basis of explosion and blast injury processes. *J R Army Med Corps* 2013;**159** (Supp I):i4–i9. doi:10.1136/jramc-2013-000030.
7. Newell N, Neal W, Pandelani T, et al. The dynamic behaviour of a vehicle floor in under body blast, *J Mater Sci Res*;**5(2)**; 2016, 59–67.
8. Proud WG, Nguyen T-T N, Bo C. et al. The high-strain rate loading of structural biological materials. Metallurgical and Materials Transactions A.
9. Butler BJ, Williams A, Tucker WJ, et al. *Comparative quasi-static mechanical characterization of fresh and stored procine trachea specimens. Eur. Phys. J. Special Topics.* https://doi.org/10.1140/epjst/e2018-00104-5.
10. Cloete TJ, Paul G. and Ismail EB. *Hopkinson bar techiques for the intermediate strain rate testing of bovine coritcal bone. Phil Trans R Soc A 2014;***372**; 20130210. http://dx.doi.org/10.1098/rsta.2013.0210.
11. Draeger RH, Barr JS. *Blast injury. JAMA* 1946;**132(13)**: 762–767.
12. Ramasamy A, Masouros MD, Newell N, et al. In-vehicle extremity injuries from improvised explosive devices: current and future foci. *Phil Trans R Soc B* 2011; **366**:160–170.
13. Eiband M. *Human tolerance to rapidly applied accelerations: a summary of the literature.* Cleveland, OH: Memo 5-19-59E, NASA, Lewis Research Center, 1959.
14. Bowen IG, Fletcher ER, Richmond DR. *Estimate of man's tolerance to direct effects of air blast.* 1968 October, Report: DASA-2113.

15. Richmond DR, Yelverton JT, Fletcher ER. New airblast criteria for man. USA: Los Alamos National Laboratory; 1986 Aug Report: LA-UR-86.

16. Phillips YY, Mundie TG, Yelverton JT, et al. Cloth Ballistic vest alters response to blast. *J Trauma* 1988; **28**:S149–S152.

17. Crucq WJB. *The WB2D and computer phantom wound ballistics computer codes*. 14th International Symposium on Ballistics; 26–29 September 1993, QC, Canada, 777–784.

18. Drapela Ph, Lorenzo R, Lampert S. *How to quantify the effects of non-lethal kinetic weapons*. 24th International Symposium on Ballistics; 23–27 September 2008, New Orleans, USA, 1284–1290.

19. van Bree JLMJ, Gotts P. *The twin peaks of BABT*. Personal Armour Systems Symposium, Colchester, UK, September 2000.

20. Cronin DS, Worswick MJ, Ennis AV, et al. Behind Armour Blunt Trauma for Ballistic Impacts on Rigid Body Armour. In: *Proceedings 19th International Symposium on Ballistics*; 7–11 May 2001, Interlaken, Switzerland, 1003–1010.

21. Schanz B. Aspects on the choice of experimental animals when reproducing missile trauma. *Acta Chir Scand* 1979;**489**:121–130.

22. Fackler ML, Malinowski JA. Ordinance gelatin for ballistic studies. *Am J Forensic Med Pathol* 1988;**9**: 218–219.

23. Pirlot M, Dyckmans G, Bastin I. Soap and Gelatine for Simulating Human Body Tissue: An Experimental and Numerical Evaluation. In: *Proceedings 19th International Symposium on Ballistics*; 7–11 May 2001, Interlaken, Switzerland, 1011–1017.

24. Lewis EA, Horsfall I, Watson C. Pencilling: A Novel Behind Armour Blunt Trauma Injury. In: *Proceedings 22nd International Symposium on Ballistics*; 14–18 November 2005, Vancouver, BC, Canada, 1326–1333.

25. Pervin F, Chen WW, Weersooriya T. Dynamic compression response of the renal cortex. *Int J Struct Changes Solid* 2010;**2**:1–7.

26. Brown KA, Bo C, Masouros SD, et al. Prospects for studying how high-intensity compression waves cause damage in human blast injuries. In: *Proceedings Shock Compression of Condensed Matter 2011, AIP Conf. Proc. 1426* (2012):131–134.

27. Bo C, Balzer J, Hahnel JM, et al. Cellular characterization of compression-induced damage in live biological samples. In: *Proceedings Shock Compression of Condensed Matter 2011, AIP Conf. Proc. 1426* (2012):153–156.

28. Ramasamy A, Masouros SD, Newell N, Hill AM, Proud WG, Brown KA, et al. In-vehicle extremity injuries from improvised explosive devices: current and future foci. *Philos Trans R Soc Lond B Biol Sci* 2011;**366**:160–170. doi:10.1098/rstb.2010.0219.

29. Ramasamy A, Hill AM, Phillip R, Gibb I, Bull AMJ, Clasper JC. The modern 'deck-slap' injury--calcaneal blast fractures from vehicle explosions. *J Trauma* 2011;**71**: 1694–1698. doi:10.1097/TA.0b013e318227a999.

31. Boutillier J et al. 'A critical literature review on primary blast thorax injury and their outcomes'. *J Trauma Acute Care Surg* 2016;**81(2)**:371–379.

32. Gondusky JS, Reiter MP. 'Protecting military convoys in Iraq: an examination of battle injuries sustained by a mechanized battalion during Operation Iraqi Freedom II'. *Military Med.* 2005;**170(6)**:546–549.

33. Mellor SG, Cooper GJ. 'Analysis of 828 servicemen killed or injured by explosion in Northern Ireland 1970–84: the Hostile Action Casualty System'. *Brit J Surg.* 1989;**76(10)**:1006–1010.

34. Ritenour AE, et al. 'Incidence of primary blast injury in US military overseas contingency operations: a retrospective study'. *Ann Surg.* 2010;**251(6)**:1140–1144.

35. Smith JE. 'The epidemiology of blast lung injury during recent military conflicts: a retrospective database review of cases presenting to deployed military hospitals, 2003–2009'. *Philos Trans R Soc Lond B Biol Sci.* 2011;**366(1562)**:291–294.

36. Combs CC. *Terrorism in the twenty-first century*. New York: Routledge, 2017.

37. National Consortium for the Study of Terrorism and Responses to Terrorism (START). Global Terrorism Database. 2017. url:https://www.start.umd.edu/gtd (visited on Aug. 15, 2017).

38. Almogy G, et al. Suicide bombing attacks: can external signs predict internal injuries? *Ann Surg* 2006;**243(4)**:541.

39. Almogy G, et al. Can external signs of trauma guide management?: Lessons learned from suicide bombing attacks in Israel. *Arch Surg.* 2005;**140(4)**: 390–393.

40. Brismar BO, Bergenwald L. The terrorist bomb explosion in Bologna, Italy, 1980: an analysis of the effects and injuries sustained. *J. Trauma* 1982;**22(3)**:216–220.

41. Cooper GJ, et al. Casualties from terrorist bombings. *J Trauma* 1983;**23(11)**:955–967.

42. Hogan DE, et al. Emergency department impact of the Oklahoma City terrorist bombing. *Ann Emerg Med.* 1999;**34(2)**:160–167.

43. Katz E, et al. Primary blast injury after a bomb explosion in a civilian bus. *Ann Surg.* 1989;**209(4)**:484.

44. Miller ISM, McGahey D, Law K. The otologic consequences of the Omagh bomb disaster. *Otolaryngol Head Neck Surg.* 2002;**126(2)**:127–128.

45. Odhiambo WA, et al. Maxillofacial injuries caused by terrorist bomb attack in Nairobi, Kenya. *Int J Oral Maxillof Surg.* 2002;**31(4)**:374–377.

46. Patel HDL, et al. Pattern and mechanism of traumatic limb amputations after explosive blast: experience from the 07/07/05 London terrorist bombings. *J Trauma Acute Care Surg.* 2012;**73(1)**:276–281.

47. Persaud R, et al. Otological trauma resulting from the Soho nail bomb in London, April 1999. *Clin Otolaryngol.* 2003;**28(3)**:203–206.

48. Radford P, et al. Tympanic membrane rupture in the survivors of the July 7, 2005, London bombings. *Otolaryngol Head Neck Surg.* 2011;**145(5)**:806–812.

49. Rodoplu Ü, et al. Impact of the terrorist bombings of the Neve Shalom and Beth Israel Synagogues on a hospital in Istanbul, Turkey. *Acad Emerg Med.* 2005;**12(2)**:135–141.

50. Rodoplu Ü, et al. Impact of the terrorist bombings of the Hong Kong Shanghai Bank Corporation headquarters and the British Consulate on two hospitals in Istanbul, Turkey, in November 2003. *J Trauma Acute Care Surg.* 2005;**59(1)**:195–201.

51. Singh AK, et al. Radiologic features of injuries from the Boston Marathon bombing at three hospitals. *Am J Roentgenol.* 2014;**203(2)**:235–239.

52. Turégano-Fuentes F, et al. Injury patterns from major urban terrorist bombings in trains: the Madrid experience. *World J Surg.* 2008;**32(6)**:1168–1175.

53. Walsh RM, et al. Bomb blast injuries to the ear: the London Bridge incident series. *Emerg Med J.* 1995; **12(3)**:194–198.

54. Yazgan C, Aksu NM. Imaging features of blast injuries: experience from 2015 Ankara bombing in Turkey. *Brit. J. Radiol.* 2016;**89(1062)**: 20160063.

55. Zafar H, et al. Suicidal bus bombing of French nationals in Pakistan: physical injuries and management of survivors. *Eur J Emerg Med.* 2005;**12(4)**: 163–167.

56. Richmond DR, Yelverton JT, Fletcher ER. *New airblast criteria for man. Tech. rep.* Alexandria, Virginia: Los Alamos National Lab NM Life Sciences Div, 1986.

57. Proud WG, Goldrein HT, Williamson DM, et al. A review of the wound Ballistics part 1: non-penetrative injuries. *Explosives Eng* 2010:6–9.

58. Stuhmiller J, Philips YY, Richmond DR. The physics and mechanism of primary blast injury. Chapter 7. In: Bellamy RF, R. Zajtchuk Z, Buescher TM, eds. *Conventional warfare: ballistic, blast, and burn injuries.* Washington, DC: Walter Reed Army Institute of Research, 1991.

Damage Control Resuscitation 3

Mark Midwinter

DAMAGE CONTROL RESUSCITATION (DCR) IN RESOURCE-LIMITED ENVIRONMENT

Damage Control Resuscitation is a trauma care bundle aimed to prevent (or minimise the progression) the 'lethal triad' of hypothermia, acidosis, and coagulopathy after major traumatic injury. It is usually considered to consist of three elements: permissive hypotension, haemostatic resuscitation, and damage control surgery (DCS). There is a lack of solid evidence for DCR as an approach as so much of the established practice is from less robust studies and 'expert' opinion who are often embedded in well-resourced civilian and military trauma systems. This needs to be borne in mind when extrapolating to resource-limited environments (RLE).

To determine which patients require a DCR approach, some are applicable to all (such as keeping warm, stopping bleeding, etc.), but not everyone will need permissive hypotension or DCS (indeed may be harmed if immediate definitive care is not provided). It is also important in RLE to be selective in the full application of DCR to preserve resources. Therefore, how can patients who require a full DCR package be identified in RLE? The following is based on anatomic physiologic and laboratory parameters, but these are only a guide – clinical acumen and context is required (Table 3.1).

Damage controlled surgery will be addressed fully in subsequent chapters.

As a strategy, DCR elements should be introduced as temporally near the point of injury as possible and continuing through the chain of care. When considering DCR, resource limitation becomes a critical distinction in terms of both evidence base and application (Figure 3.1). The physiological constraints and goals of DCR may differ for well-developed and resourced trauma systems, where they are capable to move injured patients to an environment effective for definitive control of haemorrhage (either surgically or radiologically) in a timely manner. In establishments with prolonged timeline and the consequences of the approach of, for example, continuing permissive hypotension, may be detrimental (not disrupting the initial clot; however, prolonged poor tissue perfusion can cause accumulation of metabolic debt and acidosis). It is important to be cognisant of the constraints of the overall trauma system one is operating in, rather than just the limitations at a single point in the chain.

This has been explored by the Trauma Hemostasis and Oxygenation Research Network (THOR Network) and the Damage Control Resuscitation Organisation. The former has defined the specific concept of *remote* DCR (RDCR). This is not necessarily synonymous with resource limitation, as advanced retrieval services can deliver interventions into remote locations; less geographically remote areas may be temporally remote and resource-limited because of external limitation on the ground. The THOR Network concede that the limited evidence, sparse as it is, is mainly from well-developed trauma systems that have the capacity to capture and analyse data. This has been extrapolated to RDCR, supported by findings from work in animal models.

DCR is usually instigated commonly in an RLE of the point of injury, remote or otherwise, but progressively moves towards better-resourced facilities. This will determine what can be applied at a given time, so application may necessarily be incremental

Table 3.1 Damage control resuscitation potential predictors

Laboratory parameters	Physiological parameters	Anatomical parameters
Lactate >2.5 mmol L^{-1}	Weak/absent peripheral pulse	Penetrating abdominal or thoracic injury
Platelet count <90,000 mL^{-1}	Core temperature <35 °C	Multicavity injury
Fibrinogen <1.5 g dL^{-1}	Systolic BP <100 mmHg	Open pelvic fracture
INR > 1.5, PT > 16 seconds	Heart rate >100	Long bone fracture with head injury
ph < 7.2	PaO$_2$/FiO$_2$ < 250	
Base deficit <−6 mEq L^{-1}		

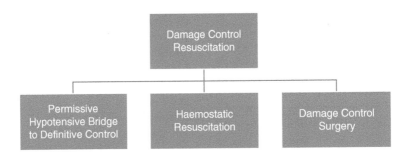

Figure 3.1 DCR potential management algorithm.

from pre-hospital to different echelons of medical treatment facilities (MTFs). The projection of more advanced interventions from the hospital to pre-hospital environment (such pre-hospital blood-based resuscitation, fluid warmers, etc.) with advanced retrieval services will augment care in the RLE.

The DCR bundle elements include preventing environmental exposure and keeping the patient warm; minimising cold, non-haemostatic fluid replacement, controlling compressible haemorrhage; maintaining blood pressure to perfuse vital organs but not aiming for normotension that could dislodge clot; early replacement of clotting factors and prevention of fibrinolysis with the use of tranexamic acid (within three hours of injury), and early planning and arrangement for DCS. Most of these interventions are deliverable in RLEs with low technology requirements (warming/protecting blankets, pelvic splint, compression bandaging and tourniquets, tranexamic acid). Supplemental oxygen has been shown to be beneficial also.

More logistically challenging is the delivery of blood products (debate continues about whole blood versus fractionated products) and surgical and critical care capability. Each RLE has its own specific limitation (from no designated MTF to a resuscitative MTF; limited retrieval to advanced retrieval). A checklist (Table 3.2) to determine the particular trauma system's physical vulnerabilities to aid in planning and understanding the operative constraints in RLE can be helpful. This needs to be considered with the timelines for patient movement through the trauma system.

Permissive Hypotension as a Bridge to Definitive Control

The level at which the systolic blood pressure (SBP) should be maintained with permissive hypotension remains a subject of debate (and clearly is not based on actual knowledge of patient's pre-injury blood pressure but is an arbitrary value for the

Table 3.2 DCR capability checklist	
Permissive hypotension	Monitoring SBP
	Point of care blood gas monitoring for serial pH and base excess measurement
Haemostatic resuscitation	Compressible haemorrhage control haemostatic ladder including haemostatic dressings tourniquets and pelvic binder
	Non-compressible haemorrhage control REBOA
	Blood products (whole, component, lyophilised, concentrate)
	Tranexamic acid
	Point of Care monitoring (viscoelastic, INR, PT)
Damage control surgery	Resuscitative packing, shunting
	Critical care transfer

individual from a population value). Consensus for target SBP of 100 mmHg has gained acceptance. If the constraint of resources or environment is such that blood pressure cannot be measured (e.g., prehospital at point of injury), then a palpable radial pulse can be used but, in an otherwise healthy adult, more closely approximates to SBP of 80 mmHg.

This implementation of permissive hypotensive strategy inevitably leads to the question of acceptable timelines, recognising that any delay will have physiological cost in response to injury and the effectiveness of DCR. The impact of prolonged permissive hypotension needs to be considered with the metabolic debt effect and in contribution to the acidosis arm of the lethal triad. This has been the driver for the concept of hybrid resuscitation where after one hour of permissive hypotension, the pressure is raised to more normotensive profile, but this has only been explored to any degree in military injuries with a blast component to the mechanism and relies on evidence from an animal model experiment. While this 'hybrid' resuscitation profile is theoretically an attractive concept in other traumatic mechanisms, it has not been tested in any clinically meaningful way.

The other question that needs to be considered is a multi-trauma patient with concomitant head injury. A balance between surviving and preserving brain perfusion to minimise the secondary brain injury needs to be considered. Here, the evidence base is even more sparse. The Brain Trauma Foundation 2016 guidelines are for *in-hospital* management. They state that there is a linear relationship between increasing SBP and reduced mortality and no SBP inflexion point between 40 and 119 mmHg to suggest a target blood pressure resuscitation endpoint. They suggest age-adjusted goals of ≥100 mmHg between 50 and 60 years old; ≥110 mmHg for 15–49- or >70-year-old patients. How this should be applied in the DCR setting in RLE is unclear.

Haemostatic Resuscitation

The priority is haemorrhage control; it may be considered compressible or non-compressible. Compressible haemorrhage control should be obtained according to a haemostatic ladder with direct pressure – a simple dressing progressing with the addition of a haemostatic dressing (e.g., Chitosan, zeolite, or kaolin-based dressing) and then, if still uncontrolled, use some device to restrict blood flow (such as a tourniquet). In some specific circumstances, it may be possible to directly control the injured vessel with a surgical clip/haemostat. Non-compressible haemorrhage (NCH) is unable to be controlled using this stepwise approach. NCH control relies more on promoting stable clot formation by permissive hypotension with haemostatic resuscitation, subsequently by definitive control measures such as surgery or interventional radiology in some circumstances. Newer techniques such as resuscitative endovascular balloon occlusion of the aorta (REBOA) is not widely adopted yet.

Effective coagulation depends on avoiding hypothermia, acidosis, and dilution coagulopathy.

Avoiding hypothermia by active warming may not be possible in a resource-limited environment; if available, they should be instigated. Avoiding cold fluids is also important (either by minimising the use of fluids as discussed earlier or, if required and resources allow, using fluid warmer). The avoidance of non-haemostatic fluids (e.g., crystalloids) will also reduce the risk of dilution of clotting factors. Using clotting factors containing fluid replacement (whole blood, fresh frozen plasma, lyophilised plasma) will help maintain clotting factors. Using fibrinogen concentrate has also been advocated.

The management of Trauma-Induced Coagulopathy (TIC) depends on recognising the two aspects contributing to the problem; (i) the exogenous factors of acidosis, hypothermia, and dilution of clotting factors that affect the normal coagulation pathways of platelets and enzyme reactions, and (ii) endogenous factors leading to the Acute Coagulopathy of Trauma (ATC) likely to be driven by tissue hypoperfusion and activated protein C mechanisms, decreasing fibrin production, and promoting fibrinolysis. Management of ATC is aimed at reversing or reducing these effects.

Replacing lost blood with whole blood has been advocated – this is hard to deliver except in well-resourced trauma systems. Whole blood in RLE can be circumvented to an extent with a donor panel but this requires both measures to assure blood safety, minimise risk, and access the donation equipment and laboratory facilities to test compatibilities.

Keeping a safe supply chain for red cells and plasma (more so platelets) is logistically demanding, particularly for transfer out of hospital environments. This may be an important capability for protracted retrieval timelines for transfer of patients to a medical treatment facility (MTF) and alternatives such as lyophilised plasma and fibrinogen concentrate become potentially useful.

Lyophilised plasma or fibrinogen concentrate can be delivered with little requirement for complex resources and are potentially useful adjuncts, along with tranexamic acid, to address fibrinolysis when planning a resource-limited trauma system.

In monitoring coagulation in RLE, this may be severely constrained. However, to preserve blood product usage may be invaluable. Viscoelastic measures of coagulation have gained wider acceptance and can be performed in more remote MTF but should not necessarily delay the execution of products earlier if the timeline dictates. Platelet provisions remain challenging even in well-resourced facilities. In an RLE, they are unlikely to be available but, in some contexts, frozen platelets can be supplied and projected forward in military operations.

Damage Control Surgery

This is more fully covered elsewhere but as an integral part of DCR, some consideration must be given in planning how the trauma system is to operate, especially in an RLE.

Any form of surgery will require an MTF – basic or mobile. DCS incorporates a critical care phase for physiological optimisation and this will most likely be unavailable, at least for a considerable time, in an RLE. The RLE DCS will be resuscitative but will require a high degree of physiological support post-intervention – to have utility requires arrangements that are in place for the timely transport of the patient with escalating management (such as a well-equipped and staffed retrieval system) to move patients to higher degrees of care and resources.

Procedures for RLE DCS will be aimed at haemorrhage control by packing, ligation, suture or shunt, and contamination control by removing gross contamination, obvious necrosis, and leaving wounds/incisions open and dressed.

Monitoring

While in severe RLE this may not be available, as the patient moves through the trauma system, early monitoring (certainly at forward MTF) will help conserve resources. Blood pressure and standard clinical vital signs, and the use of viscoelastic coagulation monitoring or point of care coagulation (PT, INR) may help the unnecessary use of blood product and conserve resources. Regular blood gas estimation to assess acidosis can also assist in determining the trajectory of the patient and help with decision regarding prolonging permissive hypotension and metabolic debt.

FURTHER READING

Philip C Spinella. *Damage control resuscitation. Identification and treatment of life-threatening haemorrhage.* Springer, 2019. ISBN 9783030208196.

Donald H Jenkins, Joseph F Rappold, John F Badloe, Olle Berséus. THOR Position Paper on Remote Damage Control Resuscitation: Definitions, Current Practice and Knowledge Gaps. *COL*, 2014.

Lorne Blackbourne, Karim H Brohi, Frank K Butler, LTC Andrew P. *Cap Shock*. 2014 May; **41(1)**: 3–12. doi:10.1097/SHK.0000000000000140.

No Blood ... What to Do?

Fluid Administration in Austere Environments

Avi Benov, Roy Nadler, Avishai M. Tsur, Ori Yaslowitz, Andrew P. Cap, Mark H. Yazer and Elon Glassberg

HAEMORRHAGE

Haemorrhage remains a major cause of trauma mortality, responsible for most pre-hospital death and is the most common aetiology of preventable death. Bleeding should be stopped as quickly as possible; once haemorrhage is controlled, efforts should be made to restore circulating volume. However, data have shown that many preventable deaths from haemorrhage involve the trunk – also known as non-compressible torso haemorrhages. Controlling such bleeding requires surgical interventions that sometimes are unavailable outside of the hospital. To bridge this gap in capabilities and maintain end-organ perfusion and oxygenation, alternative and supplemental treatment methods are needed. Volume resuscitation using intravenous fluids is aimed at expanding the intravascular volume, increasing pre-load and cardiac output, and ultimately improving tissue perfusion, regardless of whether the cause of shock is a compressible or non-compressible haemorrhage.

The optimal resuscitation fluid should be safe, cheap, easily available, can carry oxygen, be able to promote haemostasis, and be stable under a variety of storage conditions and temperatures without special preparation before use. Over the last decades, crystalloid-based solutions have been the mainstay of volume resuscitation. The use of crystalloids was advocated by most surgical and emergency medicine societies worldwide, and numerous volume resuscitation protocols have been developed. However, published data indicate that crystalloid based resuscitation is detrimental for patient outcomes. Damage control resuscitation principles supporting

the early transfusion of blood products featuring packed red blood cells (PRBC), plasma, and platelets are now widely accepted for in-hospital care at ratios as similar as possible to 1:1:1. Current data also support the use of PRBCs and plasma in prehospital environment, despite the challenges involved with the use of blood products. Although data from randomised trials comparing the use of stored whole blood with balanced component therapy are not currently available, the 2009 US National Trauma Data Bank data set was used to evaluate the relationship between transfusion type and mortality in adult patients with major trauma (n = 1,745). Logistic regression analysis identified three independent predictors of mortality: Injury Severity Score, emergency medical system transfer time, and type of blood transfusion: whole blood or components. Transfusion of whole blood was associated with reduced mortality; thus, it may provide superior survival outcomes in this population. It is expected to be at least as good as conventional component therapy, with a trend towards lower mortality and faster correction of an abnormal lactate concentration amongst the whole blood-recipients.

TREATMENT OPTIONS IN THE PREHOSPITAL ARENA

Whole Blood

Stored whole blood (SWB) and fresh whole blood (FWB) provide FFP: RBC: PLTs in a physiologic ratio. SWB is most provided as low titre group O whole blood (LTOWB). The AABB (formerly known as the American Association of Blood Banks) requires any facility using LTOWB to locally determine the number of units that a patient can receive, the nature of the patients, and the maximum anti-A and anti-B titre threshold. Civilian and military practices of LTOWB vary in terms of these parameters. Also, the length of time that an LTOWB unit can be stored and transfused varies, but the duration can never exceed that specified by the nature of the anticoagulant in which the whole blood was collected. LTOWB offers a more 'concentrated' product compared to reconstituted whole blood using conventional components, as whole blood is collected into 70 mL of storage solution/anticoagulant whereas each conventional RBC unit transfused contains up to 110 mL of additive solution that permits the extended storage of the RBCs up to 42 days; the additive solution does not carry oxygen, nor does it promote haemostasis. FWB is also collected into 70 mL of solution, but it is not stored for a prolonged period before its transfusion. FWB is not normally permitted for civilian use as it is not tested for transmissible diseases before transfusion. Both LTOWB and FWB offer several other advantages over separated blood products, including convenience in transportation than separate units of RBCs, plasma, and platelets and reduced risk of bacterial contamination compared to conventional warm stored platelets and simplifying the logistics of the resuscitation by offering all three components in one bag. In fact, in a study of paediatric trauma patients, the use of LTOWB was shown to provide balanced resuscitation quicker than when only conventional components were used, even though a massive transfusion protocol that included the immediate provision of platelets was available at the hospital where the study was conducted.

The evidence to support the use of LTOWB, especially in early resuscitation, is mounting, albeit indirectly. In a secondary analysis of a randomised controlled trial that demonstrated the superiority of adding two units of plasma transfusion to the standard of care during the helicopter evacuation of trauma patients to a hospital, receipt of any blood product during pre-hospital resuscitation yielded a significantly improved 30-day survival rate compared to patients who received crystalloids alone. A greater survival benefit was demonstrated amongst those who received RBCs and plasma compared to those who received plasma alone. While this study did not involve the transfusion of LTOWB directly, the combination of RBC and plasma transfusion would have been provided by LTOWB, in addition to a small dose of cold-stored platelets (which might be hyper-functional compared to their room temperature-stored). During the recent conflicts in Iraq and Afghanistan, for casualties presenting haemorrhagic shock, a transfusion strategy that included FWB with RBCs and plasma was associated with improved survival compared to the use of stored components only (FFP, RBCs, and PLTs). Compared to SWB or component therapy, FWB is available in austere conditions (requires only the presence of donors and collection equipment), has no loss of clotting factor or platelet activity that is often associated with storage, and has no red blood cell 'storage lesion'.

PACKED RED BLOOD CELLS

The main advantage of a packed red blood cell (PRBCs) transfusion is the replenishment of oxygen-carrying capacity. Emergency transfusion of PRBC when the recipient blood group is unknown should be performed using only type O units. In the past, resuscitation of bleeding trauma patients was based on the transfusion of high volumes of PRBCs, in ratios reaching 10:1 between PRBCs and plasma. However, recent data suggest that imbalanced transfusion ratios with high ratios of PRBCs have a detrimental effect on patient outcomes. Thus, most resuscitation protocols now instruct a balanced transfusion of PRBCs with plasma and platelets. In prehospital scenario, the use of PRBCs is hindered by the need for cold storage and controlled temperature capability, so most prehospital systems do not provide PRBCs at the point of injury. Some systems, however, provide PRBCs during transport for patients suffering from haemorrhagic shock. The positive effect of prehospital PRBCs transfusion was demonstrated in a retrospective analysis of US military combat casualties treated during aeromedical evacuation; early transfusion of PRBCs was associated with improved survival.

PLASMA

The use of plasma as a resuscitation fluid holds many theoretical advantages – plasma has a high oncotic pressure which allows effective intravascular volume preservation, a physiologic pH level for mitigation of trauma-related acidosis, and a normal concentration of clotting factors that can potentially reduce the lethal trauma-induced coagulopathy. Emergency transfusion of plasma to patients of unknown blood group should be performed with group AB or A plasma. Abundant data support the beneficial effect of early plasma-based resuscitation. Most of these data are derived from in-hospital care; however, in recent years, prehospital systems are adopting the use of plasma as a resuscitation fluid, replacing the classic crystalloids-based resuscitation with some preliminary data supporting the beneficial effect of prehospital plasma use already available. The main obstacle to prehospital plasma use remains the logistical challenge. The most used plasma is either thawed fresh frozen plasma (FFP) or liquid, never-frozen plasma. These fluids require refrigeration, and unless being used in a high-volume environment, will result in a high wastage rate. A possible solution to the logistical constraints of liquid plasma transfusion is freeze-dried plasma (FDP). FDP has similar biochemical properties of thawed FFP or liquid plasma, can be stored at ambient temperatures, has a shelf life of 18–24 months, and can be reconstituted and ready to use within minutes. These characteristics of FDP make it an ideal product for plasma administration in prehospital scenario and point of injury care. Several FDP products are currently available worldwide.

CRYSTALLOIDS

These are solutions of water and electrolytes, including 0.9% normal saline (NS), lactated Ringer's solution (LR), and Hartmann's solutions (HS). NS is slightly hypertonic, containing equal amounts of sodium and chloride, causing it to be both hypernatremic and hyperchloremic. Replenishing extracellular fluid volume with a large volume of saline was previously advocated, especially during the wars in Korea and Vietnam. However, the widespread use of isotonic fluids was not without harmful effects,

such as the so-called Da Nang lung (later termed acute respiratory distress syndrome or ARDS), compartment syndrome, coagulopathy, hyperchloremic metabolic acidosis, immune dysfunction, kidney injury, and eventually, increased mortality.

An important study that investigated outcomes of trauma patients who were resuscitated using large volumes of crystalloid was published in 1994 by Bickell et al. In this study, hypotensive patients with gunshot or stab wounds to the torso were randomised to receive crystalloid therapy before surgery, including during transport to the hospital (early), or to only receive fluids during their surgical procedure (delayed). The randomisation was effective: the patients in the early fluid intervention group received an average of 870 ± 667 mL of crystalloid fluid in the pre-hospital phase of their resuscitation compared to an average of 92 ± 309 mL in the delayed resuscitation group ($p < 0.001$). Similarly, the volume of crystalloid administered after arrival at the trauma centre and before the surgery was also significantly higher in the early intervention group compared to the delayed intervention group ($1608 \pm 120l$ vs. 283 ± 722 mL, respectively, $p < 0.001$). There was an 8% reduction in mortality in the group that only received fluids during their surgical intervention compared to the early fluid resuscitation group; patients in this group also had a significantly shorter average hospital length of stay, without an increase in postoperative complications.

LR and HS more closely resemble plasma as they contain potassium, calcium, and lactate – with less sodium and chloride than 0.9% NS – and seemed reasonable alternatives for NS, especially for trauma patients. Indeed, LR was found superior to NS for haemorrhagic shock resuscitation since NS caused a more severe metabolic acidosis, worsened coagulopathy, and led to increased blood loss. However, LR still contributes to coagulopathy by hemodilution and does not provide oxygen-carrying capabilities.

COLLOIDS

Colloids are aqueous solutions that also contain electrolytes and organic macromolecules. These macromolecule constituents are unable to cross the endothelial membrane of the blood vessels, remaining within the intravascular space, exerting higher oncotic pressure than the electrolytes contained in crystalloids. Several types of colloids are in use, differing in the type of macromolecules contained in each. The most common options include albumin, hydroxyethyl starch (HES), gelatins, and dextrans. Despite the presumed rationale for colloid, compared with crystalloid use, the expected greater intravascular volume expansion was not shown to improve the prognosis of patients suffering from haemorrhagic shock. Furthermore, colloids were shown to increase kidney injury, impair immune function, and worsen coagulopathy.

TRANEXAMIC ACID

Tranexamic acid (TXA) inhibits the enzymatic breakdown of fibrin blood clots (fibrinolysis) and is expected to reduce bleeding. The CRASH 2 trial, a large prospective interventional trial, showed that in trauma patients suffering from major bleeding, early administration (under 3 hours from injury) of TXA reduces mortality. Subsequent analysis showed that delay in treatment (beyond 3 hours) increase mortality. The MATTERS study reinforced the results of the CRASH 2 trial, a retrospective analysis conducted on haemorrhaging combat casualties in a military hospital. The results of these studies led to widespread implementation of TXA administration both in prehospital scenario – by military and civilian systems – as well as in trauma bays. The recently published CRASH-3 study demonstrated that TXA is also effective in reducing mortality in patients with mild to moderate isolated traumatic brain injury.

HOW DO I STOP THINKING ABOUT THE FUTURE AND TREAT THE PATIENT NOW?

To provide casualties with optimal care, austere environment providers must not only overcome the challenge of choosing the ideal of the worst options available but also deal with the fact that the best resuscitative protocol is yet to be determined and supported by high-quality studies. One should treat patients using practical means – making sure that compressible bleeding has stopped, using a single

infusion bag at a time, aiming for a restored radial pulse, mental status, or systolic blood pressures – depending on the specific protocol used. These boluses are to be repeated if necessary.

The decision to use blood products is a medical decision and, in most countries, it must be made only by a physician. In an austere environment, the medical provider should have full knowledge of both the clinical situation and the availability of compatible blood products. Establishing a Walking Blood Bank (WBB) Program before treatment, based on risk assessment and potential for casualties, is recommended.

Patients in shock need resuscitation. Patients who have mechanisms of injury likely to produce shock (traumatic amputation, penetrating injury to the thorax or abdomen) will probably require transfusion prior to shock. Transfusions should be prioritised in patients clearly in shock and then to those who will need blood, based on injury patterns and volume lost, but who are not yet in shock. The goal, if resources permit, is to keep the latter patients out of shock:

- Where and when possible – whole blood (fresh or stored)
- Plasma, RBCs, and platelets in a 1:1:1 ratio
- Plasma and RBCs at a 1:1 ratio
- Any of the blood products available – RBCs/plasma
- Freeze-dried/reconstituted dried plasma
- Combination of solutions with physiologic activity: Albumin + Fibrinogen concentrate
- If all you have left is NS – Let's face it, in the RDCR/austere environment context, if this is all you have, you better have some training in palliative care as well

WHENEVER SHOCK IS DIAGNOSED, ADMINISTER TRANEXAMIC ACID (TXA)

Administer 1 g of tranexamic acid in 100 mL Normal Saline or Lactated Ringers as soon as possible but NOT later than 3 hours after injury. When given, TXA should be administered over 10 minutes by IV infusion.

KEY POINTS

1. Follow preceding algorithm.
2. Initiate hypothermia prevention that should occur along with treatment.
3. Blood products induce hypocalcemia. Treatment should start early. Give 2 g CaCl or 6 g Ca gluconate EARLY (<4 U transfused).
4. Documentation.
5. Follow adverse effects.

FURTHER READING

1. Standards for blood banks and transfusion services. 31st ed. Bethesda, Maryland: AABB, 2018.
2. Yazer MH, Spinella PC. The use of low-titer group O whole blood for the resuscitation of civilian trauma patients in 2018. *Transfusion* 2018;**58**:2744–2746.
3. Yazer MH, Spinella PC. Review of low titer group O whole blood use for massively bleeding patients around the world in 2019. *ISBT Sci Seri.* 2019;**14**:276–281.
4. Seheult JN, Anto V, Alarcon LH, *et al.* Clinical outcomes among low-titer group O whole blood recipients compared to recipients of conventional components in civilian trauma resuscitation. *Transfusion* 2018;**58**:1838–1845.
5. Seheult JN, Bahr MP, Spinella PC, *et al.* The Dead Sea needs salt water… massively bleeding patients need whole blood: The evolution of blood product resuscitation. *Transfus Clin Biol.* 2019.
6. Yazer MH, Cap AP, Spinella PC. Raising the standards on whole blood. *J Trauma Acute Care Surg.* 2017.
7. Leeper CM, Yazer MH, Cladis FP, *et al.* Use of uncrossmatched cold-stored whole blood in injured children with hemorrhagic shock. *JAMA Pediatr.* 2018;**172**:491–492.
8. Sperry JL, Guyette FX, Brown JB, *et al.* Prehospital plasma during air medical transport in trauma patients at risk for hemorrhagic shock. *N Engl J Med.* 2018;**379**:315–326.
9. Guyette FX, Sperry JL, Peitzman AB, *et al.* Prehospital blood product and crystalloid resuscitation in the severely injured patient: a secondary analysis of the prehospital air medical plasma trial. *Ann Surg.* 2019.
10. Reddoch KM, Pidcoke HF, Montgomery RK, *et al.* Hemostatic function of apheresis platelets stored at 4 degrees c and 22 degrees c. *Shock* 2014;**41 Suppl. 1**: 54–61.
11. Pidcoke HF, McFaul SJ, Ramasubramanian AK, *et al.* Primary hemostatic capacity of whole blood: a comprehensive analysis of pathogen reduction and refrigeration effects over time. *Transfusion* 2013;**53 Suppl. 1**: 137S–149SS.
12. Bickell WH, Wall MJ, Jr., Pepe PE, *et al.* Immediate versus delayed fluid resuscitation for hypotensive patients with penetrating torso injuries. *N Engl J Med* 1994;**331**:1105–1109.
13. Cap AP, Pidcoke HF, Spinella P, Strandenes G, Borgman MA, Schreiber M, Holcomb J, Tien HC, Beckett AN, Doughty H, Woolley T, Rappold J, Ward K, Reade M, Prat N, Ausset S, Kheirabadi B, Benov A, Griffin EP, Corley JB, Simon CD, Fahie R, Jenkins D, Eastridge BJ, Stockinger Z. Damage control resuscitation. *Mil Med.* 2018 Sep 1;**183(suppl. 2)**:36–43. doi:10.1093/milmed/usy112.
14. Guyette FX, Sperry JL, Peitzman AB, Billiar TR, Daley BJ, Miller RS, Harbrecht BG, Claridge JA, Putnam T, Duane TM, Phelan HA, Brown JB. Prehospital blood product and crystalloid resuscitation in the severely injured patient: a secondary analysis of the prehospital air medical plasma trial. *Ann Surg.* 2019 Apr 13. doi: 10.1097/SLA.0000000000003324. [Epub ahead of print]
15. Sperry JL, Guyette FX, Adams PW. Prehospital plasma during air medical transport in trauma patients. *N Engl J Med.* 2018 Nov 1;**379(18)**:1783. doi: 10.1056/NEJMc1811315. No abstract available.
16. Shakur H, Roberts I, Bautista R, Caballero J, Coats T, Dewan Y, El-Sayed H, Gogichaishvili T, Gupta S, Herrera J, Hunt B, Iribhogbe P, Izurieta M, Khamis H, Komolafe E, Marrero MA, Mejía-Mantilla J, Miranda J, Morales C, Olaomi O, Olldashi F, Perel P, Peto R, Ramana PV, Ravi RR, Yutthakasemsunt S. Effects of tranexamic acid on death, vascular occlusive events, and blood transfusion in trauma patients with significant haemorrhage (**CRASH-2**): a randomised, placebo-controlled trial. *Lancet.* 2010 Jul 3;**376(9734)**:23–32. doi: 10.1016/S0140-6736(10)60835-5. Epub 2010 Jun 14.
17. Roberts I, Shakur H, Afolabi A, Brohi K, Coats T, Dewan Y, Gando S, Guyatt G, Hunt BJ, Morales C, Perel P, Prieto-Merino D, Woolley T. The importance of early treatment with tranexamic acid in bleeding trauma patients: an exploratory analysis of the **CRASH-2** randomised controlled trial. *Lancet.* 2011 Mar 26;**377(9771)**:1096–1101, 1101.e1-2. doi: 10.1016/S0140-6736(11)60278-X.
18. Morrison JJ, Dubose JJ, Rasmussen TE, Midwinter MJ. Military application of tranexamic acid in trauma emergency resuscitation (**MATTERs**) study. *Arch Surg.*

2012 Feb;**147(2)**:113–119. doi: 10.1001/archsurg.2011.287. Epub 2011 Oct 17. PMID: 22006852.

19. Studer NM, April MD, Bowling F, Danielson PD, Cap AP. Albumin for prehospital fluid resuscitation of hemorrhagic shock in tactical combat casualty care. *J Spec Oper Med.* Summer 2017;**17(2)**:82–88. PMID: 28599038.

20. CRASH-3 trial collaborators. *Effects of tranexamic acid on death, disability, vascular occlusive events and other morbidities in patients with acute traumatic brain injury (CRASH-3): a randomised, placebo-controlled trial. Lancet.* 2019 Oct 14. pii: S0140-6736(19)32233-0. doi: 10.1016/S0140-6736(19)32233-0. [Epub ahead of print].

21. Roberts I, Belli A, Brenner A, Chaudhri R, Fawole B, Harris T, Jooma R, Mahmood A, Shokunbi T, Shakur H; CRASH-3 trial collaborators. Tranexamic acid for significant traumatic brain injury (The CRASH-3 trial): Statistical analysis plan for an international, randomised, double-blind, placebo-controlled trial. Version 2. *Wellcome Open Res.* 2018 Sep 26 [revised 2018 Jan 1];*3*:86. doi: 10.12688/wellcomeopenres.14700.2. eCollection 2018.

22. Cap AP. *CRASH-3: a win for patients with traumatic brain injury. Lancet.* 2019 Oct 14. pii: S0140-6736(19)32312-8. doi: 10.1016/S0140-6736(19)32312-8. [Epub ahead of print] No abstract available. PMID: 31623893.

Point-of-Care Ultrasound 5

Carlos Augusto M. Menegozzo and Bruno M. Pereira

INTRODUCTION

In mentioning the Resource-Limited Environment (RLE), we are narrowing our focus to pre-hospital care scenario with few resources or critical care conditions. These are usually clinical situations in remote or hard to reach areas, rescue in wild areas, battlefield, and space flights – among others. It is important to mention that one of the main missions of pre-hospital care in this scenario is to provide fast, high-quality care, and subsequently transport patients quickly from the remote site to definitive care, avoiding delays and negative outcomes.

To increase the quality of care in a distant/critical environment and reduce mortality, recent advances in point-of-care ultrasound (POCUS) in pre-hospital care stands out. Historically, POCUS has its first reports of military use as a screening tool in harsh environments and remote locations. This fact is corroborated by articles and consensus statements that choose POCUS as a priority in the care of critically ill patients in this scenario. POCUS is, therefore, supposed to be focused on specific issues such as traumatic and non-traumatic acute pulmonary changes, presence of cavity fluids, aetiology of shock and acute neurological damage—in other words, identification of acute life-threatening conditions. While POCUS has several applications in austere environment, three protocols are the most comprehensive in this scenario: E-FAST, RUSH, and Optic Nerve Sheath Diameter (ONSD).

RESOURCE LIMITATION CONCERN

POCUS has gained widespread utilisation due to its several advantages over other image gadgets. It is low-cost, does not expose patients to radiation, and yields real-time images. However, one of the main reasons why healthcare providers working in austere environments should master POCUS is its portability and accuracy as a diagnostic tool. Indeed, the development of pocket-sized ultrasound machines has revolutionised the patients' bedside assessment. Probes are now used as an extension of physical examination by trained physicians, enhancing diagnostic accuracy without the need for further testing. By applying POCUS as an adjunct to interventional procedures, patients can be more safely managed. POCUS outperforms conventional radiographs in several life-threatening situations in terms of diagnostic accuracy, while displaying portability and procedure-guidance advantages. Computerised tomography (CT) yields better results in terms of diagnostic accuracy, although it presents several cumbersome features such as the use of ionising radiation, the need to transport patients to dedicated suites, higher costs, and greater equipment size. These features render POCUS an invaluable tool in the assessment, management, and triage of patients in remote locations.

In an RLE, triage decisions are critical. Scarce resources push healthcare providers to make decisions based on the best evidence available. In that sense, POCUS offers advantages with its wide range of applications in the fields of Emergency, General Surgery, and Trauma, as an adjunct for life-saving decision-making. It is a small, pocket-size machine which provides excellent diagnostic and interventional results.

BRIEF REVIEW OF MATERIAL

In an RLE scenario, portability and size matter. There are several ultrasound machines with such characteristics in the market. It is also important to bear in mind the basic ultrasound principles, temperature and battery concerns, and the specifications of each transducer. The principles of ultrasound are not the scope of this chapter and can be found in several textbooks and articles. Due to climate extremes, it is imperative to optimise storage and usage requirements to reduce the impact of extreme environmental conditions on equipment functionality and durability. Since each transducer has its own characteristics and advantages, having only one probe available may jeopardise a broader applicability of point of care ultrasound. Ideally, at least two probes—a low- and a high-frequency transducer—should be available to make the most of this tool in the frontline. Normally, the linear probe exhibits a 7–12 MHz frequency and is ideal for superficial structures scanning and procedures such as foreign objects identification, soft tissue evaluation, and vascular accesses. The low-frequency (3–5 MHz) probes, such as the curvilinear or the phased array, are used to evaluate deep structures and to guide interventional procedures. Hence, E-FAST should be performed using these probes.

Box 5.1 Essentials of Austere Environment POCUS

- Clinical situations in remote or hard to reach areas, rescue in wild areas, battlefield, space flights among others are defined as remote/austere environment. Such scenarios demand fast and objective evaluation using portable equipment.
- POCUS use on the military frontline should initially focus on life-threatening conditions. Therefore, E-FAST, RUSH, and ONSD are the essential applications of POCUS.
- POCUS has a wide range of applications that may help the clinician make critical decisions based on the best available evidence in low-resource settings.
- At least one high- and one low-frequency transducer should be available to perform the essential applications of POCUS.

RESOURCE-LIMITED ENVIRONMENT POCUS

E-Fast

The *Extended Focused Assessment Sonography for Trauma* (E-FAST) evaluation aims to identify free intraperitoneal fluid, pericardial effusion, and pneumothorax or haemothorax in trauma patients. To perform the E-FAST exam, the physician should use a curvilinear or phased array transducer to evaluate the four abdominal views and four thoracic views (apex and basal views, bilaterally). The clinician may choose to use a higher-frequency linear probe to evaluate the thoracic windows, as it yields sharper images of superficial structures.

HOW TO PERFORM THE EXAM

To obtain a good subxiphoid view, the examiner should place the transducer horizontally, almost parallel to the skin (Figure 5.1C and Video 5.1: Subxyphoid). The optimal image will show liver parenchyma between the skin and the right ventricle (the most anterior cardiac chamber). All cardiac chambers are displayed in an almost complete coronal view, and the physician may search for pericardial fluid anteriorly or posteriorly.

VIDEO CONTENT

 The videos referenced in this chapter can be accessed at https://www.routledge.com/ 9780367435592, under Support Material, or by viewing the QR code to the left.

The hepato-renal space (Morrison's Pouch) may be evaluated by putting the probe longitudinally at the level of the 11th–12th rib on the midaxillary line. It is important to scan the whole hepato-renal surface, as fluid may accumulate at the tip of the inferior margin of the liver (Figure 5.1A; Video 5.2: Morrisons positive). Approximately 70% of the positive FAST exams will display free fluid in this space. The physician may also look for fluid in the suprahepatic space.

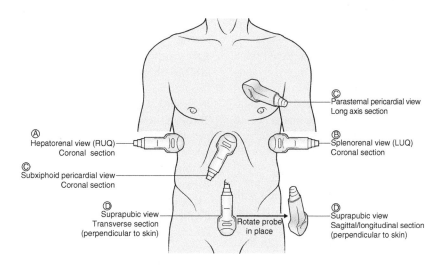

Figure 5.1

VIDEO CONTENT

The videos referenced in this chapter can be accessed at https://www.routledge.com/ 9780367435592, under Support Material, or by viewing the QR code to the left.

The splenorenal space is evaluated similarly, but slightly cranially (10th–11th rib) and posteriorly (Figure 5.1B; Video 5.3: Splenorenal positive). It is imperative to scan the subdiaphragmatic region on this side, as fluid accumulates in that space more often than in the splenorenal.

The pelvic window is obtained by placing the transducer horizontally, 1–2 cm above the pubis. The examiner should basculate the transducer caudally in approximately 45° to facilitate the bladder visualisation. One should scan the whole bladder surface to minimise missing a positive exam (Figure 5.1D). The physician may also perform this evaluation with the transducer in the longitudinal position, obtaining a sagittal view of the bladder.

The thoracic views of the E-FAST may be more cumbersome, although the results are more reliable.

POCUS can identify tiny amounts of fluid in the thoracic cavity, and the interpretation of the exam is similar to the abdominal views (anechoic images representing fluid surrounded by structures with different echogenicity). However, while looking for pneumothorax, the healthcare provider should also be familiar with lung ultrasound artefacts. It is imperative to evaluate sings such as lung sliding, A-lines and B-lines, and actively look for the lung point, in cases where pneumothorax may be a differential diagnosis. Studies show that POCUS outperforms chest radiographs, with an 86–100% sensitivity and a 92–100% specificity for the diagnosis of pneumothorax, making it an excellent tool for ruling out that condition. When analysing the diagnostic performance of ultrasound to identify pleural effusion, evidence shows a sensitivity of 82–94% and a specificity of 97%, also outperforming chest X-rays. Moreover, ultrasound can be used to follow stable patients undergoing unpressurised aircraft transfer.

RUSH (Rapid Ultrasound for Shock)

The RUSH protocol is a complete and fast-running protocol that assesses the various probable causes of shock. It divides shock assessment into three broad groups: the pump, the tank, and the pipes. The 'pump' is the part that corresponds to the cardiac evaluation; the 'tank' represents the evaluation of the lung, the great vessels and the abdomen, and the 'pipes' stand for the vessels, more specifically the aorta and femoral vein. The protocol recommends the use of two probes—the phase matrix (3.5–5 MHz) for thoracoabdominal evaluation and the linear matrix (7.5–10 MHz) for venous and pneumothorax evaluation.

PUMP EVALUATION

For this evaluation, four cardiac ultrasound windows are used: parasternal long and short axis, apical, and subxiphoid. The first is obtained by placing the phased array transducer at the level between the third and fifth ribs, with the probe marker pointing to the right shoulder (Videos 5.4–5.7). This view will provide an adequate evaluation of the left ventricle, the interventricular septum, and the aortic and mitral valves. The optimal view is obtained when the image displays the right ventricle outlet and descending aorta. The parasternal short axis view is obtained by rotating the probe 90° clockwise, aiming the probe marker to the left shoulder of the patient. This view displays the relationship between the left and the right ventricles and may be used to estimate the contractility of the former when visualising both papillary muscles. The apical view is obtained by placing the transducer horizontally at the tip of the heart, yielding a coronal view of the four chambers. As such, the physician can assess size, contractility, presence of pericardial effusion, or intracardiac thrombi. The last view is the subxiphoid, the same sonographic window present in the FAST exam.

VIDEO CONTENT

 The videos referenced in this chapter can be accessed at https://www.routledge.com/9780367435592, under Support Material, or by viewing the QR code to the left.

In the cardiac evaluation, the RUSH protocol recommends the evaluation of three variables: pericardial effusion, left ventricular dysfunction, and right ventricular dysfunction. Thus, it is possible to identify three plausible causes of shock—cardiac tamponade, myocardial ischemia, and pulmonary hypertension with right ventricular involvement. Through these windows, it is possible to evaluate the pericardium, confirm or rule out the presence of cardiac effusion and tamponade, evaluate the contractility of both ventricles, and estimate the degree of dysfunction. If present, left dysfunction is suggestive of myocardial ischemia, while right dysfunction suggests pulmonary hypertension as a result of possible embolism. In the latter, a massive event may result in enlarged right cardiac chambers and a leftward insinuation of the interventricular septum.

TANK EVALUATION

The tank is composed of the lungs, abdomen, and large vessels known to be reservoirs of blood. During this evaluation, the thoracic cavity is evaluated for pneumothorax or pleural effusion, following the same principles as the E-FAST exam. The thoracic evaluation should also aim to identify patients with pulmonary oedema. This can be achieved by observing B-lines at the intercostal spaces, which arise due to interlobular septal thickening. These lines are sonographic artefacts due to reverberation of the sound waves. B-lines are hyperechoic and bright images that arise from the pleural line and stream downwards to the end of the image. They are different from the 'comet tail' artefact, which are more commonly distributed along the pleural line and are not as long as the B-line. The presence of B-lines, especially of more than three in an intercostal space, is often pathological and may be associated with pulmonary oedema when diffused, or focal pathologies if more restricted (i.e. pneumonia) (Video 5.7). It is important to note that the number of B-lines and intercostal spaces displaying this sonographic sign is associated with the severity of the condition and can be used to evaluate the clinical response to treatment.

In the abdominal part, FAST is performed to search free fluid in the cavity, indicating leakage in the tank. This examination may be useful for patients in remote scenarios (to facilitate decision-making), immediate postoperative period of an abdominal surgery (i.e. frontline surgery team), or those recovering in the ICU bed who develops persistent hypotension.

In relation to the great vessels, the inferior vena cava (IVC) will be evaluated to define its collapsibility during the breathing cycle and yield an estimate of intravascular volume – whether the patient will respond to volume infusion. The IVC view may be obtained by placing the curvilinear or phased array transducer longitudinally in the epigastric or right flank (like the e-FAST view) areas. The optimal view should display the IVC and the right atrium inlet. The identification of the 'kissing walls' sign (i.e. when the IVC collapses until its walls touch each other) should be interpreted as hypovolemia in an adequate clinical context, especially when the available cardiac windows corroborate this finding. Studies demonstrate a positive correlation between IVC measurements and central venous pressure (CVP). IVC measurements are better performed using the M-mode to identify the inspiratory and expiratory phases of ventilation. It is important to complement the IVC evaluation with a horizontal view of the vessel to avoid underestimation due to cylinder effect. The collapsibility index is calculated dividing the IVC diameter during inspiration and by its diameter during expiration. Roughly, ≤2 cm IVC with ≥50% collapsibility correlates with a CVP of less than 10 mmHg. When the IVC diameter is ≥2 cm displaying <50% collapse during inspiration, the estimated CVP is higher than 10 mmHg. These measurements may also be used to monitor clinical response to treatment.

PIPE EVALUATION

The pipes will be evaluated for aneurysm, dissection, and rupture of the aorta by scanning the sites with the highest incidence of these abnormalities—the suprasternal, parasternal, epigastric, and supraumbilical. The ideal transducer for this assessment is the phased array, and the examiner may identify aortic enlargements, intraluminal flaps, and periaortic hematomas. The aorta is evaluated by placing the probe in at least four regions. The aortic root is visualised by placing the transducer horizontally on the suprasternal area. The

physician should then obtain a parasternal long-axis view to evaluate the descending aorta. Further down, the examiner should place the transducer horizontally in the epigastric and periumbilical areas to cover the abdominal aorta. Abdominal compression may be necessary to obtain a clearer image of the aorta by displacing intraluminal gas. Since most of the aortic ruptures and hematomas are in the retroperitoneum, this specific evaluation may be limited with ultrasound. However, the presence of aortic aneurysm in a hypotensive patient should prompt the need for urgent investigation of a possible rupture. The sensitivity of ultrasound to detect aortic aneurysms vary from 93-100%. Aortic dissection may be identified by aortic root enlargement or an intimal flap. The suprasternal, parasternal long axis, epigastric, and periumbilical views may cover the most common areas of dissection. By using the colour Doppler, it may be possible to identify two distinct lumens in some cases.

In the venous part, healthcare providers will evaluate the femoral and the popliteal veins with the linear transducer, actively searching for thrombi. The examiner should start by obtaining a transverse view of the common femoral vein just below the inguinal ligament, followed by images of the superficial femoral vein distally to the great saphenous vein confluence. The examiner should then pursue a transverse view of the popliteal vein in the posterior aspect of the knee. The transverse view facilitates identification of the vessel, but the examiner should also use the longitudinal view. There are three key features associated with intraluminal thrombi: absence of collapsibility during compression, presence of a hyperechoic intraluminal material, and absence of flow on colour imaging. The evaluation of the pipes may help manage the patient who will be urgently operated on and has a risk factor for thrombosis. The evidence of thrombi may help the clinician to decide, for example, whether to place a vena cava filter prior to the operation.

Optic Nerve Sheath Diameter (ONSD)

The gold standard for diagnosing high intracranial pressure (ICP) after a traumatic brain injury (TBI) is through the insertion of an intraventricular catheter that allows ICP monitoring. However, it is an invasive method not universally available, and associated with complications such as infection, bleeding, and neurological dysfunction. Because of this, clinical examination and CT of the head are used when high ICP is suspected. However, in a remote setting, tomography is unavailable and the use of POCUS ONSD becomes a perfect tool. High ICP is suspected through typical signs such as headache, vomiting, optic papilla oedema, and Cushing's response, characterised by a reflex increase in blood pressure, bradycardia, and changes in respiratory rhythm. Once clinical suspicion is present, POCUS ONSD for the diagnosis of high ICP has been proved to be a safe, reliable, and practical diagnostic method for rapid therapeutic action.

Due to the anatomical relationship of the optic nerve complex with the entire cerebral subarachnoid space, an increase in ICP results in distension of the sheath and a consequent increase in its thickness. Thus, the diameter of the optic nerve sheath (ONSD) directly translates to ICP.

A high frequency (7–10 MHz) linear transducer is used, and ultrasound is configured to visualise structures up to 5–6 cm deep. The transducer is placed over the closed eyelid, horizontally or longitudinally, after generous gel application. The optic nerve is identified as a hypoechoic structure traversing along a regular course behind the eyeball. For measurement, a vertical line is drawn from the junction between the optic nerve and the eyeball. This line is for reference only and should be 3 mm long. Once the 3-mm length is established, a horizontal line is drawn across the optic nerve sheath (Figure 5.2). This second line provides the measurement of the optic nerve sheath in mm. To lessen the effect of intraobserver variability, it is proposed that the final measurement should be the mean of the three measurements (Video 5.8).

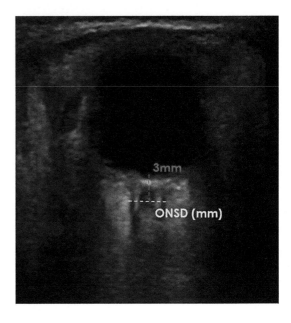

Figure 5.2

radiation, proving to be an extremely promising and efficient exam to evaluate critically ill patients in a remote or austere scenario.

VIDEO CONTENT

 The videos referenced in this chapter can be accessed at https://www.routledge.com/9780367435592, under Support Material, or by viewing the QR code to the left.

POCUS ONSD is a low-cost, accurate, fast, portable, non-invasive exam that does not use ionising

---

Box 5.2 Main POCUS Uses in the Austere Environment

- The *Extended Focused Assessment Sonography for Trauma* (E-FAST) evaluation aims to identify free intraperitoneal fluid, pericardial effusion, and pneumothorax or haemothorax in trauma patients.
- The RUSH protocol is a complete and fast-running protocol that assesses the various probable causes of shock. It divides shock assessment into three broad groups: the pump, the tank, and the pipes.
- POCUS ONSD for the diagnosis of high ICP has been proven to be a safe, reliable, and practical diagnostic method for rapid therapeutic action. An increase in ICP results in distension of the sheath and a consequent increase in its thickness.

OTHER POCUS RANGE IN THE RESOURCE-LIMITED ENVIRONMENT

There are several situations in which point of care ultrasound can enhance the quality of care and safety of the patient, serving as an excellent triage tool for critical decisions in the RLE. Although these may be considered as 'non-life-saving' applications, POCUS may provide an objective assessment and help with the decision to urgently evacuate the patient to a more complex facility. In that sense, POCUS can provide the diagnosis of inflammatory conditions such as acute appendicitis, cholecystitis and diverticulitis, and intra-abdominal hypertension (IAH) in critical scenarios. Pneumoperitoneum may be identified using POCUS with a much higher accuracy than X-rays or physical signs. Patients with acute scrotal pain may be urgently operated on for a testicular torsion, based on ultrasound results. Signs of intestinal obstruction may be confirmed with a simple ultrasound scanning. Moreover, studies show that POCUS may be used for tube thoracotomies, airway access, and other interventional procedures.

Box 5.3 Other Uses of POCUS

- POCUS may provide an objective assessment and help with the decision to urgently evacuate the patient to a more complex facility. Moreover, POCUS may be used to guide interventional procedures.
- POCUS may be used to diagnose appendicitis, cholecystitis, diverticulitis, small bowel obstruction, pneumoperitoneum, testicular torsion, pulmonary diseases, and other conditions. It can be used as an adjunct for procedures (i.e. tube thoracotomies, thoracocentesis, paracentesis, airway access, and others).

TEN RESOURCE-LIMITED ENVIRONMENT POCUS KEY POINTS

1. Austere environment is the pre-hospital care scenario with few resources or critical care conditions.

2. POCUS is a powerful tool to improve care on remote scenario.
3. Must POCUS knowledge for austere environment: E-FAST, RUSH, and ONSD.
4. POCUS is a portable and accurate diagnostic tool.
5. At the frontline scenario, both low- and high-frequency probes are needed.
6. E-FAST displays a high positive predictive value for intraabdominal free fluid, and a high accuracy for both pneumothorax and haemothorax diagnosis.
7. RUSH may be used for differential diagnosis of SHOCK.
8. ONSD rules out high ICP and can also assess TBI severity quantitatively.
9. POCUS can provide significant help in the acute care surgery diagnosis on a faraway scenario.
10. POCUS has a valuable role in invasive procedures in the remote environment.

FURTHER READING

1. Abu-zidan F, Cevik A. Diagnostic point-of-care ultrasound (POCUS) for gastrointestinal pathology: state of the art from basics to advanced. *World J Emerg Surg.* 2018;**13(47)**:1–14.
2. Ball CG, Williams BH, Wyrzykowski AD et al. A caveat to the performance of pericardial ultrasound in patients with penetrating cardiac wounds. *J Trauma Acute Care Surg.* 2009;**67(5)**:1123–1124.
3. Bekerman I, Sigal T, Kimiagar I, Ben Ely A, Vaiman M. The quantitative evaluation of intracranial pressure by optic nerve sheath diameter/eye diameter CT measurement. *Am J Emerg Med.* 2016;**34(12)**:2336–2342.
4. Blaivas M, Kuhn W, Reynolds B, Brannam L: Change in differential diagnosis and patient management with the use of portable ultrasound in a remote setting. *Wilderness Environ Med.* 2005;**16(1)**:38–41.
5. Ding W, Shen Y, Yang J, He X, Zhang M: Diagnosis of pneumothorax by radiography and ultrasonography. *Chest* 2011;**140(4)**:859–866.
6. Komut E, Kozaci N, Sönmez BM, Yilmaz F, Komut S, Yildirim ZN, et al. Bedside sonographic measurement of optic nerve sheath diameter as a predictor of intracranial pressure in ED. *Am J Emerg Med.* 2016;**34(6)**: 963–967.
7. Lapostolle F, Petrovic T, Lenoir G, et al: Usefulness of hand-held ultrasound devices in out-of-hospital

diagnosis performed by emergency physicians. *Am J Emerg Med.* 2006;**24**:237–242.

8. Lichtenstein D. BLUE-protocol and FALLS-protocol: two applications of lung ultrasound in the critically ill. *Chest* 2015;**147(6)**:1659–1670.

9. Ma O, Mateer J. Trauma ultrasound examination versus chest radiography in the detection of hemothorax. *J Trauma.*

10. Menegozzo CAM, Meyer-Pflug AR, Utiyama EM. How to reduce pleural drainage complications using an ultrasound-guided technique. *Rev Col Bras Cir.* 2018;**45(4)**:e1952

11. Menegozzo CAM, Utiyama EM. Steering the wheel towards the standard of care: Proposal of a step-by-step ultrasound-guided emergency chest tube drainage and literature review. *Int J Surg.* 2018;**56**:315–319

12. Menegozzo CAM, Artifon ELA, Meyer-Pflug AR, Rocha MC, Utiyama EM. Can ultrasound be used as an adjunct for tube thoracostomy? A systematic review of potential application to reduce procedure-related complications. *Int J Surg.* 2019;**68**:85–90.

13. Menegozzo CAM, Utiyama EM. Getting out of the comfort zone with point-of-care ultrasound. *Am J Surg.* 2019;**217(1)**:190–191

14. Nelson BP, Chason K: Use of ultrasound by emergency medical services: a review. *Int J Emerg Med.* 2008;**1(4)**:253–259.

15. Nicol A, Navsaria P, Beningfield S et al. Screening for occult penetrating cardiac injuries. *Ann Surg.* 2015;**261(3)**:573–578.

16. Pereira BM, Dorigatti AE. Current specialist awareness on ultrasound use for central venous catheterization. *Emerg Med Open J.* 2016;**2(1)**:1–4.

17. Pereira BM, Pereira RG, Wise R, Sugrue G, Zakrison TL, Dorigatti AE, Fiorelli RK, Malbrain MLNG. The role of point-of-care ultrasound in intra-abdominal hypertension management. *Anaesthesiol Intensive Ther.* 2017;**49(5)**:373–381

18. Perera P, Mailhot T, Riley D, Mandavia D. The RUSH exam: rapid ultrasound in shock in the evaluation of the critically ill. *Emerg Med Clin N Am* (2010);**28**:29–56.

19. Polk JD, Fallon WF, Kovach B: The "Airmedical F.A.S.T." for trauma patients—the initial report of a novel application for sonography. *Aviat Space Environ Med* 2001;**72(5)**:432–436.

20. Rebik K, Wagner JM, Middleton W. Scrotal ultrasound. *Radiol Clin N Am.* 2019;**57(3)**:635–648.

21. Rozanski TA, Edmonson JM, Jone SB: Ultrasonography in a forward-deployed military hospital. *Mil Med.* 2005;**170(2)**:99–102.

22. Russel T, Crawford P: Ultrasound in the Austere environment: a review of the history, indications, and specifications. *Military Med.* 2013;**178(1)**:21–28.

23. Rozycki GS, Ballard RB, Feliciano DV, et al. Surgeon-performed ultrasound for the assessment of truncal injuries: lessons learned from 1540 patients. *Ann Surg.* 1998;**228(4)**:557–567.

24. Stengel D, Bauwens K, Rademacher G, et al. Association between compliance with methodological standards of diagnostic research and reported test accuracy: meta-analysis of focused assessment of US for trauma. *Radiology* 2005;**236(1)**:102–111.

25. Williams S, Perera P, Gharahbaghian L. The FAST and E-FAST in 2013: trauma ultrasonography. Overview, practical techniques, controversies, and new frontiers. *Crit Care Clin.* 2014;**30(1)**:119–150.

26. Zafren K: How useful is on-mountain sonography? *Wilderness Environ Med.* 2001;**12(4)**:230–231.

27. Zanobetti M, Coppa A, Nazerian P. Chest abdominal-focused assessment sonography for trauma during the primary survey in the emergency department: the CA-FAST protocol. *Eur J Trauma Emerg Surg.* 2015;**44(6)**:805–810.

Thoracic Injury Management 6

David R. King and James V. O'Connor

INTRODUCTION

The reported range of operative mortality following emergent thoracic exploration varies but, in general, is about 30% – tractotomy 13%, wedge resection 30%, lobectomy 43%, and pneumonectomy 50% – and is consistent with other published reports.

Analysis of the outcomes following cardiac injury is challenging for several reasons, as many patients die in the field, especially in austere settings as the time to definitive care is prolonged due to the terrain and hostilities. The survival for those *in extremis* requiring a trauma bay thoracotomy remains low, with many studies combining both blunt and penetrating cohorts in the analysis. The reported mortality rates for patients after penetrating cardiac trauma organic on arrival at hospital is about 33%. Precordial penetrating injuries are especially worrisome, and a cardiac injury must be excluded by ultrasound, imaging, pericardial window, or simply exploration if the ultrasound examination is in any way unsatisfying or non-diagnostic.

Tracheobronchial and oesophageal injuries are uncommon, typically occurring in the neck than the true thorax, and may result from either blunt or penetrating mechanisms. Compromise or loss of the airway is a dreaded complication with the potential for rapidly fatal consequences. Promptly securing the airway requires sound judgement and advanced airway skills. Because these injuries occur infrequently and most published series include both blunt and penetrating injuries, in addition to grouping both cervical and thoracic injured groups,

outcomes are difficult to interpret. But, even with the inherent limitations of these studies, several key principles can be formulated.

- Penetrating injuries occur more commonly in the neck and are often diagnosed by physical examination.
- Conversely, blunt airway injuries are more commonly intra-thoracic with almost two-thirds occurring in proximity to the carina.
- A continuous air leak or a large persistent pneumothorax following tube thoracostomy should prompt further investigation (bronchoscopy is the modality of choice in the civilian setting but may require operative intervention at a Role 2 facility if ventilation proving problematic and inability to transfer to a higher level of care).

In general, tracheobronchial injuries require operative repair, and delayed repair is associated with a higher mortality and morbidity. The operative mortality for all tracheobronchial injuries is between 15–19%. Similarly, oesophageal injuries are uncommon and almost universally the result of penetrating trauma. Cervical oesophageal injury is more easily diagnosed and treated, with a much lower morbidity and mortality. An intra-thoracic oesophageal injury is decidedly more difficult to diagnose and treat. A missed intra-thoracic oesophageal injury results in mediastinitis, sepsis, and shock – associated with high mortality. Mediastinal air seen on plain radiograph requires further investigation, which may mean operative exploration if facilities allow; otherwise, insertion of large chest drains, and aggressive antibiotic and antifungals is required. Operative mortality varies between 6–19% but increases dramatically with delay in surgical intervention. Because of the high morality associated with a delay in definitive treatment, it is imperative that the clinician rapidly excludes these injuries if suspected. If an intra-thoracic oesophageal injury is diagnosed, then a prompt, definitive operation is required.

Great vessel injuries (aorta, aortic arch, and its great branches) are daunting, with full thickness disruptions constantly not surviving to reach surgical care. Life-threatening haemorrhage, challenging surgical exposure, and a lack of experience treating these infrequent injuries all contribute to their lethality. Over half the patients die prior to reaching hospital and operative mortality rates are up to 40%. Adverse resource-limited environment associated effects on outcomes include

- Longer transport times
- Degree of shock
- Combined great vessel arterial and venous injuries

Rapid evaluation of patients presenting in shock is imperative. Physical examination should concentrate on cardiorespiratory status and upper extremity neurovascular evaluation. An ultrasonographic exam (FAST), with both abdominal and pericardial views, and a portable chest x-ray complete the evaluation. Supradiaphragmatic and infradiaphragmatic large bore venous access should be obtained in ideal circumstances, since ballistic trajectories are impossible to predict based on exterior wounds and venous injuries may be present above and below the diaphragm. Surgical exposure is best obtained via a clamshell thoracotomy for most thoracic injuries. Except for the superior vena cava (SVC) and inferior vena cava (IVC), the great thoracic veins may be ligated if injured. Arterial injuries may be repaired primarily or with interposition grafting, with ligation reserved only for those *in extremis* if shunting is not feasible. In the battlefield, or other resource-limited environments, open surgical repair remains the gold standard.

A fundamental question the surgeon needs to address when operating for thoracic trauma is the role of *damage control*, which has demonstrated a survival benefit. The principles of damage control were first described for penetrating abdominal trauma. They include

- Rapid control of haemorrhage and contamination;
- Resuscitation in the intensive care unit (with blood and blood products) including establishing normothermia; and
- Planned, definitive surgery once normal physiology is restored.

These principles have also been successfully applied to vascular and orthopaedic surgery, and more recently, damage control thoracic surgery has been described. The decision to use damage control thoracic surgery is based on a few guiding principles:

- Overall injury burden
- Thoracic injury severity
- Coagulopathy
- Hypothermia
- Degree of acidosis (reflects depth of shock)
- The need for concomitant surgery (e.g., laparotomy, orthopaedic, extremity vascular)

Rapid control of lung *parenchymal haemorrhage* is achieved initially by manual compression, then definitively by a stapler. Often, multiple loads are necessary to perform a non-anatomic resection. As described earlier, large veins (except SVC and IVC) may be ligated if injured and arteries repaired or shunted (for damage control). The pleural space is drained, and packs may be placed on the raw pleural surface and a temporary closure used. Once normal physiology is restored (typically 2–3 days), the patient is returned to the operating room. The packs are removed, the plural spaces irrigated, and the chest formally closed. A couple of points are worth emphasising:

- *Packs adjacent to the heart and mediastinum should not be packed too tightly.*
- *Posteriorly placed large bore chest drains are essential and must be in the dependent position.*

If done correctly and appropriately, damage control thoracic surgery will not cause additional cardior-espiratory compromise.

LEFT ANTEROLATERAL THORACOTOMY

The left anterolateral thoracotomy can be per-formed rapidly and provides adequate exposure to the left pleural space, which may be further ex-tended into a clamshell thoracotomy (bilateral anterolateral thoracotomy) for greater exposure of the mediastinum and right hemithorax. The major disadvantage of the left anterolateral ap-proach is its limited exposure of the posterior chest structures but is the most used approach for a resuscitative thoracotomy in patients presenting *in extremis*.

Place a bump under the back to elevate the chest by 20–30° and extend the ipsilateral arm out of the field afford better visualisation (Figure 6.1). Position the patient in this manner to allow the incision to be carried further posteriorly (right down to the gurney/bed), allowing improved ex-posure of the pleural space. The incision follows the inferior border of the *pectoralis major* muscle, which corresponds to the fifth intercostal space, just in-ferior to the nipple. In women, the landmark is the infra-mammary fold. Do not count ribs, as you will get it wrong – it wastes time and causes confusion. The incision starts at the middle of the sternum on the left sternal border, follows the curve of the rib and extends as far posteriorly as possible. The fifth intercostal muscle is incised on the superior rib border, avoiding the intercostal bundle on the rib's inferior surface. A Finochietto chest retractor is positioned with the handle *towards the axilla*. This allows the incision to be extended into a clamshell thoracotomy, if necessary, without needing to re-position the retractor. With the retractor widely opened, the heart and left pleural space are easily accessed (Figure 6.2). Incising the inferior pul-monary ligament (fused parietal and visceral pleura) will mobilise the lung.

The pericardium is opened anterior (stay high on the heart) and parallel to the phrenic nerve in a

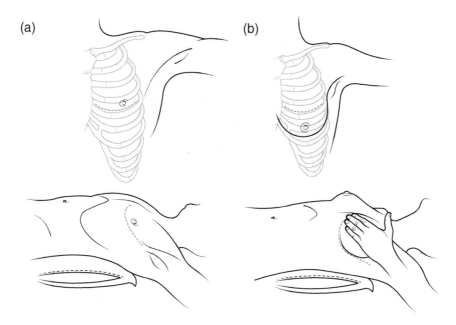

(a)   (b)

Figure 6.1 Anterolateral thoracotomy. Exposure is improved by placing a bump under the back and the fully extended ipsilateral arm.

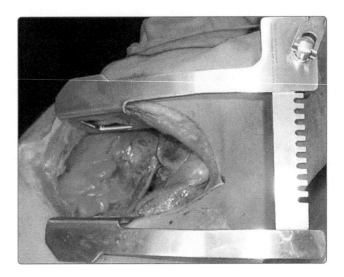

Figure 6.2 Chest exposure with an anterolateral thoracotomy. The retractor's handle is positioned towards the axilla to facilitate extending the incision to a clamshell thoracotomy.

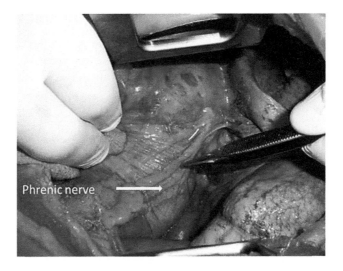

Phrenic nerve

Figure 6.3 Pericardiotomy. The pericardium should be opened anterior and parallel to the phrenic nerve (arrow).

longitudinal fashion (Figure 6.3). The heart is then delivered out of the pericardium (make sure the pericardial opening is long enough) and open cardiac massage may be performed if necessary. If needed, the descending thoracic aorta may be crossed clamped. This manoeuvre may be challenging, as the aorta is typically collapsed if hypotensive/ hypovolaemic. Rapidly incising the inferior pulmonary ligament improves exposure (taking care not to injure the vessels at the inferior part of the left hilum) and, if time permits, placing a nasogastric tube will assist in identifying and distinguishing the aorta from the oesophagus. The distal mediastinal pleura overlying the descending thoracic aorta must be opened and the aorta bluntly dissected, allowing the operator's left hand to encircle it while the cross clamp is placed with the right (Figure 6.4). Take care not to injure an intercostal branch, which will lead to additional bleeding. The pleura must be removed from the aorta (about 1–2 cm) to ensure effective cross-clamping of the correct structure and to prevent additional injury (especially intercostal branches).

CLAMSHELL THORACOTOMY

This incision affords superb exposure to the anterior mediastinum and both pleural spaces, and is ideally suited as the resuscitative thoracotomy of choice. As mentioned earlier, a left anterolateral thoracotomy can be extended as a clamshell. Using a Lebsche knife, sternal saw, and trauma shears or bone cutters, the sternum is divided horizontally. The incision is then extended as a right anterolateral mirror-image thoracotomy (Figure 6.5). There are several key technical details:

- **For maximal exposure, the incision must come across the body of the sternum – at its middle and not the xiphoid. There is a tendency to place the incision too inferiorly, which will seriously hamper exposure.**
- **The divided bilateral internal mammary arteries must be ligated, both proximally and distally, as they will bleed. In the profoundly hypotensive patient, these vessels may not be appreciated immediately but still require ligation. If not ligated at the initial operation, they will be when re-explored for bleeding.**

Fully opening bilateral rib spreaders yields excellent exposure to the anterior mediastinum and both hemithoraces (Figure 6.6). Almost all surgical procedures can be accomplished through this incision, including pulmonary resection, cardiorrhaphy, great vessel, and most tracheal repairs. There is, however, limited exposure of posterior mediastinal structures.

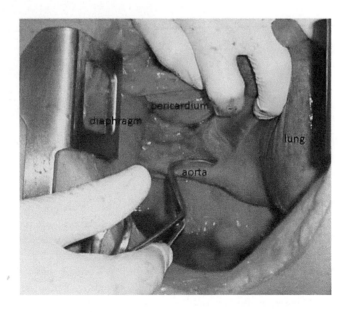

Figure 6.4 Aortic cross-clamping. To place an aortic cross clamp, the mediastinal pleura is bluntly dissected fully mobilised the aorta. The cross clamp is placed, achieving aortic occlusion. It is easy to misidentify the aorta in a hypotensive patient.

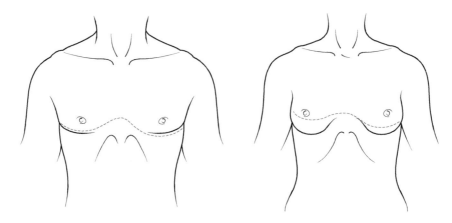

Figure 6.5 Clamshell thoracotomy. It is important to place the incision across the sternum, not the xiphoid. Placing the incision too inferiorly will hamper exposure.

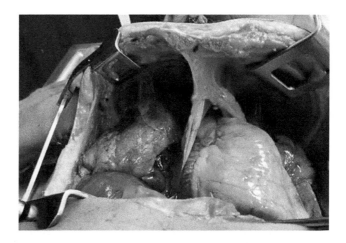

Figure 6.6 Clamshell thoracotomy. Bilateral retractors provided excellent exposure of pleural spaces and the mediastinum.

CARDIAC INJURIES

Cardiac injuries should be suspected when there is any penetrating injury within the *cardiac box*, which is bounded superiorly by the clavicles, inferiorly by the costal margin, and laterally by the midclavicular line (Figure 6.7). *The absence of hypotension does not exclude a possible cardiac injury* as the patient, especially if young, initially may be in compensated shock. The classic description of tamponade with Beck's triad (hypotension, distended neck veins, and muffled heart sounds) is infrequently present and unreliable. A rapid bedside cardiac ultrasound exam is accurate, sensitive, and specific – unless there is a concomitant haemothorax (especially left-sided). The patient presenting in shock with a precordial wound warrants immediate operation. The anterior position of the heart puts it at risk with a penetrating injury. In decreasing frequency, the cardiac chambers involved are the right ventricle, left ventricle, right atrium, and left atrium.

The chest is opened through a left anterolateral incision, with extension as a clamshell. Compared to

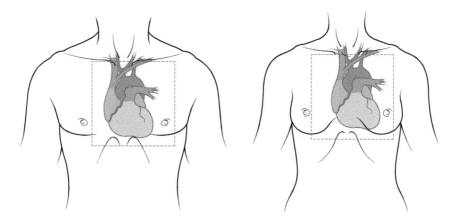

Figure 6.7 The cardiac box. The borders are inferior to the clavicles, superior to the costal margin and medial to both midclavicular lines. Penetrating injuries in the location must be evaluated for a cardiac injury.

the anterolateral incision, the clamshell affords superior cardiac exposure, especially of the SVC, IVC, and right atrium. It also allows the heart to be more easily delivered out of the pericardium.

Once a myocardial injury is encountered, there are several techniques to obtain temporary bleeding control; however, *the author's choice is direct, gentle digital pressure*. Staples may make the definitive repair more challenging and, if the Foley is placed under tension, it may pull out of the heart – creating an even larger wound to repair. Once the injury is identified and temporary control obtained, plans for definitive repair are formulated. This also affords time for the anaesthesia team to 'catch up' with blood and blood product loss. In general, lower pressure structures – the right atrium and ventricles – are easier to repair. The left atrium, although a relatively low-pressure chamber, is challenging to repair because of its more posterior position within the chest. While both the IVC and SVC are low pressure, high flow structures, the intrathoracic IVC is quite short – presenting a technical challenge to control and repair.

Right atrial and SVC injuries may immediately be controlled using a curved vascular clamp (Figure 6.8) and the injury closed with a running 4-0 or 5-0 Prolene suture. If a more secure closure is necessary, then a two-layer closure is used: a deeper horizontal mattress suture and superficial running suture (author's preferred technique). The left atrium's posterior location can, as mentioned, present a challenge; a small, curved vascular clamp is especially

useful in maintaining control. The heart may need to be gently rotated to facilitate its repair. In doing this, warn the anaesthetic team, as manipulating the heart, especially with rotation, may cause severe haemodynamic compromise, particularly in the acidotic patient in severe shock. Care must be exercised during this manoeuvre, and close communication with the anaesthesia team is essential.

The right ventricular pressure is about one quarter that of systemic – it facilitates the repair but its myocardium is thinner compared with the left ventricle, making it prone to tearing (suture may 'cheesewire' through) if not carefully sutured. The left ventricle is under systemic pressure and has a thicker myocardium. Although there is much written about using pledgets to bolster the repair, there are no fixed rules. Pledgets will distribute the suture's tension more uniformly, which may be beneficial with a thinner or more friable myocardium. Attention to detail is paramount when repairing a ventricular wound.

It is essential that the needle engages the ventricular wall at right angles, suture placement is timed to the ventricular contraction, and the bite follows the curve of the needle. Placing all the sutures prior to tying is also a useful technique.

Injuries adjacent to a coronary artery present a particular challenge. Small, distal coronary arterial branches can be ligated with minimal morbidity. However, ligation of a large, proximal coronary artery may prove fatal (massive myocardial infarction). Precise suture placement deep to the vessel will avoid

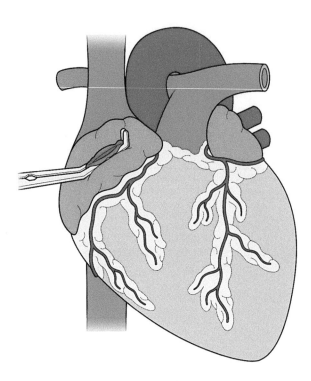

Figure 6.8 Control of a right atrial injury with a vascular clamp.

narrowing or occlusion of the artery (Figure 6.9). Injuries involving the posterior wall can also be problematic since the heart needs to be rotated to visualise the posterior surface. During this man-oeuvre, there is frequently a precipitous drop in blood pressure, and ventricular fibrillation is common. For any cardiac operation, always have internal defibrillation paddles in the field. The ap-proach to these injuries needs to be well-thought-out with a precise, deliberative repair. Once the posterior injury is rapidly identified, the heart is returned to its normal position. The sutures should be loaded on needle holders and placed through pledgets, if they are to be used. The heart is then manipulated, allowing visualisation of the injury and, the suture rapidly – but precisely – placed. The heart is again returned to its normal position with resolution of profound hypotension. This process is repeated until all the sutures are in place, and then repeated when tying. If an intra-cardiac injury (atrial septal defect, ventricular septal defect) is diagnosed by in-traoperative trans-oesophageal echocardiography, repair is deferred. There is almost no need for car-diopulmonary bypass when managing a traumatic cardiac injury. *The management of penetrating cardiac*

injuries demands rapid assessment, optimal exposure, a precise repair, and close coordination with the anaes-thesia team.

HILAR INJURIES

Hilar injuries are severe injuries, often requiring a formal anatomic pulmonary resection, and are asso-ciated with significant mortality and morbidity. The major concern with a hilar injury is life-threatening haemorrhage and less commonly air embolism. In either case, *hilar control* is essential. There are two common methods to rapidly control the hilum:

1. Pulmonary hilar twist
2. Direct manual control (author's preferred manoeuvre)

With the pulmonary hilar twist, the inferior pul-monary ligament is incised to allow mobility of the lung, and the lobes are rotated clockwise for hilar control (Figure 6.10). For direct manual control, a rapid blunt dissection enables the operator to con-trol the hilum between the thumb and forefinger,

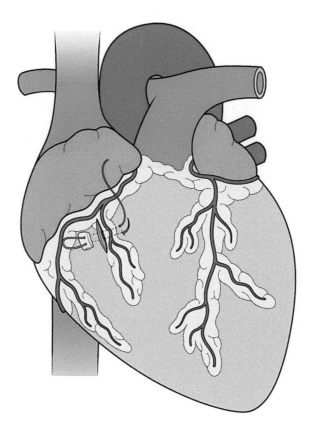

Figure 6.9 Ventricular injury in proximity to a coronary artery. The sutures are carefully placed deep to the vessel avoiding stenosis or occlusion.

and then a vascular clamp is placed for definitive control (Figure 6.11). *The authors' preference is for direct manual control as opposed to hilar twist.*

Whichever technique is used, there may be sudden and dramatic haemodynamic changes due to loss of preload and rapid increase in pulmonary resistance (50% of the pulmonary vascular space is acutely removed). Once haemorrhage has been controlled, a detailed evaluation of the injury may be performed. Occasionally, a hilar injury can be primarily repaired, but more typically, an anatomic resection, lobectomy, or pneumonectomy is necessary.

When performing a lobectomy or pneumonectomy, it is preferable to isolate the pulmonary artery, pulmonary vein, and bronchus separately. They can be individually divided using surgical staplers. Reinforcing the bronchial stump with a vascularised muscle pedicle (e.g., intercostal or diaphragm) will decrease the risk of a bronchial stump suture line

dehiscence (bronchopleural fistula), which is associated with significant morbidity and mortality.

PULMONARY INJURIES

There are several techniques to manage pulmonary parenchymal injuries and choosing the appropriate one depends on the severity of injury (typically depth of injury) and the patient's physiologic state. In the presence of profound shock, severe metabolic acidosis, coagulopathy, and hypothermia, a damage control strategy is the optimal approach. Lung parenchymal trauma ranges from minimal (treated by suture repair) to severe (requiring a pneumonectomy). Simple, superficial pulmonary lacerations can be closed by pneumonorrhaphy (Figure 6.12). Through and through, pulmonary injuries are managed by tractotomy. This is a simple, well-described, rapid method to control deeper lung

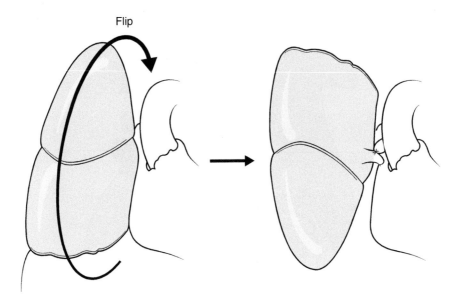

Figure 6.10 Pulmonary hilar twist. The lobes are rotated clockwise occluding the hilar vessels. The acute increase in pulmonary vascular resistance and decrease pre-load may result in cardiovascular collapse.

lacerations not involving the hilum. A stapler is placed through the injury tract and fired (Figure 6.13). Once the tract is opened, air leaks from small airways and bleeding vessels are controlled with suture ligation. This is an excellent damage control technique. A non-anatomic wedge resection is another rapid method to address more extensive parenchymal injuries and is particularly suited to peripheral lung injury. The lung is grasped with a lung clamp and a stapler fired to excise the injured lung. For a larger, non-anatomic resection, multiple reloads are necessary (Figure 6.14). The staple line is inspected for bleeding or air leak, which is then controlled by over-sewing the staple line. This technique is not appropriate if there is hilar involvement. In these instances, an anatomic resection, either lobectomy or pneumonectomy, is necessary.

If an anatomic resection is performed, it is crucial to understand the pulmonary arterial and venous anatomy. A detailed description of all these procedures is beyond the scope of this chapter, but the operative principles include careful dissection of the pulmonary arterial branches to the injured lobe, double-ligation before dividing them (or ligation and suture ligation which is the author's practice),

and individually dividing the pulmonary vein and bronchus with a stapler. The steps are the same for a pneumonectomy; however, the vessels and bronchus can be individually divided using a stapler. Muscle coverage of the bronchial stump is advised.

POSTERIOR MEDIASTINAL INJURIES

The posterior structures at risk are

- Descending thoracic aorta;
- Oesophagus; and
- Tracheobronchial tree.

Aortic Control

As discussed earlier, thoracic aortic exposure is enhanced by dividing the inferior pulmonary ligament, retracting the lung anteriorly, and widely opening the mediastinal pleura overlying the aorta. This can expose the thoracic aorta from the left subclavian artery origin to diaphragm. Haemorrhage is initially controlled with gentle digital pressure or by applying a partial occluding

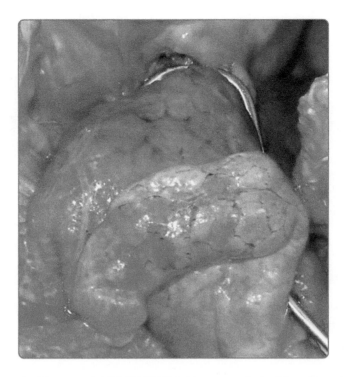

Figure 6.11 Hilar control with a vascular clamp. The lung is retracted, the hilum (arrow) bluntly dissected, and a vascular clamp applied. Hemodynamic compromise may occur.

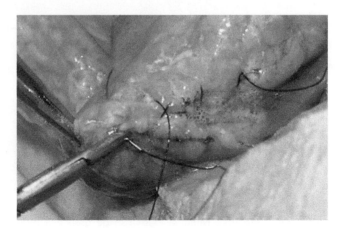

Figure 6.12 Pneumonorrhaphy with a running suture for a superficial lung laceration.

vascular clamp. Once temporary control is obtained, the definitive repair can be accomplished using interrupted 3-0 or 4-0 Prolene sutures. Even though the vessel has a relatively large lumen, it is important not to stenose during repair.

Tracheobronchial Injury

Management of tracheobronchial injuries depends on the site of injury. Proximal intra-thoracic airway injuries can be repaired through a collar incision.

(a)

(b)

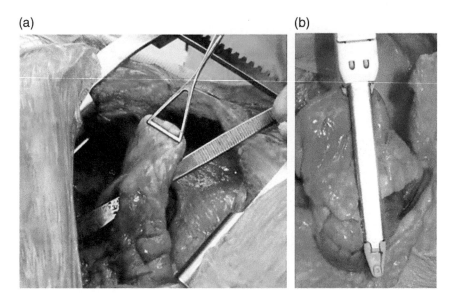

Figure 6.13 Panel A demonstrates a through and through lung injury; panel B depicts a tractotomy performed with a stapler.

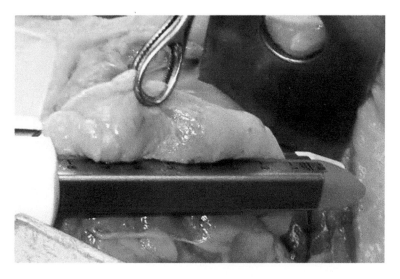

Figure 6.14 A stapled wedge resection. Multiple loads can be used if a more extensive non-anatomic resection is required.

Distal tracheal, including the carina, all right bronchial and proximal left bronchial injuries, are repaired through a right postero-lateral thoracotomy. Conversely, distal left bronchial injuries are explored through a left postero-lateral thoracotomy. Tracheo-oesophageal injuries are difficult to repair through a clamshell thoracotomy. This is the incision of choice for emergent bi-pleural surgical exploration but not well-suited for repair of posterior structures. The postero-lateral thoracotomy exposure is ideal for a definitive repair as opposed to the initial exploration for haemorrhage control.

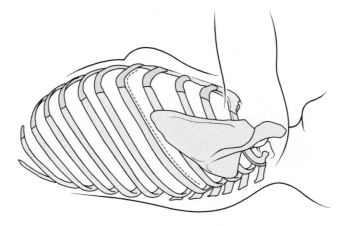

Figure 6.15 A postero-lateral thoracotomy. This is a useful incision to repair tracheobronchial and oesophageal injuries but is not the incision of choice for thoracic exploration.

Single lung ventilation with a double lumen endotracheal tube will greatly facilitate exposure in patients being operated for trachea-oesophageal injuries but has no role in those in haemorrhagic shock or *in extremis*. In the absence of double lumen tubes, selective lung ventilation can be assisted by the surgeon with intra-thoracic manipulation of the ET tube. The patient is positioned in the lateral decubitus, situated with an axillary role in place. A standard curvilinear thoracotomy incision is made starting 2–3 finger breadths below the nipple, passing two finger breadths below the scapular tip, and ending midway between the scapula and spine (Figure 6.15). The serratus and latissimus muscles are divided with a cautery (a muscle sparing approach can also be used). The ribs are counted, and the pleural space entered in the fifth intercostal space. Since most tracheobronchial injuries are exposed from the right side, that approach is discussed. The azygos vein is isolated, doubly ligated, and divided. Then, the mediastinal pleura is widely incised and can be tacked back to provide better exposure. This will provide exposure to the tracheobronchial tree (Figure 6.16). A nasogastric tube will facilitate definition of the plane between the oesophagus and trachea. Care must be taken when mobilising the trachea, as its blood supply is segmental. The trachea is debrided back to healthy tissue and repaired with interrupted absorbable sutures. Extreme care must be exercised to avoid puncturing the endotracheal tube balloon or catching the endotracheal tube with a suture. Early post-operative extubation is the goal.

Oesophageal Injury

A delayed diagnosis and/or management of an intra-thoracic oesophageal injury is associated with an extremely high mortality, secondary to mediastinitis and sepsis. Mediastinal air on chest radiograph warrants further investigation, particularly following penetrating trauma since oesophageal injury from blunt trauma is extraordinarily rare. Given the proximity of the trachea and oesophagus, both should be evaluated. All but the most distal intra-thoracic oesophageal injuries (those near the oesophago-gastric junction) are approached through a right postero-lateral thoracotomy. The technical details in exploring the mediastinum are identical to those of a tracheobronchial injury. Oesophageal blood supply is sub-mucosal, so the oesophagus can be widely mobilised. Its lack of a serosal layer demands a precise repair to avoid post-operative leak.

Following debridement of non-viable tissue, a two-layer closure is performed. Attention to detail is essential. The mucosa must be precisely reapproximated, the muscular layer sutures placed at a slightly oblique angle, and all the knots tied on the outside. Corner stay sutures and performing the

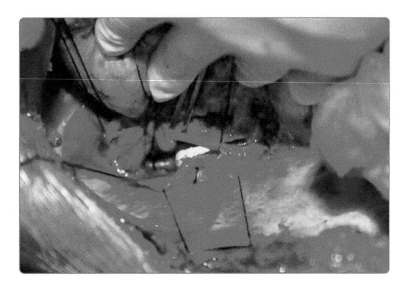

Figure 6.16 Intra-operative photograph of a severe tracheal injury. The exposure is through a right thoracotomy, the mediastinal pleura is retracted by tacking sutures, and the endotracheal tube is plainly visible through the tracheal defect.

repair over a nasogastric (NG) tube may be helpful adjuncts. Figure 6.17 demonstrates a right postero-lateral approach to an intra-thoracic oesophageal injury, with the NG tube clearly visible. Wide drainage, distal feeding access, NPO, and antibiotics are essential. The drains remain in until an oesophagram can be performed at a higher level of care.

Combined Tracheobronchial Injuries

The proximity of the trachea, oesophagus, and great vessels make combined injuries likely. The strategy for dealing with this situation is to manage each injury as if it were isolated, with attention to vascular injuries almost always coming first. The fundamental principle to combined injuries is to position a vascularised muscle buttress between any adjacent suture lines. This will nearly eliminate fistula formation between the adjacent suture lines, which could be a fatal complication.

CLAMSHELL THORACOTOMY AND EXPOSURE OF ARCH VESSELS

Injury to the great vessels and the aortic arch can be particularly formidable. These injuries result in rapid, massive haemorrhage, and obtaining adequate exposure and control is challenging. There are two common surgical exposures of the arch and great vessels:

1. Median sternotomy
2. Clamshell thoracotomy

Each has its advantages and disadvantages. Clamshell thoracotomy has already been discussed. If the incision is properly placed, it affords adequate exposure of the superior mediastinum (Figure 6.6); however, if placed too inferiorly (a frequent problem), exposure will be less optimal. Median sternotomy provides excellent exposure of the heart and great vessels; however, to aid consistency, only clamshell thoracotomy and exposure are discussed. The major disadvantages are the surgeon's experience and the need for specialised equipment (e.g., sternal saw or Lebsche knife and mallet).

Once exposure is obtained, the vessels are explored. The gatekeeper to the region is the left innominate vein, which crosses anterior to the aortic arch and its branches. Once mobilised (or ligated, which can be done with absolute impunity), the arch vessels can be individually isolated and

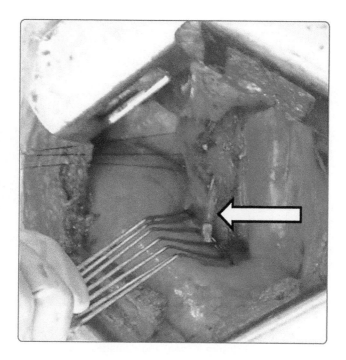

Figure 6.17 Intra-thoracic oesophageal injury. Exposure is through a right postero-lateral thoracotomy, tacking sutures retract the mediastinal pleura, and the lung is retracted. The NG tube (arrow) is seen outside the oesophageal lumen.

controlled. Apart from the SVC and IVC, the great veins can be ligated. It is important to ensure that veins to be ligated do not have a central line within them. Arterial injuries initially may be controlled with gentle digital pressure until vascular clamps are applied. In the damage control situation, vascular shunts can be used, and definitive reconstruction delayed, until haemodynamic and physiologic stability is restored. Depending on the extent of the arterial injury, primary repair or interposition graft is utilised.

There are a few key anatomic points:

- *It is important to appreciate the location of the recurrent laryngeal nerves; the right encircles the proximal right subclavian artery and the left passes around the aortic arch between the left carotid and subclavian arteries.*
- *There is also variation in the origin of the arch vessels; the most frequent variant is a common origin of the innominate and left common carotid arteries (bovine arch).*

CLOSURE AND DRAINS

The first decision is whether the thoracic cavity should be closed. If in damage control mode (profound shock, severe metabolic acidosis, coagulopathy, and hypothermia), the chest may be packed open (Figure 6.18). Concerns that packing the pleural space will result in cardiac tamponade or compromised pulmonary function are unfounded. The technique is straightforward: pleural and mediastinal drains are placed; the pleural surfaces are packed with laparotomy pads and a dressing is applied. An airtight seal is helpful and necessary if utilising a modified vacuum dressing, as described in the following. Posteriorly positioned, large bore (38 or 40 Fr) chest drains are essential. A smaller mediastinal drain (24 or 28 Fr), either straight or angled, is placed in the mediastinum. The authors' approach is to place an angled mediastinal tube in the pericardium. Coagulopathic bleeding from the raw pleural surfaces are controlled with the laparotomy pads; avoid tightly packing against the mediastinum. A sterile 10 × 10 Steri-Drape (3M) is

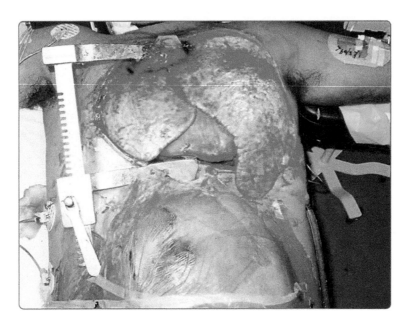

Figure 6.18 Damage control thoracic surgery. This patient sustained severe blunt trauma requiring a damage control laparotomy (modified closure is seen) and damage control clamshell.

fenestrated and placed over the chest and mediastinal contents, including the lungs and heart. Moist towels are placed over the Steri-Drape, two NG tubes are positioned on the towels, and a large Ioban (3M) adhesive drape secures the dressing. A vacuum seal is achieved by applying suction to the NG tubes.

Following correction of the metabolic derangements (restoration of normal pH, clotting factors, and temperature), the chest may be formally closed. This is typically performed on the second or third day following damage control. Generally, these patients are significantly volume overloaded, and once physiologically replete, diuresis begins, which facilitates chest closure. Upon return to the operating room, the modified vacuum dressing and packs are carefully removed, and the pleural spaces irrigated removing fibrin deposits or retained haemothorax. Routine closure of the bony thorax is performed (Figure 6.19). The chest wall musculature may require debridement prior to closure and the skin is generally left open.

ANTEROLATERAL THORACOTOMY

If the patient is stable enough for chest closure, it is accomplished like in an elective procedure. The

pleural space is irrigated, and haemostasis achieved. Generally, two pleural tubes are placed, anterior and posterior, with the tips near the apex. If there is concern for fluid accumulating inferiorly, an angled tube is positioned in the costophrenic angle. They are connected to individual collecting systems and placed on suction. The skeletal thorax is closed with interrupted, large (0 or #1) absorbable or non-absorbable sutures. Tension can be taken off the chest wall by pulling the sutures together prior to tying or by using a Bailey rib approximator. The muscle groups are closed in layers with running absorbable sutures and the skin closed with staples or sutures. Obtaining a portable chest radiograph prior to leaving the operating room is also preferable.

CLAMSHELL

Clamshell closure is like closing an anterolateral thoracotomy with a few significant differences. The sternum, which was divided horizontally, is closed with stainless steel wire, as a simple closure or figure of eight. Remember to ensure that the bilateral internal thoracic (mammary) arteries are

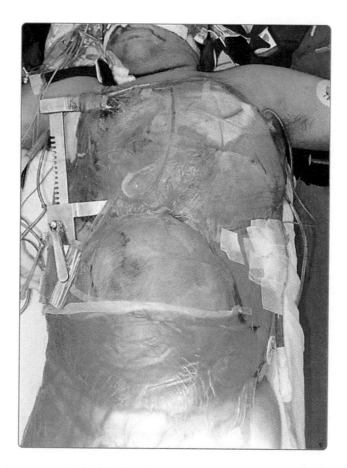

Figure 6.19 Modified vacuum closure of the thorax. Attempts to remove the chest retractor prior to modified closure resulted in profound hypotension; therefore, it was incorporated in the modified closure. Definitive chest closure was performed 3 days after the index operation. Following a prolonged hospitalisation, the patient made a full recovery.

ligated (proximally and distally). These vessels may not be bleeding briskly in the hypotensive patient and may be overlooked. Finally, the chest wall musculature becomes attenuated toward the midline and, occasionally, local advancement of the pectoralis is necessary to permit a tension-free closure.

ADDITIONAL READING

Asensio JA, Berne JD, Demetriades D et al. One hundred give penetrating cardiac injuries: a 2-year prospective evaluation. *J Trauma* 1998;**44**:1073–1082.

Asensio JA, Chahwan S, Forno W et al. Penetrating esophageal injuries: multicenter study of the American Association for the Surgery of Trauma. *J Trauma* 2001;**50(2)**:289–296.

Asensio JA, Garcia-Nunez LM, Petrone P. Trauma to the heart. In Feliciano DV, Mattox KL, Moore EE, eds. *Trauma*. 6th ed. New York, NY: McGraw-Hill Medical, 2008: 569–586.

Asensio JA, Murray J, Demetriades D et al. Penetrating cardiac injuries: a prospective study of variables predicting outcomes. *J Am Coll Surg* 1998;**186**: 24–34.

Cassada DC, Munyikwa MP, Moniz MP, Dieter RA, Schuchmann GF, Enderson BL. Acute injuries of the trachea and major bronchi: importance of early diagnosis. *Ann Thorac Surg* 2000;**69**:1563–1567.

Cothren C, Moore EE, Biffl WL, Franciose RJ, Offner PJ, Burch JM. Lung-sparing techniques are associated with improved outcome compared with anatomic resection for severe lung injuries. *J Trauma* 2002;**53**: 483–487.

DuBose J, O'Connor JV, Scalea TM. Lung, trachea and esophagus. In Feliciano DV, Mattox KL, Moore EE, eds. *Trauma*. 7th ed. New York: McGraw Hill, 2013; 468–484.

Fulton JO, de Groot KM, Buckels NJ, von Oppell UO. Penetrating injuries involving the intrathoracic great vessels. *S Afr J Surg* 1997;**35**:82–86.

Goins WA, Ford DH. The lethality of penetrating cardiac wounds. *Am Surg* 1996;**62(12)**:987–993.

Hajarizadeh H, Rohrer MJ, Cutler BS. Surgical exposure of the left subclavian artery by median sternotomy and left supraclavicular extension. *J Trauma* 1996;**41**:136–139.

Huh J, Wall MW Jr, Estrera AL, Soltero ER, Mattox KL. Surgical management of traumatic pulmonary injury. *Am J Surg* 2003;**186**:620–624.

Karmy-Jones R, Jurkovich GJ, Nathens AB et al. Timing of urgent thoracotomy for hemorrhage after trauma. *Arch Surg* 2001;**36**:513–518.

Karmy-Jones R, Jurkovich GJ, Shatz DV et al. Management of traumatic lung injury: a western trauma association multicenter review. *J Trauma* 2001;**51**:1049–1053.

Mandal KS, Sanusi M. Penetrating chest wounds: 24 years experience. *World J Surg* 2001;**25**:1145–1149.

Martin MJ, McDonald JM, Mullenix PS, Steele SR, Demetriades D. Operative management and outcomes of traumatic lung resection. *J Am Coll Surg* 2006; **203**:336–344.

Meredith JW, Hoth JJ. Thoracic trauma: when and how to intervene. *Surg Clin North Am* 2007;**87**:95–118.

O'Connor JV, DuBose JJ, Scalea TM. Damage control thoracic surgery: management and outcomes. *J Trauma Acute Care Surg* 2014;**77(5)**:660–665.

O'Connor JV, Scalea TM. Penetrating thoracic great vessel injury: impact of admission hemodynamics and preoperative imaging. *J Trauma* 2010;**68(4)**:834–837.

Rhee PM, Acosta J, Bridgeman A, Wang D, Jordan M, Rich N. Survival after emergency department thoracotomy: review of published data from the past 25 ears. *J Am Coll Surg* 2000;**190**:288–298.

Rossbach MM, Johnson SB, Gomez MA, Sako EY, Miller OL, Calhoon JH. Management of major tracheobronchial injuries: a 28-year experience. *Ann Thorac Surg* 1998;**65**:182–186.

Rotondo MF, Schwab CW, McGonigal MD et al. 'Damage control': an approach for improved survival in exsanguinating penetrating abdominal injury. *J Trauma* 1993;**35(3)**:375–382.

Smakman N, Nicol AJ, Walther G, Brooks A, Navsaria PH, Zellweger R. Factors affecting outcome in penetrating oesophageal trauma. *Br J Surg* 2004;**91(11)**: 1513–1519.

Tominaga GT, Waxman K, Scannell G, Annas C, Ott RA, Gazzaniga AB. Emergency thoracotomy with lung resection following trauma. *Am Surg* 1993;**59(12)**:834–837.

Tyburski JG, Astra L, Wilson RF, Dente C, Staffes C. Factors affecting prognosis with penetrating wounds of the heart. *J Trauma* 2000;**48**:587–590; discussion 590–591.

Von Oppell UO, Bautz P, De Groot M. Penetrating thoracic injuries: what we have learnt. *Thorac Cardiovasc Surg* 2000;**48**:55–61.

Junctional and Extremity Vascular Trauma

7

David S. Kauvar and Mohammed Mar'ae Asieri

JUNCTIONAL AND EXTREMITY VASCULAR TRAUMA

Epidemiology

The extremities and junctional regions (groin and axilla) are the most frequently injured body areas in military and civilian trauma and correspondingly sustain the greatest number of vascular injuries. Junctional and extremity vascular injuries can present threats to both life (through haemorrhage) and limb (through distal ischaemia) and must be diagnosed and managed expeditiously as part of the initial operative care of an injured patient. In general, proximal arterial injuries present greater risk of exsanguination, while distal injuries present a greater risk for limb loss. Regardless of the level of trauma, most vascular injuries mandate early haemorrhage control and restoration of distal flow, and their management should be considered as part of the initial damage control resuscitation and surgical care of an injured patient. Junctional and extremity vascular injuries can occur via penetrating and blunt mechanisms as well as from crush injuries and explosions. Amputation is more common in blunt, crush, and explosive injuries due to the compounding effect of multiple nonvascular tissue injuries (fractures, nerve injuries, and soft tissue defects) and the disruption of collateral blood flow pathways, especially in the lower extremity. High-energy projectiles such as military rifle rounds can produce tissue disruption out of proportion to externally visible wounds. A high index of suspicion for vascular injury should be maintained in limbs with rifle and other high-energy wounds and any clinical sign of vascular injury.

Presentation and Initial Workup

The clinical presentation of a junctional or extremity vascular injury determines the urgency and nature of workup and initial intervention. The traditional distinction between 'hard' and 'soft' clinical signs of limb arterial injury is of limited utility in blunt trauma cases and does not inherently suggest an appropriate management strategy. An equally sensitive and more operationally relevant scheme in identifying the presence of a limb arterial injury is classifying clinical signs as haemorrhagic or ischaemic (Box 7.1). Haemorrhagic signs are indicative of potentially life-threatening bleeding, mandating urgent early haemorrhage control prior to consideration of vascular reconstruction. A limb presenting with predominantly haemorrhagic signs may require urgent preoperative temporary haemostasis measures such as sustained direct pressure, tourniquet, or intravascular balloon placement – particularly if systemic hypotension or shock is present. These measures should be rapidly followed by an expeditious imaging workup (if available) and urgent operative exploration of the vascular injury. A presentation with predominantly ischaemic signs requires an estimation of the total limb ischemic time, as this will influence the urgency of operative

---

Box 7.1 Hemorrhagic and Ischemic Signs of Extremity Vascular Injury

Haemorrhagic Signs	Ischaemic Signs
Active haemorrhage (especially pulsatile) from a limb wound	Diminished or absent distal pulse
History of large volume of limb haemorrhage	Monophasic or absent distal Doppler signal
Systemic hypotension not accounted for by other injuries	Injured extremity-brachial index <1.0
Pulsatile mass in proximity to the suspected area of injury	Cool limb distal to suspected injury
Palpable thrill in proximity to the suspected area of injury	Pallor distal to suspected injury
Haematoma (especially expanding) or limb circumference discrepancy	Impaired motor or sensory function distal to suspected injury

---

intervention, vascular imaging, operative sequencing, and the use of vascular damage control and other adjunctive procedures such as fasciotomy (Chapter 17). Regardless of the presenting clinical signs of vascular injury and the extensiveness of the imaging workup, both should be used to develop a pre-operative plan for vascular control and reconstruction which should include the items in Box 7.2.

Box 7.2 Elements of Preoperative Extremity Vascular Surgical Plan

Sequencing	• Temporary shunting • Fracture reduction • Vascular reconstruction • Fasciotomy
Vascular Control	• Tourniquet vs. Pressure • Proximal & distal vessels • Systemic vs. local anticoagulation
Vascular Exposures	• Incisions • Patient positioning • Inflow and outflow vessels
Conduit	• Prep and draping • Degree of contamination • Graft course (tunnelling)
Tissue coverage	• Adequacy of available perfused soft tissue • Local flap (skin, muscle) • Negative pressure dressing

Pathology

Physical injury to blood vessels can take two general forms: occlusive or disruptive, which roughly correspond to the ischaemic and haemorrhagic presentations noted (Box 7.3). Occlusive pathologies result predominantly from blunt mechanisms and are associated with varying degrees of distal ischemia (ischaemic signs) at presentation. Mural disruption with resulting luminal loss or focal thrombosis and kinking due to orthopaedic injury comprise the principal occlusive traumatic vascular pathologies. Even intact arteries that are not directly injured but are in proximity to high-energy tissue disruptions are prone to focal spasm, which can produce ischaemic signs. This phenomenon is difficult, if not impossible, to detect without conventional or CT angiography (CTA). Disruptive vascular pathologies arise more commonly from penetrating mechanisms and are associated with haemorrhage from the injured vessel (haemorrhagic signs). Laceration and partial and complete vessel transection are the primary forms of disruptive vascular pathology and can result in segmental loss of vessel length – the degree of which has implications for the choice of a repair strategy. Vascular injuries resulting from explosions are to be noted as such mechanisms can produce both disruptive vessel pathology from fragment penetration (secondary blast injury) and occlusive pathology from blunt injury (tertiary blast injury). A high index of suspicion for complex vascular pathology should be maintained in these cases.

CONSIDERATIONS FOR VASCULAR SURGERY IN AUSTERE CONDITIONS

Priorities in the Multiply Injured Patient

Extremity vascular injuries should be considered in the context of the entire complex of a patient's injuries and their physiologic status. The goal of vascular reconstruction is limb salvage, but operative procedures are time- and resource-intensive and should not take precedence over life-saving manoeuvres. This is especially true when dealing with mangled extremities, which may require numerous procedures to salvage a limb that may not be fully or partially functional. In general, the threshold for primary amputation of a mangled lower extremity should be lower than that for an upper extremity. Multidisciplinary planning before initial surgical intervention is essential to properly prioritise vascular reconstruction in the multiply injured patient. Box 7.3 contains a list of prioritisation concerns relevant to junctional and extremity vascular injuries.

Injury Diagnosis and Imaging

Computed tomography angiography (CTA) has become the gold standard for imaging of vascular injuries in the trauma centre environment but is unlikely to be available in far environments. As such, the diagnosis and characterisation of junctional and extremity vascular

---

Box 7.3	Non-vascular Prioritisation Concerns in the Multiply Injured Patient
Concomitant Injuries	• Closed or open head injury • Solid-organ injury • Need for thoracotomy and/or laparotomy
Physiological Status	• Haemodynamic stability • Base deficit and trend • Responsiveness to resuscitation
Situational	• Triage of multiple patients • Available blood products • Available surgical teams • Evacuation timing and plan

injuries in these circumstances rely on the clinical exam supplemented with available bedside testing. A careful extremity vascular examination will make apparent most of the haemorrhagic and ischemic signs noted earlier. If a pulse cannot easily be palpated distal to a suspected arterial injury, then the examination should be supplemented with continuous-wave Doppler interrogation. Any distal Doppler signal that is not strongly multiphasic should increase suspicion for proximal arterial injury. The addition of the injured extremity index (IEI – the ratio of the Doppler-derived distal injured extremity systolic blood pressure to the higher brachial pressure) can provide additional information regarding arterial perfusion distal to an occlusive injury. If the equipment and expertise are available, duplex ultrasound can also be helpful in characterising the vascular anatomy and physiology of an injured extremity, especially in ruling out a significant vascular occlusion. In cases of complex trauma to multiple tissue types (crush and blast injuries) with any haemorrhagic or ischaemic signs, vascular injury should be ruled out during wound exploration by exposure and direct inspection of named vessels around the injury.

In limbs with ischaemic signs where the level and nature of the arterial disruption is unclear from the clinical exam (particularly in blunt trauma), an 'on table' angiogram may be useful in localising and characterising the injury. While digital subtraction provides the best vascular imaging, it is not required – angiography and using non-subtracted fluoroscopy can demonstrate relationships between the imaged vessels and any orthopaedic injuries that may be present. Angiography may be performed with any continuous fluoroscopy-capable C-arm and the limb on a radiolucent surface. An angiogram can also provide valuable information regarding the presence of collateral circulation around the injured arterial segment, but to do so, the contrast injection must be performed above the level of the primary collateral donor vessel and the native inflow must be kept open during the angiogram. This is simpler in the lower extremity, requiring only a direct antegrade puncture of the ipsilateral common femoral artery (CFA) and placement of a short introducer for the injection. We recommend using ultrasound-guided access of the midportion of the CFA using a micropuncture system. For stability, the 0.018″ wire can be advanced into the superficial femoral artery (SFA) and a small (<4 French) introducer placed, then withdrawn until ultrasound confirms the introducer tip is within the CFA.

Injection is performed through the introducer and contrast fills both the SFA and the profundal femoris artery (PFA), allowing for collateral visualisation. Use of a micropuncture system allows for direct removal and haemostasis via external direct pressure, requiring no cut-down and separate vascular repair. The primary proximal upper extremity collateral circulation arises from branches of the subclavian artery and, therefore, cannot be visualise through angiography via direct arterial puncture. The axillary and proximal brachial arteries are also not recommended for percutaneous access due to their depth and relative incompressibility. A small cut down in the proximal bicipital groove will allow direct exposure of the brachial artery, and a micropuncture system can be used for direct arterial puncture as described earlier. This arteriotomy should require only a single longitudinally oriented suture for repair. The introducer can be directed distally for antegrade injection of the vessels of the forearm, wrist, and hand or proximally for retrograde injection into the axilla-subclavian arteries.

Surgical Equipment and Supplies

Many items specific to the practice of hospital-based vascular surgery will likely be unavailable in austere field conditions. Surgeons operating in such circumstances should be prepared to perform basic open vascular operative procedures. Box 7.4 contains fundamental equipment and supply set for the reconstruction of junctional and extremity vascular injuries.

Orthopaedic Injury

Fractures and dislocations are commonly present in limbs sustaining major vascular injuries. Prior to operative vascular intervention, it is vital that the affected limb be brought to length and the vascular examination repeated. In some cases, this manoeuvre relieves an arterial kink or spasm with normalisation of the vascular exam, precluding the need for a vascular intervention or operative exploration. In cases where haemorrhage control requires vascular occlusion, this should be performed before orthopaedic manipulation, and in most cases, a vascular shunt placed (see the following discussion). External fixators, especially those spanning the knee, can impair the ability to easily perform vascular exposure, and it

---

Box 7.4   Suggested Supplies and Equipment for Extremity Vascular Surgery

Retractors	• Beckman-Weitlaner, Adson • Henley retractor set • Meyerding or appendiceal
Vascular Clamps	• Small Satinsky • Bulldog clamp set • Profunda • Angled DeBakey
Supplies	• Polypropylene sutures (4–0 through 7–0), RB, BV, C needles • Thick and thin silastic vessel loops • Rummel tourniquet & umbilical tape • Heparin for local injection • Syringes, sterile IV tubing, IV contrast, micropuncture introducer set • Tunnelling system (i.e. Scanlan) • Externally reinforced ePTFE vascular graft (6 and 8 mm)

---

is generally preferable to place them once vessels have been exposed and a shunt placed. This is particularly true for popliteal injuries, which are most readily exposed with the knee bent and a bump placed under the distal thigh and knee. Once flow has been restored via the shunt, the decision can be made to proceed with bony fixation prior to or following definitive vascular reconstruction. When fixation follows vascular repair, it is important to keep the eventual limb length in mind while reconstructing the vessels.

Vascular Damage Control

Temporary vascular shunts are placed for one of two indications: to consider the effect of concomitant orthopaedic injuries (as described earlier) or due to a patient's tenuous physiologic status. Placement of a shunt restores distal arterial perfusion, allowing time for orthopaedic manipulation or fixation, harvest of vein conduit, further resuscitation, or other necessary operations to be performed prior to formal vascular reconstruction. Arterial shunting which restores perfusion will also precipitate outflow from the injured extremity, aiding in identification of venous injuries which may require ligation for haemorrhage control. Doppler confirmation of shunt flow is essential. If an arterial shunt thrombosis develops a resistant (water-

hammer) Doppler signal, a major venous outflow occlusion may be present, which can threaten the patency of an arterial reconstruction. This suggests that limb outcome may be improved with venous reconstruction with or without temporary venous shunting.

Though any appropriately sized tube with a lumen can be used as a vascular shunt, it is preferable to use a device designed for the purpose. Thin tube shunts (Argyle) are easily placed and can be secured entirely inside an artery, reducing dislodgement risk. These generally extend into uninjured artery proximally and distally, potentially placing branches at risk of thrombosis. Longer flexible shunts with bulb tips (Sundt) are secured close to the vessel injury and can bridge long distances, which may allow greater limb manipulation while they are in place. Shunts should be secured within the vessel with circumferential proximal and distal ligatures or doubled vessel loops pulled to tension (Figure 7.1). The more distal the outflow vessel of an arterial shunt (i.e. forearm and calf arteries), the worse the expected patency. Arterial shunts will generally remain patent in the absence of systemic anticoagulation for at least 1 hour in a normotensive patient. If an arterial shunt is to be left in place for longer than 1–2 hours, consideration should be given for systemically anticoagulating the patient.

Ligation as a vascular damage control manoeuvre is rarely the first choice for major junctional or

(a)

Vascular clamp

(b)

Shunt placed
upstream

3–4 cm

Bevelled end to
prevent intimal
flap creation

(c)

3–4 cm   3–4 cm

(d)

Shunt
in situ

Suture to hold
shunt in situ

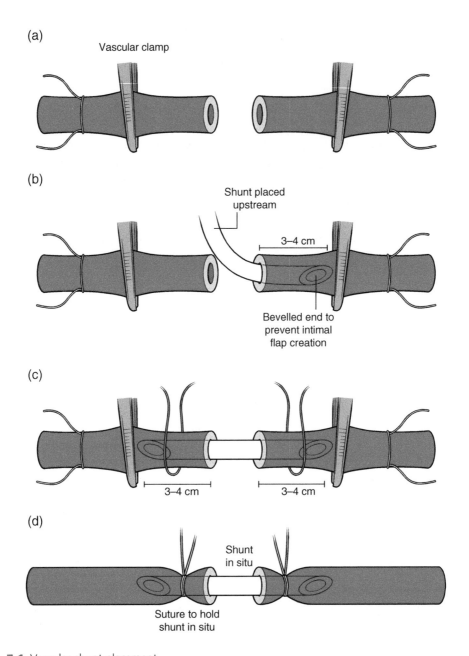

Figure 7.1 Vascular shunt placement.

extremity arterial injuries. Some arterial injuries may be safely ligated as a definitive vascular procedure. In the upper extremity, generous collateral circulation can permit ligation of the distal axillary and brachial arteries with preservation of Doppler signals in the palmar arch. Most upper extremities are ulnar-dominant, meaning that the radial artery can be ligated without producing hand and digital ischaemia. Confirmation of a Doppler signal in the distal radial artery with the proximal vessel occluded (Allen test) is mandatory if the vessel is to be definitively ligated. In the lower extremity, secondary and more distal branches of the profunda femoris artery (PFA) and single tibial arteries may generally be safely ligated. Definitive ligation of other named lower extremity arteries is likely to produce clinically significant distal ischaemia.

Vein Injury Management

Major junctional and extremity venous injury occurs concomitant with 25–50% of arterial injuries but is rarely reported in isolation, reflecting the less dramatic clinical manifestations of venous disruption. When present, however, extremity venous injury (whether repaired or ligated) is a consistent predictor of poor limb outcomes. There is no consensus on whether ligation of injured proximal limb veins (axillary, femoral, popliteal) worsens limb outcomes, but generous collateral venous circulation generally allows for ligation of injured brachial, forearm, and calf veins. In a crushed or mangled extremity, collateral outflow pathways may be disrupted, and a venous reconstruction may provide the sole source of limb outflow. Venous reconstruction provides the short-term advantages of decreasing venous hypertension with reduced bleeding, compartment pressure, and likely improved arterial graft patency. Extremity venous reconstructions are technically demanding with poor long- and medium-term patency, and it is generally appropriate to ligate venous injuries if time, expertise, or patient physiological tolerance will not allow for reconstruction.

Fasciotomy

To prevent compartment syndrome, four compartment fasciotomies of the calf are generally recommended to be performed immediately before or following revascularisation of a limb that has been ischaemic for more than 2 hours (including tourniquet time; see Chapter 17). The impact of this prophylactic approach to compartment decompression on limb and patient outcomes is controversial, but prophylactic fasciotomy is considered a standard practice in austere circumstances in which compartment pressures cannot be closely monitored following revascularisation. The greater collateral circulation typically present in upper extremities with arterial injury renders the recommendation for prophylactic forearm fasciotomy less stringent.

Postoperative Assessment and Monitoring

A patient with a revascularised extremity requires close monitoring after vascular reconstruction. In most cases, a properly performed arterial reconstruction should result in a palpable radial or pedal pulse and a strongly multiphasic Doppler signal. If these are not present immediately following reconstruction, then there may be arterial spasm in the outflow vessels and an 'on table' angiogram should be performed to confirm patency of the reconstruction and the diagnosis of spasm. Arterial spasm appears angiographically as one or more tapering arterial stenoses, producing a waxing and waning Doppler signal. A revascularised limb should be kept warm (i.e. with an externally applied warming blanket) for 6–12 hours following reconstruction to minimise arterial spasm and promote vascular outflow. During this period, hourly checks of clinical perfusion and Doppler signal should be performed to rapidly identify a failure of the reconstruction necessitating a return for exploration and possible revision.

GENERAL VASCULAR RECONSTRUCTION TECHNIQUES

Vascular Control

The first step in surgically addressing any vascular injury is obtaining control of the inflow and outflow of the zone of injury. It is always more expeditious to gain inflow and outflow vessel control using an anatomic vascular exposure (see the following discussion) through non-disrupted tissue planes than to directly explore the zone of injury. This is particularly true in haemorrhagic cases, where temporary haemostasis via direct pressure, pressure dressing, or tourniquet can be used while anatomic inflow control is obtained. In selected purely ischaemic cases, direct exploration of the area of suspected vascular injury may be possible, but haematoma, disrupted muscle, and bone fragments in the injured area often significantly disrupt the expected anatomy. Additionally, direct exposure of an injured vessel presenting with ischaemia may disrupt local tamponade and thrombus, precipitating haemorrhage. If direct exposure of the injured area for vascular control is necessary, temporary proximal

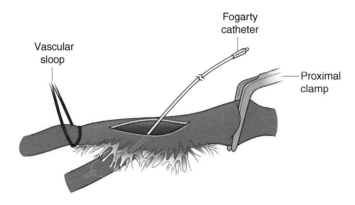

Figure 7.2 Intra-luminal balloon inflation for distal control.

and/or distal control can be obtained using intraluminal balloon(s) inserted into the injured vessel, permitting time for additional vascular dissection and clamping (Figure 7.2).

Gaining proximal control for junctional (axillary or common femoral) injuries can be a significant challenge. Endovascular balloon control is an option (if available), but this capability is frequently lacking in austere environments. For proximal axillary injuries, the distal subclavian artery must be controlled; while this is most often performed through a proximal lateral thoracotomy (left) or median sternotomy (right), it is also possible to encircle the subclavian artery from the supraclavicular approach. The supraclavicular space is small, and care must be taken to avoid injury to the phrenic nerve, subclavian vein, and brachial plexus. Supraclavicular subclavian control is only recommended for those familiar operating in the area. For proximal common femoral injuries, the distal external iliac artery (EIA) must be controlled. While it is possible to expose the distal EIA through an inguinal incision, this requires division of the inguinal ligament. Some of the fibres of the ligament can be safely divided to aid proximal inguinal retraction, but complete division of the inguinal ligament carries significant morbidity. An oblique flank incision with division of the external and internal oblique muscles gives straightforward access to the retroperitoneum, where the distal EIA can be controlled and used as an inflow vessel for an interposition or bypass graft, if necessary.

Injury Exposure

Once inflow and outflow control have been obtained, the zone of injury can be directly exposed and assessed. Existing traumatic wounds should be extended so a complete evaluation of the extent of vessel injury can be made. The injured area should be dissected circumferentially and opened longitudinally to examine the proximal, distal, and circumferential extent of intimal and luminal disruption. Local inflow and outflow sources for the eventual reconstruction are selected at this point and, if possible, existing proximal and distal vascular clamps moved closer to the injury. The inflow source should be proximal to all arterial disruptions and the outflow to a named vessel patent to the level of the hand or foot.

Thrombectomy and Anticoagulation

An assessment of inflow and outflow quality should be made and if pulsatile flow is not present proximally and/or there is little or no backbleeding, antegrade and retrograde balloon-catheter thrombectomy should be performed to assess and retrieve any thrombus (Figure 7.3). If no thrombus is present, the proximal arterial system should be assessed, usually with an 'on-table' angiogram. A lack of backbleeding does not always indicate inadequate outflow in a long ischaemic time or considerable haemorrhage. Circumferential compression of the

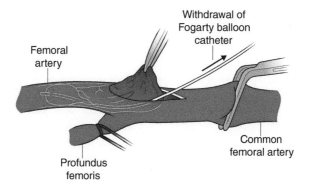

Figure 7.3 Thrombectomy.

distal portion of the limb should elicit a small amount of backbleeding in these cases, confirming outflow patency.

A decision must be made regarding anticoagulation. Systemic anticoagulation with heparin (60–80 μ/kg) is preferred but often contraindicated in the face of concomitant haemorrhagic injuries. If this is the case, local anticoagulation should be performed by injecting 10 mL of dilute heparinised normal saline (100 units mL^{-1}) directly into the planned inflow and outflow vessels. This manoeuvre should prevent local intravascular thrombosis in most cases.

Focal Repairs

A primary repair represents the simplest and most localised vascular reconstruction and is appropriate only for very focal vessel disruptions such as an arteriotomy from iatrogenic puncture and for some venous injuries. Full-thickness, interrupted sutures should be placed in the direction of the longitudinal axis of the vessel to avoid luminal narrowing (Figure 7.4). The exception is in the case of a simple vein laceration, which can be repaired with a lateral venorrhaphy via a running suture primarily closing the injury. Patch angioplasty, where autologous vein or prosthetic material is sutured in place to close a longitudinal defect without luminal narrowing, is also possible for focal arterial disruptions but is not recommended if there is more than minimal intimal injury. Finally, some arteries are longitudinally mobile and can be repaired via end-to-end anastomosis after resection of a short-injured segment. This is sometimes the case with focal brachial and SFA injuries. Care must be taken to ensure there is enough vascular mobility to allow spatulated anastomosis that will remain tension-free through the entire extremity range of motion.

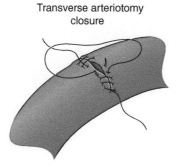

Figure 7.4 Transverse arteriotomy closure.

Interposition and Bypass Grafts

An interposition graft is most commonly required for reconstruction of short-segment vascular injuries, while a bypass graft may be required for longer segment injuries. There are five critical aspects to vascular graft procedures:

1. Inline inflow to the graft
2. Adequate outflow from the graft
3. A suitable graft conduit
4. Generous, spatulated anastomoses
5. A graft course free of twisting or kinking.

Establishing adequate inflow and outflow is covered above. In general, reversed greater saphenous vein (GSV) provides the most versatile, durable, and infection-resistant conduit for traumatic extremity vascular injuries. The standard dogma is that lower extremity outcomes are improved if the GSV is harvested from the extremity contralateral to the reconstruction, but this is debatable considering current evidence. Using contralateral GSV can make it easier for multiple surgical teams to perform exposure and control and vein harvest simultaneously. A properly spatulated GSV will accommodate most extremity vessels in terms of size match; however, the jugular vein can be used for large-diameter, short-segment reconstructions. The use of femoral vein for extremity vascular bypass is not recommended. Enough vein should be harvested so the bypass anastomoses will remain free of tension throughout

the entire extremity range of motion. With the knowledge that a harvested vein will foreshorten until it is pressurised, it is wise to use suture length to measure the eventual intended graft length and to harvest more vein than may be needed. Due to the contaminated nature of most traumatic vascular wounds, prosthetic conduit is not recommended except in very well-selected cases such as 'clean' simple stab wounds which can be copiously irrigated. It may be appropriate to perform a temporary prosthetic bypass to formally revise to a GSV conduit within a few days. The prosthetic graft material of choice in this case is expanded polytetra-fluoroethylene. For short interposition grafts of straight vessels such as the mid brachial and SFA, it can help to leave a bridge of native tissue in place during placement of the graft to avoid vessel retraction and give a true measurement of the defect to be grafted.

All extremity vascular anastomoses should be generously spatulated and the distance required for the overlap of the spatulated areas accounted for in harvesting the conduit. One to 2 cm of spatulation is generally adequate and the entire anastomotic area should consist of uninjured vascular tissue. In some areas (particularly the proximal axillary and above and below knee popliteal), the anastomosis may be difficult to see with the graft in place. In these areas, a 'parachute' technique of placing the first few sutures at the heel without pulling the stitch taut can aid with visualisation (Figure 7.5). Bypass grafts should be completely free of twists and kinks. This is best

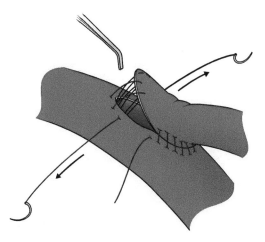

Figure 7.5 Spatulated repair.

ensured by pressurising the graft after completion of the proximal anastomosis, which will untwist the conduit. Under pressurisation, the graft can then be marked with a single, continuous line to ensure that it is not twisted during tunnelling, and cut at an appropriate length. A tunnelling device specific for the purpose is always recommended for use, preferably one with a sheath that remains in place to protect the graft as it is drawn through the tunnel. The most frequently employed tunnel is from the above to the below knee popliteal. It is critical to ensure that this tunnel is created between the femoral and tibial condyles to prevent extrinsic graft compression. Blunt finger dissection should be used to guide the tunnelling device in and out of the tunnel.

Tissue Coverage

All vascular reconstructions must be copiously irrigated and covered by perfused soft tissue to prevent further contamination and infection and forestall desiccation and possible graft or anastomotic breakdown. A plan for tissue coverage should be made preoperatively, especially in limbs that sustained significant soft tissue loss, such as those with explosive or crush injuries. If the limb lacks sufficient soft tissue for adequate coverage of the planned vascular reconstruction, then primary amputation should be considered early, rather than after completion of a reconstruction that cannot be covered. A temporary shunt placed early in the operation may assist in evaluating the adequacy of the available soft tissue. Local muscle, skin, or combined tissue flaps are frequently required for vascular coverage and will likely be successful as long as tissue perfusion can be maintained. Complex rotational or free flap coverage methods require considerable time and specialised surgical expertise which are likely restrictive in austere circumstances.

COMMON VASCULAR EXPOSURES AND RECONSTRUCTIONS

Upper Extremity

Radiolucent arm table
  Arm should be abducted to 90°
  Circumferential prep with exposed wrist and hand

1. Axillary Vessels

   - Transverse incision between pectoralis major and minor laterally on anterior shoulder in deltopectoral groove, dividing clavipectoral fascia (Figures 7.6 and 7.7).

     o Pectoralis major may be divided.
     o Preserve brachial plexus branches.

   - Typically requires interposition graft (GSV or 6 mm prosthetic).
   - Axillary vein injuries should be repaired if possible, unless basilic vein is intact and ligation is distal to the basilic–brachial confluence.

2. Brachial Vessels

   - Longitudinal incision medial upper arm inferior to biceps muscle.

     o Paired brachial veins crossing over brachial artery.
     o Median nerve in close proximity.
     o Superficial and easily accessible, just proximal to elbow deep to antebrachial fascia.
     o Brachial artery extends a few centimetres distal to the elbow joint and then bifurcates into radial and ulnar arteries.

   - If a forearm outflow target is required, the ulnar artery is preferred.

   - Short segment injuries may be circumferentially mobilised for end-to-end spatulated anastomosis.

     o Shoulder must be abducted to 90° and elbow fully extended to ensure anastomosis free of tension.

   - Brachial vein injuries can generally be ligated without significant consequences.

Lower Extremity
  One or both legs circumferentially prepped (depending on vein harvest).
  Foot and ankle exposed for exam.
  Sterile bump and/or external rotation helpful.

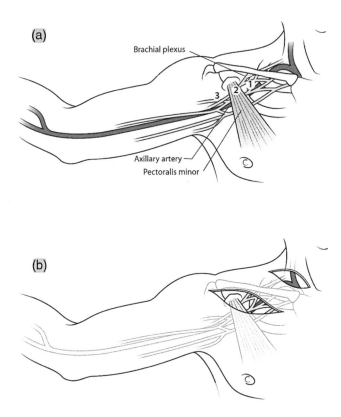

Figure 7.6 Axillary artery. (a) The pectoralis minor muscle is the gatekeeper to the axillary artery and is divided to gain access to the axillary artery and vein. The cords of the brachial plexus are intimately associated with the vessel and must be protected. (b) Axillary artery exposure. The axillary artery may be approached about 1 cm below and parallel to the clavicle. With severe injury, proximal control may be approached above the clavicle at the SCA (as described earlier).

1. External Iliac Vessels

- Preferred retroperitoneal exposure via oblique pelvic flank incision with division of external/internal oblique and transversus abdominus muscles, sweeping peritoneum superomedially (Figure 7.8).

  o Ureter crosses from proximal external iliac from lateral to medial.

- Alternative EIA exposure through cephalad extension of longitudinal femoral incision.

  o Distal fibres of the inguinal ligament may be divided to permit additional proximal retraction of the inguinal incision.

  o If inguinal ligament is completely divided, avoid violating peritoneum.

- Ligament should be reapproximated using permanent sutures.

  o One or more large circumflex iliac vein courses from lateral to medial over distal EIA. Injury from the inguinal approach will precipitate difficult to control bleeding.

- Typically requires interposition graft (proximal GSV or 8 mm prosthetic).
- If used as inflow for bypass to femoral, tunnel should course in peri-adventitial plane beneath inguinal ligament.

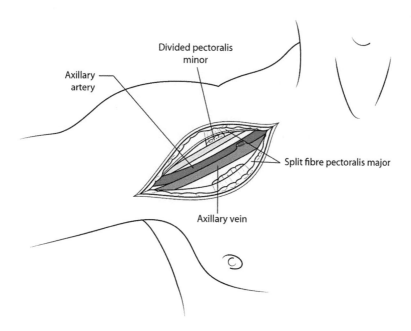

Figure 7.7 The fibres of the pectoralis major muscle are split (rather like a grid iron) to gain access to the pectoralis minor muscle (gate keeper to the axillary artery). This smaller muscle is encircled and divided with electrocautery. The axillary artery and vein (more anterior) and the cords of the brachial plexus are the identified.

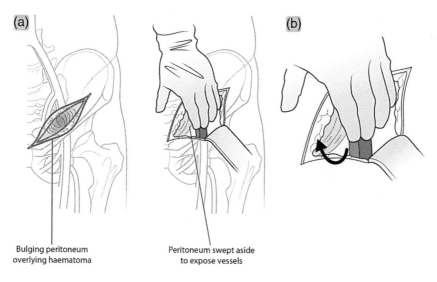

Figure 7.8 (a) An oblique incision over the lower quadrant, but parallel to and about 2 cm above the inguinal ligament is made. The external sheath is incised parallel to its fibres and the muscle of the anterior wall divided. (b) Once inside the true pelvis, the peritoneum is swept upwards away from the pelvis, revealing the iliac vessel underneath. If a haematoma is present, often the peritoneum will be dissected free from the pelvic side wall and the surgeon may enter this natural plane to control the vessels.

- Repair of external iliac vein injuries should be considered, though ligation may be tolerated if femoral veins are intact.

  o Lateral venorrhaphy or interposition graft (for injuries >50% diameter).

2. Femoral Triangle

- Longitudinal incision directly overlying CFA (approximately 2 cm lateral to pubic tubercle) (Figures 7.9 and 7.10).

  o Proximal extent cephalad to inguinal ligament, vessels lie immediately deep.
  o Small Satinsky clamp useful for clamping distal EIA under inguinal ligament.

- CFA injuries usually require control of proximal SFA and PFA.

  o CFA calibre change indicates SFA origin (control SFA about 2 cm distal).
  o Lateral/deep CFA dissection exposes thin-walled PFA (1–3 main branches can arise from CFA).
  o Circumflex femoral veins lie between SFA and PFA.
  o PFA can be controlled by exclusion using dissections of the distal CFA and proximal SFA.

- Dissection beyond its first 1–2 branches is not recommended as PFA dives deep into the vastus lateralis muscle.

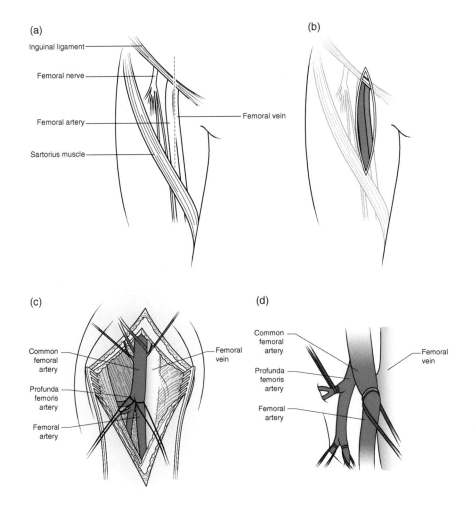

Figure 7.9 Femoral vessel exposure.

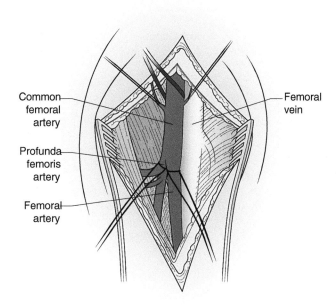

Common femoral artery

Profunda femoris artery

Femoral artery

Femoral vein

Figure 7.10 Femoral artery and vein exposure.

- Distal to the first PFA bifurcation, PFA branches may typically be ligated.

- Focal CFA injuries may be repaired with a prosthetic or vein patch – larger injuries typically require interposition graft.

  o CFA injuries extending to/involving SFA and/or PFA origin can be managed by including branch origins into the distal CFA patch or graft anastomosis.
  o More extensive femoral bifurcation injuries can be reconstructed with interposition graft to SFA and short vein bypass or reimplantation of PFA.

- Common femoral vein injuries should be repaired.

  o Lateral venorrhaphy or interposition graft (for injuries > 50% diameter).

3. **Superficial Femoral Artery**

- Longitudinal medial thigh incision posterior palpable bulk of rectus femoris/vastus medialis muscle complex.

  o Muscular fascia divided, sartorius muscle reflected (easiest anteriorly in proximal thigh, posteriorly in distal thigh).

  o Distal SFA exposure easier than the above-knee (AK) popliteal exposure; SFA is appropriate inflow source for bypass to below-knee (BK) popliteal.

- SFA injuries usually require interposition graft with vein or appropriately sized prosthetic.
- Femoral vein injuries can generally be ligated with preserved venous outflow if PFV and CFV are intact.

4. **Popliteal Vessels**

- Popliteal artery behind the knee surgically inaccessible from medial approach. Exposure through AK and BK incisions is recommended (Figure 7.11).

  o Deep, adjustable self-retaining retractor (Henley, Beckman-Weitlaner, Adson) helpful.
  o Vessel loops can be used to elevate vessel into surgical field

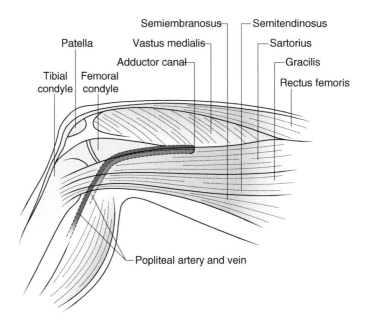

Figure 7.11 Above and below knee vessel exposure.

- AK popliteal vessels exposed with medial thigh incision similar to distal SFA (Figure 7.12).

  o Adductor hiatus identified and vastus medialis muscle is reflected anteriorly as popliteal courses deep into popliteal space.
  o Adductor magnus tendon lies across exposure here and may be mobilised and/or divided.
  o Neurovascular bundle lies anteriorly in the distal thigh, deep to femur.

- AK popliteal artery, a single popliteal vein(s), and large tibial nerve.
- Vein usually encountered first from and moblised to access the artery.

- BK popliteal vessels exposed through a medial proximal calf incision 1–2 cm medial to medial tibial border (Figure 7.13a–d).

  o Superficial fascia divided, and gastrocnemius muscle reflected posteriorly, exposing proximal popliteal space and neurovascular bundle.

- BK popliteal artery, paired (usually) popliteal veins, and tibial nerve.

  o Distal BK popliteal exposure requires division of soleus muscle from the medial tibial border with electrocautery.

- Exposure can be carried down to anterior tibial artery origin (coursing deep-laterally within incision) and the tibioperoneal trunk.

- Surgically accessible AK and BK popliteal artery are short – injuries usually require injured segment exclusion via proximal and distal ligation and interposition graft from the distal SFA/AK popliteal to the BK popliteal or tibioperoneal trunk. Recommended conduit is GSV.

  o Preserve geniculate vessels as possible.
  o AK-to-BK popliteal reconstruction typically required in three common injury patterns associated with popliteal injury.

- Posterior knee dislocation.
- Severe tibial plateau fracture.

(a)

Vastus
medialis

Incision
line

Adductor canal
leading to adductor
hiatus

Sartorius

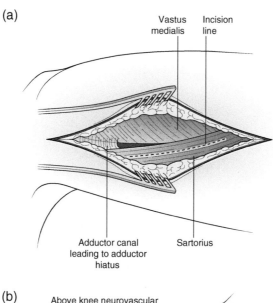

(b)

Above knee neurovascular
bundle

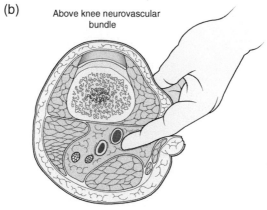

(c)

Above knee vasculature

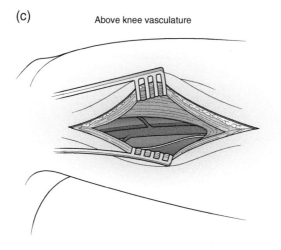

Figure 7.12 Above knee vascular exposure.

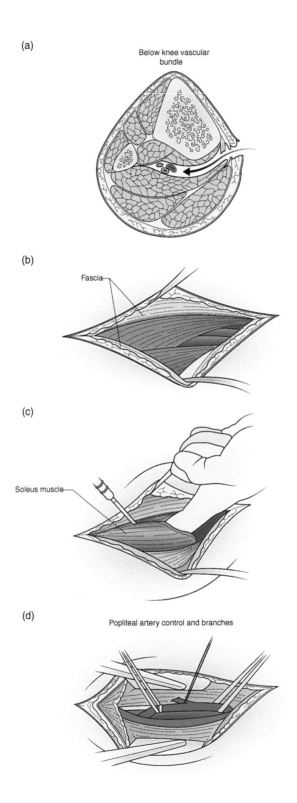

Figure 7.13 Below knee vascular exposure.

- Distal femur and proximal tibia fracture ('floating knee').

- Repair of popliteal vein injuries is controversial; repair (lateral venorrhaphy or interposition graft for >50% diameter) should be considered if collateral outflow (GSV) is disrupted or significant soft tissue injury is present.

5. **Tibial Vessels**

- Generally accepted that a single in-line patent tibial vessel to the foot with palpable pulse and/or ABI > 1.0 is adequate for limb salvage.

  o Single tibial artery injuries may be ligated.
  o Angiography helpful with severe limb trauma (crush, explosion).

- Multiple tibial artery injuries imply high-energy injury with likely segmental, circumferential tissue destruction.

  o Poor limb salvage rates with or without revascularisation.
  o Beware of 'segmental ischaemia' with bypass to distal tibial artery from femoral/popliteal – intervening tissues may not be adequately perfused.

- Tibial veins may be ligated.

KEY POINTS

1. Injuries to extremity and junctional blood vessels present potential threats to life, limb, and function.
2. Junctional and extremity vascular injuries present with predominantly haemorrhagic or ischaemic signs which correspond to disruptive and occlusive vascular pathology.
3. Careful bedside examination, including an injured extremity index, are primary diagnostic modalities.
4. Multidisciplinary planning including assessment of available personnel, time, and resources is essential in cases of severely injured (mangled) extremities.
5. Arterial and/or venous shunting should be considered when formal reconstruction will be delayed.

6. Most major extremity venous injuries and some distal and branch artery injuries may be safely ligated.
7. Fasciotomy should be considered at the time of revascularisation unless the patient can be consistently and closely monitored postoperatively.
8. On-table angiography and balloon catheter thrombectomy should be used if there is a question in inflow and outflow quality.
9. Standard vascular operative principles should be used: anatomic exposures, inflow and outflow control, simplest repair, or shortest possible conduit (autologous preferred) with spatulated anastomosis.
10. All vascular reconstructions should have viable tissue coverage.

FURTHER READING

Alarhayem AQ, Cohn SM, Cantu-Nunez O, Eastridge BJ, Rasmussen TE. *Impact of time to repair on outcomes in patients with lower extremity arterial injuries. J Vasc Surg.* 2018; **5**:1–5. doi:10.1016/j.jvs.2018.07.075.

Chong VE, Lee WS, Miraflor E, Victorino GP. Applying peripheral vascular injury guidelines to penetrating trauma. *J Surg Res.* 2014; **190(1)**:300–304. doi:10.1016/j.jss.2014.03.035.

deSouza IS, Benabbas R, McKee S, et al. Accuracy of physical examination, ankle-brachial index, and ultrasonography in the diagnosis of arterial injury in patients with penetrating extremity trauma: a systematic review and meta-analysis. *Acad Emerg Med.* 2017; **24(8)**:994–1017. doi:10.1111/acem.13227.

Doukas WC, Hayda RA, Frisch HM, et al. The military extremity trauma amputation/limb salvage (METALS) study: outcomes of amputation versus limb salvage following major lower-extremity Trauma. *J Bone Jt Surg Ser A.* 2013; **95(2)**:138–145. doi:10.2106/JBJS.K.00734.

Dua A, Patel B, Desai SS, et al. Comparison of military and civilian popliteal artery trauma outcomes. *J Vasc Surg.* 2014; **59(6)**:1628–1632. doi:10.1016/j.jvs.2013.12.037.

Fortuna G, DuBose JJ, Mendelsberg R, et al. Contemporary outcomes of lower extremity vascular repairs extending below the knee: a multicenter retrospective study. *J Trauma Acute Care Surg.* 2016; **81(1)**:63–70. doi:10.1097/TA.0000000000000996.

Guice JL, Gifford SM, Hata K, Shi X, Propper BW, Kauvar DS. *Analysis of limb outcomes by management of concomitant vein injury in military popliteal artery trauma. Ann Vasc Surg.* 2019; *62*:1–6. doi:10.1016/j. avsg.2019.05.007.

Hemingway JF, Adjei EA, Desikan SK, et al. Lowering the ankle brachial index threshold in blunt lower extremity trauma may prevent unnecessary imaging. *Ann Vasc Surg.* 2019; *55*:9–10. doi:10.1016/j.avsg.2018.12.014.

Inaba K, Aksoy H, Seamon MJ, et al. Multicenter evaluation of temporary intravascular shunt use in vascular trauma. *J Trauma Acute Care Surg.* 2016; *80(3)*:359–365. doi:10.1097/TA.0000000000000949.

Klocker J, Bertoldi A, Benda B, Pellegrini L, Gorny O, Fraedrich G. Outcome after interposition of vein grafts for arterial repair of extremity injuries in civilians. *J Vasc Surg.* 2014; *59(6)*:1633–1637. doi:10.1016/j.jvs.2014. 01.006.

Manley N, Magnotti L, Fabian T, Cutshall M, Croce M, Sharpe J. Factors contributing to morbidity after combined arterial and venous lower extremity trauma. *Am J Surg.* 2018; *84(7)*:1217–1223.

Matsumoto S, Jung K, Smith A, Coimbra R. Outcomes comparison between ligation and repair after major lower extremity venous injury. *Ann Vasc Surg.* 2018; *54(August 2018)*:152–160. doi:10.1016/j.avsg.2018. 05.062.

Perkins ZB, Yet B, Glasgow S, Marsh DWR, Tai NRM, Rasmussen TE. Long-term, patient-centered outcomes of lower-extremity vascular trauma. *J Trauma Acute Care Surg.* 2018; *85(1S Suppl 2)*:S104–S111. doi:10. 1097/TA.0000000000001956.

Sharrock AE, Tai N, Perkins Z, et al. Management and outcome of 597 wartime penetrating lower extremity arterial injuries from an international military cohort. *J Vasc Surg.* 2019; *70(1)*:224–232. doi:10.1016/j.jvs. 2018.11.024.

Scalea JR, Crawford R, Scurci S, et al. Below-the-knee arterial injury: the type of vessel may be more important than the number of vessels injured. *J Trauma Acute Care Surg.* 2014; *77(6)*:920–925. doi:10.1097/TA. 0000000000000458.

Thomas SB, Schechtman DW, Walters TJ, Kauvar DS. Predictors and timing of amputations in military lower extremity trauma with arterial injury. *J Trauma Acute Care Surg.* 2019; *87(1)*:1. doi:10.1097/ta.0000000000002185.

Watson JDB, Houston R, Morrison JJ, Gifford SM, Rasmussen TE. A retrospective cohort comparison of expanded polytetrafluorethylene to autologous vein for vascular reconstruction in modern combat casualty care. *Ann Vasc Surg.* 2015;29(4):822–829. doi:10. 1016/j.avsg.2014.12.026.

Wlodarczyk JR, Thomas AS, Schroll R, et al. To shunt or not to shunt in combined orthopedic and vascular extremity trauma. *J Trauma Acute Care Surg.* 2018. doi:10.1097/TA.0000000000002065.

Trauma Laparotomy and Damage Control Laparotomy

8

Carrie Valdez and David Nott

INTRODUCTION

The primary goal of damage control laparotomy is to immediately treat severe haemorrhage and limit/arrest contamination in patients whose condition is likely to worsen with prolonged or extensive surgery. This can be expanded in the resource-limited environment to include situations where surgical capacity is limited. For example, in a restricted one surgical team with more than one casualty, abbreviated surgery may be undertaken to allow the arrest of haemorrhage in multiple casualties. The decision may be taken at the outset of surgery or anytime during surgery, should the patient's physiologic and metabolic condition determine.

Who Needs Damage Control Surgery?

The decision to perform a damage control trauma laparotomy is determined by several factors, including inbound trauma operative workload, anatomical and physiological factors, major incidents, and mass casualty situations. Anatomical factors include injury burden, complex injuries (likely to fail at the index procedure such as complex duodenal/pancreatic injuries, need for prolonged vascular bypass, other more compelling injuries in need of treatment (e.g., traumatic brain injury [TBI]) or any injury that may require a relook procedure, e.g. bowel of questionable viability). Physiologic factors are determined by the metabolic state of end-organ tissue perfusion, determined by the presence of

acidosis, hypothermia, and evidence of coagulopathy. For these groups of patients, an immediate surgical procedure to rapidly save a life is indicated, as a prolonged operation would worsen physiological impairment, typically ending in catastrophic failure. Patients who have lost a significant volume of blood, if not treated expeditiously, will quickly become *coagulopathic*, *hypothermic* and *acidotic* – the *trauma triad of death*. Additional decisions to perform a damage control trauma laparotomy include the number of casualties in need of surgery and your own surgical skill set.

Although there is no absolute time cut-off for damage control surgery (DCS), the surgeon should aim to have all bleeding and contamination under control within 60 minutes and be on the way to the intensive care unit (ICU) by 90 minutes. Some surgeons advocate that this is even too long in truly exsanguinating patients.

Damage Control Laparotomy

Uncontrollable bleeding within the chest or abdomen mandates immediate laparotomy. A rapid sequence of steps is followed in a methodical fashion to arrest haemorrhage, contain contamination, and improve end-organ oxygenation and perfusion. This surgery will be a temporary measure to prevent worsening of the patient's physiology while pending recovery of the haemodynamic and metabolic state to justify safe, definitive surgery later. After a period of physiological improvement in the ICU, where the hypothermia, acidosis, and coagulopathy are reversed, definitive anatomical surgery is scheduled. This may be as short as a few hours or may take up to 48 hours. The sooner definitive surgery is undertaken, the better the outcome.

The Venue

Ideally, surgery should take place in a warm operating theatre, set at 30 °C, that is well equipped for all cavity surgery — with monitoring equipment, excellent lighting, and access to blood products. **Unfortunately, this may be a luxury in a resource-limited setting, and the operating team must endeavour to do their best to mitigate this.**

As the surgical field must expose the patient from neck to knee as more than one cavity may be opened, there is a risk of aggravating hypothermia. Underwarmer bedding may be helpful, but the best way to prevent it is a warm environment. This will feel too hot for the surgeon but is better for the patient. In addition, it will serve as a constant reminder to abbreviate the surgery.

Equipment should include a major laparotomy set, a major vascular set, and a major thoracotomy set.

Most important, 20 large abdominal packs must be on the surgical field and already accounted for in the nursing pre-count, ready to use. These are placed by the scrub nurse within easy reach of the surgeon.

Patient Position

The patient is placed supine on the operating table in a T-shape configuration, with the arms outstretched (the *crucifix position*; Figure 8.1). The patient is draped from the neck to the knees with as much lateral exposure as possible. Large bore multichannel central venous line and bladder catheter may be placed, but if *in extremis*, these may be deferred until later if there are at least two wide-bore IV lines in place. The pre-operative World Health Organization checklist must also be deferred if the patient is *in extremis*.

The Technique

Remember, the clock is ticking, and the surgeon must decide as they make the first incision whether this is going to be a damage control trauma

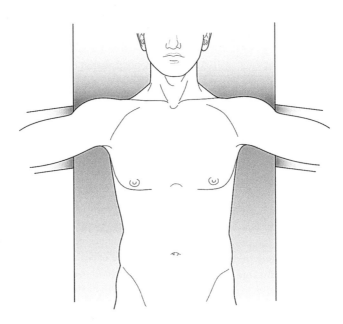

Figure 8.1 Trauma laparotomy positioning. The patient is placed supine on the operating table in a T-shape configuration with the arms outstretched.

laparotomy or a standard trauma laparotomy without the need for damage control. If DCS is indicated, a certain tempo must be maintained, remaining cognisant of rapid gross haemorrhage and contamination control, followed by temporary abdominal closure with planned re-exploration.

The Incision

A midline incision is made from the xiphoid process to the pubis, which may be extended into the chest if necessary (Figure 8.1). This follows the same procedure as any standard emergency laparotomy, but the abdominal wall is opened along its full length with only the surgical knife and in about four sweeps of the blade. The linea alba is incised, and entry into the abdomen proceeds, taking care not to damage bowel often floating within the haemoperitoneum. Once scalpel entry is made, blunt scissors can be used to open the remaining linea alba to reduce risk of bowel injury. Electrocautery will be useless as blood will be covering the tissue intended to be opened.

Once Inside

If a massive haemoperitoneum is encountered, don't panic! It's already outside of the patient's intravascular space. The best first manoeuvre is to exteriorise the small bowel in its entirety by sweeping it from the left side of the abdominal cavity outwards (Figure 8.2). This will assist in temporarily stemming any major mesenteric bleeding as the base of the mesentery tamponades against the patient's open right side of the abdominal wall. It also allows access for packing into the left abdominal cavity. In a clockwise fashion, rolled large abdominal packs are placed sequentially, starting at the upper left quadrant (the spleen is statistically the compelling source of bleeding in a blind trauma laparotomy), left paracolic gutter and intraperitoneal pelvic cavity (Figure 8.3). The small bowel is then re-mobilised to overhang the left side of the abdominal wall, and the same packing procedure followed in the right side of the abdominal cavity, upper-right quadrant (above, below, and lateral to the liver), the right paracolic gutter, and into the right side of the intraperitoneal pelvic cavity (Figure 8.4). Additional packs may then

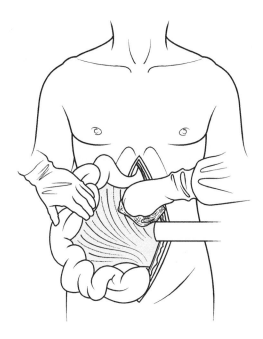

Figure 8.2 Exteriorise the small bowel from the duodenojejunal flexure to the ileocolic peritoneum. Packing begins in the upper-left quadrant, left paracolic gutter, and intraperitoneal pelvic cavity.

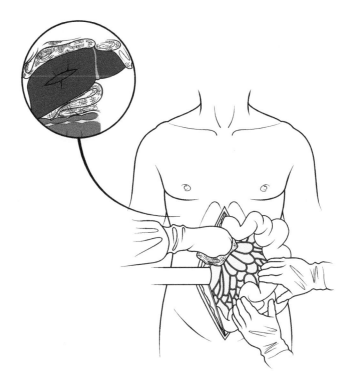

Figure 8.3 The small bowel is mobilised to overhang the left abdominal wall. Packs are placed in the upper-right quadrant above and below the right lobe of the liver.

be placed centrally overlying the retroperitoneum, in the superior and inferior aspects and the small bowel and mesentery (supra- and inframesocolic spaces), and the small bowel is then placed back into the abdomen. A large abdominal swab is placed on top of the small bowel (now back *in situ*), and the surgeon places his hands on top of this swab and compresses gently downwards, placing moderate pressure on the abdominal contents. The surgeon then stops and waits!

Then What?

The surgeon communicates with the anaesthetic team to assess the haemodynamic and haematological parameters. Once gross haemorrhage control has been achieved, this pause period also allows the anaesthetic team to 'catch up' with resuscitation using blood and blood products and limiting crystalloid. The patient's parameters are continually reassessed by both the surgeon and the anaesthetic team. If possible, serial blood gases should be sent to assess the acid–base status and the temperature should be under continuous monitoring. The team, led by the surgeon, may then decide if abbreviated damage control surgery is indicated. They must remain vigilant to the changing parameters and patient condition and be dynamic and prepared to adjust the planned surgical track to respond to the changing situation.

One pitfall is that if the packs are removed too early, it could aggravate bleeding that is potentially under control. Resist this temptation! If the bleeding has been controlled and a brief, but adequate, period of reassessment has taken place, we advocate the removal of the packs in a sequential manner – beginning at the area *least* likely injured or bleeding. By doing this, the surgeon can declare these areas in sequence 'injury-free', thereby allowing them to concentrate on the more severely injured parts of the abdomen.

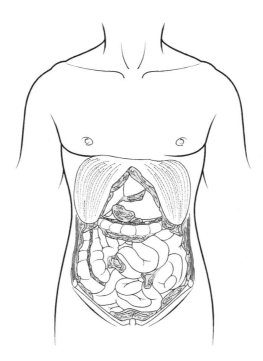

Figure 8.4 More packs are then placed in the central part of the abdomen in the superior and inferior aspect, the small bowel and mesentery are then placed back on the packs, and the packs placed on the small bowel.

Total Haemorrhage Control

If there is continuing or uncontrolled bleeding with packing, it is likely arterial. This may not be acknowledged at first if the patient is very hypotensive. At this point, a more definitive procedure must be performed. Total haemorrhage control of arterial inflow to the abdomen is typically reserved for uncontrollable haemorrhage seen with larger arterial injuries such as the aorta, in patients *in extremis*. Control is performed by compressing the supracoeliac aorta manually at first (e.g., the aorta squeezed between the thumb and index finger) or a pressure device is applied against the aorta (e.g., aortic stop) to compress it against the thoracic vertebrae, followed by application of a supracoeliac vascular clamp (if the surgeon's skills and experience allow).

The supracoeliac aorta above the visceral segment is accessed by pulling the stomach downwards (caudal direction), identifying the gastrohepatic ligament (lesser omentum), and opening a window in this ligament at its medial aspect, which allows the surgeon direct access to the aorta as it passes through the aortic hiatus of the diaphragm. This can be a challenging manoeuvre even in experienced hands, especially when time is of the essence.

A preferred option for the patient *in extremis* in need of immediate and total arterial inflow control to the abdomen is to perform a left anterolateral thoracotomy, followed by immediate cross-clamping of the descending thoracic aorta. In addition, the intra-thoracic inferior vena cava (IVC) may also be accessed and clamped from the left chest, with total loss of venous return to the heart. If you perform this manoeuvre, note that it's very important to warn the anaesthetic team and resuscitate from lines above the level of the diaphragm.

The Retroperitoneum

The retroperitoneum (RP) is carefully inspected for haematoma. This is further discussed in Chapter 10.

Hollow Viscus Injury

Small holes in the small bowel may be closed primarily in a transverse or circular fashion to prevent stenosis. Severely damaged small bowel should be rapidly oversewn or resected to manage contamination, and the ends stapled closed or tied with a heavy suture/tape. The bowel may be left in discontinuity for a few days; typically, there will be an ileus anyway. In addition, any attempt to anastomose in the face of profound shock and damage control is likely to lead to dehiscence and further sepsis known as second-hit phenomenon.

Other Important Injuries Not to Miss

All other injuries require a full exploratory laparotomy if physiology allows. The most likely positions of missed injuries which must be inspected and ruled out directly and specifically are as follows:

- Gastro-oesophageal junction
- Anterior and posterior wall of the stomach
- Pancreas and duodenum (anterior and posterior aspects)
- Transverse colon
- Ascending and descending colon
- Root of the mesentery
- Rectum

At the End of Damage Control Surgery Stage I

The abdomen is typically left open with the packs *in situ*, but if the patient is *in extremis*, a running suture just to close the skin will leave the fascial domain untouched for definitive repair later but still contribute to the abdominal tamponade and gross haemorrhage control. This is superior to other temporary closure methods (e.g., Bogota bag sutured to the aponeurosis) to preserve the oedematous aponeurosis, in addition to being a time-consuming procedure. If relatively stable at this point – or the skin cannot be approximated – we advise fashioning a laparostomy with vacuum dressing, which may be improvised using Ioban™ and surgical swabs.

Depending on the resources available, the patient may have to be kept in a location and a relook

warranted or evacuated for further procedures. This is dictated by operational tempo, resource availability, and evacuation chain.

Ten Key Points:

1. Don't panic. The patient has arrived alive.
2. If the patient has uncontrolled haemorrhage, immediately go to the operating theatre.
3. Make a decision and make an incision.
4. Control haemorrhage in a sequential, controlled fashion.
5. Give anaesthesia time to catch up.
6. Explore the abdomen in a sequential fashion starting with the LEAST likely area of haemorrhage.
7. Determine if this is definitive surgery or damage control trauma laparotomy.
8. If definitive, complete expeditiously.
9. If damage control laparotomy, control intra-abdominal spillage and haemorrhage. Place temporary abdominal dressing or just close the skin.
10. Return to OR when physiologically stable.

ADDITIONAL READING

Bowley DM, Barker P, Boffard KD. Damage control surgery – concepts and practice. *J R Army Med Corps* 2000; **146(3)**:176–182.

Brasel KJ, Weigelt JA. Damage control in trauma surgery. *Curr Opin Crit Care* 2000;**6(4)**:276–280.

Cirocchi R, Abraha I, Montedori A et al. *Damage control surgery for abdominal trauma. Cochrane Database Syst Rev* 2013**(3)**: CD007438.

Diaz JJ Jr., Cullinane DC, Dutton WD et al. The management of the open abdomen in trauma and emergency general surgery: part 1 – damage control. *J Trauma* 2010;**68(6)**:1425–1438.

Duchesne JC, Kimonis K, Marr AB et al. Damage control resuscitation in combination with damage control laparotomy: a survival advantage. *J Trauma* 2010;**69(1)**: 46–52.

Eiseman B, Moore EE, Meldrum DR, Raeburn C. Feasibility of damage control surgery in the management of military combat casualties. *Arch Surg* 2000;**135(11)**: 1323–1327.

Goldberg SR, Henning J, Wolfe LG, Duane TM. Practice patterns for the use of antibiotic agents in damage control laparotomy and its impact on outcomes. *Surg Infect (Larchmt)* 2017;**18(3)**:282–286.

Hirshberg A, Walden R. Damage control for abdominal trauma. *Surg Clin North Am* 1997;**77(4)**:813–820.

Hommes M, Chowdhury S, Visconti D et al. Contemporary damage control surgery outcomes: 80 patients with severe abdominal injuries in the right upper quadrant analyzed. *Eur J Trauma Emerg Surg* 2018;**44(1)**:79–85.

Karamarkovic AR, Popovic NM, Blagojevic ZB et al. Damage control surgery in abdominal trauma. *Acta Chir Iugosl* 2010;**57(1)**:15–24.

Kirkpatrick AW, McKee JL, Tien H et al. Damage control surgery in weightlessness: a comparative study of simulated torso hemorrhage control comparing terrestrial and weightless conditions. *J Trauma Acute Care Surg* 2017;**82(2)**:392–399.

Moore EE, Burch JM, Franciose RJ, Offner PJ, Biffl WL. Staged physiologic restoration and damage control surgery. *World J Surg* 1998;**22(12)**:1184–1190; discussion 1190–1191.

Morgan K, Mansker D, Adams DB. Not just for trauma patients: damage control laparotomy in pancreatic surgery. *J Gastrointest Surg* 2010;**14(5)**:768–772.

Myrhoj T, Moller P. Liver packing and planned reoperation in the management of severe hepatic trauma. *Annales Chirurgiae et Gynaecologiae* 1987;**76(4)**:215–217.

Parajuli P, Kumar S, Gupta A et al. Role of laparoscopy in patients with abdominal trauma at level-I trauma center. *Surg Laparosc Endosc Percutan Tech* 2018;**28(1)**:20–25.

Poortman P, Meeuwis JD, Leenen LP. Multitrauma patients: principles of 'damage control surgery'. *Ned Tijdschr Geneeskd* 2000;**144(28)**:1337–1341.

Rignault DP. Abdominal trauma in war. *World J Surg* 1992;**16(5)**:940–946.

Rotondo MF, Schwab CW, McGonigal MD et al. 'Damage control': an approach for improved survival in exsanguinating penetrating abdominal injury. *J Trauma* 1993;**35(3)**:375–382; discussion 382–383.

Scalea TM, Phillips TF, Goldstein AS et al. Injuries missed at operation: nemesis of the trauma surgeon. *J Trauma* 1988;**28(7)**:962–967.

Schellenberg M, Inaba K, Bardes JM et al. Defining the GE junction in trauma: epidemiology and management of a challenging injury. *J Trauma Acute Care Surg* 2017;**83(5)**:798–802.

Smith JE, Midwinter M, Lambert AW. Avoiding cavity surgery in penetrating torso trauma: the role of the computed tomography scan. *Ann R Coll Surg Engl* 2010;**92(6)**:486–488.

Sharrock AE, Barker T, Yuen HM, Rickard R, Tai N. Management and closure of the open abdomen after damage control laparotomy for trauma. A systematic review and meta-analysis. *Injury* 2016;**47(2)**:296–306.

Timmermans J, Nicol A, Kairinos N, Teijink J, Prins M, Navsaria P. Predicting mortality in damage control surgery for major abdominal trauma. *S Afr J Surg* 2010;**48(1)**:6–9.

Zacharias SR, Offner P, Moore EE, Burch J. Damage control surgery. *AACN Clin Issues* 1999;**10(1)**:95–103; quiz 141–142.

Damage Control for Severe Pelvic Haemorrhage in Trauma

9

Kristin Hummel and John H. Armstrong

INTRODUCTION

High-energy pelvic fractures constitute one of several potential sources of haemorrhage – up to 13% of patients sustaining blunt pelvic fractures will present in shock. Concomitant chest and abdominal trauma carry a 30% mortality rate. Distinguishing pelvic trauma as the most compelling source of bleeding or haemodynamic instability may be confounded by traumatic brain injury (TBI) or bleeding in another compartment. To save the lives of these severely injured patients, a comprehensive approach is required for haemorrhage control and the trauma team must rapidly:

- Identify the pelvis as a primary or contributing source of exsanguination.
- Intervene quickly to stop the bleeding.

In this environment we do not have the luxury of interventional radiology techniques or REBOA. Therefore, a high index of suspicion and aggressive management will be required.

Pelvic Anatomy and Haemorrhage

The bony pelvis includes three paired bones of the pubis, ilium, and ischium with a single sacrum posterior. Together, these form the anteroinferior tilted bony cavity (Figure 9.1a,b). The bones are connected anteriorly by the ligamentous public symphysis and posteriorly by the sacroiliac joints (sacrospinous,

sacrotuberous, and sacroiliac ligaments) which, if disrupted, allow a larger pelvic basin for haemorrhage. The pubis has two rami – superior and inferior – that join the ischium to form the obturator foramina. The pelvic cavity not only houses organs of the urogenital and lower gastrointestinal tracts, but also contains a dense concentration of blood vessels – including an intricate lattice of venous drainage in addition to the named transiting lower extremity neurovascular structures. The rich venous plexus lies in the presacral space posterior but closely adherent to the iliac arteries and the numerous branches of the internal iliac artery (particularly, the superior gluteal and internal pudendal arteries). The fractured surfaces of the pelvic bones themselves can bleed. Thus, there are three primary sources of pelvic bleeding:

1. Venous plexus (the commonest source of bleeding)
2. Arterial branches (occurs in 10–15% of open-book pelvic fractures and present in 75% of haemodynamically unstable pelvic fractures)
3. Cancellous bony ends at fracture sites

The pelvis is a ring that rarely breaks in one place alone. Structures in proximity to the fractures can be injured, especially the thin-walled pelvic veins. The pelvic cavity pressure is lower than the venous pressure, creating a large potential retroperitoneal space for haemorrhage and clot to fill. The pelvic organs are readily compressed or displaced upwards into the abdomen, allowing further haemorrhage into the

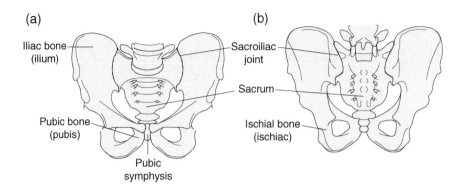

Figure 9.1 Pelvic anatomy.

enlarged potential space as it dissects away from the bony pelvis. Exsanguinating pelvic haemorrhage is typically associated with additional arterial bleeding. The pelvic bones and ligaments are sturdy structures and, therefore, require a significant amount of energy to break (e.g., high energy motor vehicle collision [MVC], falls >2 m, pedestrian versus motor vehicle). There are three broad patterns of severe pelvic fracture:

1. Lateral compression (Figure 9.2a)
2. Anterior–posterior (A-P) compression ('open book') (Figure 9.2b)
3. Vertical shear (Figure 9.2c)

In modern high-speed MVCs, it is not unusual to see a combination of pelvic injury patterns. However, if an A-P compression injury is present, this will open the pelvic ring, increasing the potential space for

blood to collect, aggravating haemorrhage, and constituting a major risk for exsanguination.

Damage Control for Pelvic Haemorrhage

As previously emphasised, recognition of exsanguinating haemorrhage in the injured patient is the first critical step in management. The mechanism of injury will define the amount and vector of energy that has caused the injury and, therefore, the potential for bleeding. A rapid diagnosis of pelvic fracture begins with clinical examination. Palpation along the pelvic margins may elicit tenderness in the lucid patient. Perineal bruising, blood at the urethral meatus, and a high-riding prostate (absent prostate on digital rectal exam) may be additional clues of pelvic fracture but in themselves are not reliable. It is not recommended to

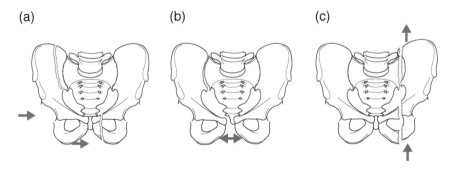

Figure 9.2 Pelvic injury patterns. (a) Lateral compression. (b) Anterior-posterior (A-P) compression (open book). (c) Vertical shear.

manually mobilise the pelvis (i.e. 'springing the pelvis' or 'open-booking the pelvis') to assess for A-P stability as this has the potential to exacerbate bleeding. A rapid anterior-posterior plain radiograph of the pelvis gives a snapshot of the fracture patterns described earlier. A FAST (focused assessment with sonography for trauma) scan may also demonstrate free fluid (i.e. blood) in the pelvis and abdomen but is not reliable to rule out pelvic bleeding.

Once an unstable or potentially unstable pelvis has been recognised, rapid application of external pelvic compression, which must be centred on the greater trochanters of the femurs, should follow. This may be accomplished with a commercial binder or a draw sheet. In the absence of a commercial pelvic binder, a draw sheet should be centred over the greater trochanters and wrapped snugly, compressing the pelvis, and secured with clamps or haemostats (Figure 9.3a–c).

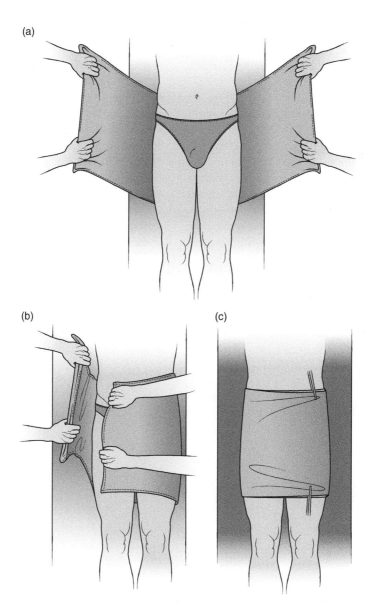

(a)

(b)

(c)

Figure 9.3 Improvised pelvic binder.

Alternatively, the sheet may be placed across the greater trochanters, twisted on itself and secured by tying a knot with the free ends and/or tucking them under the patient.

The reduction in pelvic volume following the application of the pelvic binder may help slow haemorrhage while other sources of bleeding are considered. The patient's response to resuscitation with massive transfusion protocol also guides further investigation. If the patient remains haemodynamically unstable and uncontrolled, pelvic haemorrhage remains a source. Extraperitoneal pelvic packing should be performed, where packs are placed deliberately within the extraperitoneal space, to achieve direct compression and tamponade low-pressure venous bleeding. Access to the retroperitoneal space may be achieved:

- During laparotomy (which will be required in most cases)
- Via pelvis-only packing (without laparotomy)

It must be stressed that for the majority of patients presenting with major haemorrhage and a significant pelvic fracture, 90% will have associated injuries; 50% of these cases will have a major source of bleeding outside of the pelvis itself, and 30% will be intra-abdominal. Therefore, if pelvic packing is required, there is a high chance that a laparotomy is also required for injuries within the abdomen. Consequently, extraperitoneal pelvic packing via a laparotomy is more commonly performed than pelvis-only pelvic packing (without laparotomy) when damage control surgery is indicated.

Technique of Pelvis-Only Extraperitoneal Pelvic Packing

- Make a lower midline infra-umbilical incision (or occasionally a Pfannenstiel incision) through the skin, subcutaneous fat, and linea alba (Figure 9.4a).
- The preperitoneal space is entered by manually sweeping the peritoneal reflection above in an upwards (cephalad) direction. Often in trauma, the pelvic haematoma will have done most of this dissection, and the space is easier to identify (Figure 9.4b).
- With the space exposed (anterior abdominal wall retraction peritoneum pushed upwards with the non-dominant hand), rolled laparotomy sponges are placed deep into the recesses of the pelvis,

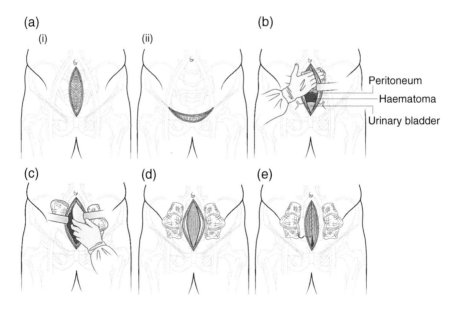

Figure 9.4 Pelvis only extra-peritoneal packing.

beginning at the sacroiliac joint posteriorly and proceeding anteriorly (Figure 9.4c).

- One may encounter large-volume haemorrhage if the pelvic haematoma has ruptured – do not panic as this blood is already outside the intravascular space but work quickly and methodically to compress any further bleeding with the laparotomy packs.
- Take care not to violate the peritoneum which will open the intra-abdominal compartment,

leading to a larger space for bleeding and allowing the small bowel to herniate into the pelvis, obscuring the surgical field for packing (Figure 9.4d).

- Repeat the same process for pack placement on the other side.
- If effective packing has taken place, the swabs on top should remain white.
- Rapidly close the skin with a running nylon suture to aid pelvic compression (Figure 9.4e).

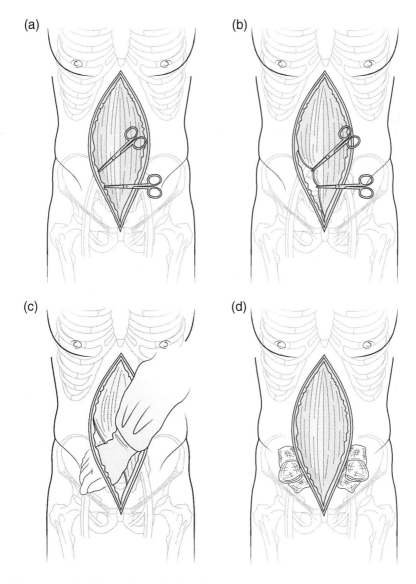

Figure 9.5 Extraperitoneal pelvic packing via the abdomen.

- Reassess patient response to resuscitation pelvic packing haemorrhage control.

Technique of Extraperitoneal Pelvic Packing via the Abdomen

- The peritoneal reflection against the pelvic sidewall is identified, then mobilised by stripping it away (hold the edge of the peritoneum with surgical clips or Littlewood graspers) off the sidewall and dissecting the plane between the peritoneum and the pelvic sidewall (Figure 9.5a).
- Typically, the pelvic haematoma has done most of this dissection already and the surgeon may only need to manually enlarge the space (Figure 9.5b).
- Ensure the pelvic space is opened widely and evacuate the haematoma (Figure 9.5c).
- Using rolled abdominal packs, pack deeply into the pelvic recesses quickly and methodically to compress any further bleeding.
- The process must be repeated on both sides (Figure 9.5d).
- Typically, the intra-abdominal cavity is also packed for damage control and the skin closed for additional tamponade.

If a non-expanding pelvic haematoma (Zone 3 retroperitoneal haematoma) is known or encountered during trauma laparotomy, it is best to leave it untouched as it is likely to be self-tamponading. Take care not to disrupt the intact overlying peritoneum. However, if expanding or pulsatile (indicative of arterial bleeding), exploration with or without pelvic packing is mandatory and may be effectively performed through the same laparotomy incision. Zone 3 retroperitoneal haematomas from penetrating trauma must be explored. In either situation, the patient should return to the ICU for further resuscitation and correction of their metabolic and physiologic derangements.

Other Strategies

Once pelvic packing has been performed, the pelvic binder may be re-applied to provide additional tamponade of the bleeding by re-apposition of the open pelvic ring. Rarely, bilateral ligation of the internal iliac arteries is required; this can be both challenging and dangerous as it necessitates opening the pelvic haematoma to identify the internal iliac arteries or its major branches. In addition, it does not control the venous bleeding which occurs in many blunt pelvic trauma cases and increases the risk of injury to the iliac veins during dissection due to their intimate relationship behind the iliac artery complex.

ADDITIONAL READING

Costantini TW, Coimbra R, Holcomb JB et al. Current management of hemorrhage from severe pelvic fractures: results of an American Association for the Surgery of Trauma multi-institutional trial. *J Trauma Acute Care Surg* 2016;**80(5)**:717–725.

Croce MA, Magnotti LJ, Savage SA, Wood GW II, Fabian TC. Emergent pelvic fixation in patients with exsanguinating pelvic fractures. *J Am Coll Surg* 2007;**204**:935–942.

Cullinane DC, Schiller HJ, Zielinski MD et al. Eastern Association for the surgery of trauma practice management guidelines for hemorrhage in pelvic fracture—update and systematic review. *J Trauma* 2011;**71**:1850–1868.

Davis JW, Moore FA, McIntyre RC Jr, Cocanour CS, Moore EE. West MA Western Trauma Association critical decisions in trauma: management of pelvic fracture with hemodynamic instability. *J Trauma* 2008;**65**: 1012–1015.

DuBose J, Inaba K, Barfmparas G et al. Bilateral internal iliac artery ligation as a damage control approach in massive retroperitoneal bleeding after pelvic fracture. *J Trauma* 2010;**69**:1507–1514.

Flint L, Cryer G. Pelvic fracture: the last 50 years. *J Trauma* 2010;**69**:483–488.

Jeske HC, Larndorder R, Krappinger D et al. Management of hemorrhage in severe pelvic injuries. *J Trauma* 2010;**68**:415–420.

Mauffrey C, Cueller DO II, Pieracci F et al. Strategies for the management of haemorrhage following pelvic fractures and associated trauma-induced coagulopathy. *Bone Joint J* 2014;**96-B**:1143–1154.

Miller PR, Moore PS, Mansell E, Meredith JW, Chang MC. External fixation or arteriogram in bleeding pelvic fracture: initial therapy guided by markers of arterial hemorrhage. *J Trauma* 2003;**54**:437–443.

Totterman A, Madsen JE, Skaga NO, Roise O. Extraperitoneal pelvic packing: a salvage procedure to control massive traumatic pelvic hemorrhage. *J Trauma* 2007;**62**:843–852.

Abdominal Injuries 10

Viktor Reva and Boris Kessel

Abdominal cavity represents a dark box filled with a variety of complex anatomical systems and structures, which might be difficult to deal with for a young surgeon, especially in austere environments with limited resources (lacking diagnostic and treatment options). While every abdominal organ is the focus of different specialists – upper gastrointestinal, colorectal, hepatobiliary, pancreatic, vascular, and others – frontline surgery mandates a common simple, effective, and reliable approach for the appropriate and available evacuation chain to be initiated.

The following are simple rules for frontline abdominal surgery:

a. Low threshold for deciding about laparotomy – 'if in doubt, open'.
b. Quick and brave surgery without flail in attempts of haemorrhage control.
c. Remove what needs to be removed; drain what cannot.
d. Ligation of what can be ligated; shunting of what cannot.
e. The simpler the technique, the better.
f. Back to basic techniques – simple manoeuvres, an educated finger, and common sense.

RESOURCE LIMITATION CONCERNS

Frontline surgery is typically deployed in resource-limited settings. A Role 2 medical treatment facility (MTF) is deployed in tents/improvised settings and is aimed towards providing resuscitative and damage control surgery. Surgery is usually performed by a forward surgical team consisting of a group of skilled healthcare professionals including surgeons and nurses with no narrowed specialists available. At this level of care, only limited equipment and diagnostic tools (i.e. portable X-Ray and ultrasound machines) are used.

The circumstances may be even more resource-limited while providing surgical care at Role 1, near (3–5 km away from) a point of injury with limited medical re-supply and blood products available. Here, surgery is usually provided by a Special Operations (Resuscitation) Surgical Team (or its analogue), consisting of 1–2 surgeons and a few more personnel. Over time, some elements of surgical care can be pushed forward to the point of injury – 'Advanced Resuscitative Care'. Far forward from a field hospital, there might be a lack of lights, monitoring opportunities, personnel, medical instruments, electricity, sterility, warming devices, imaging, and – related to abdominal injuries – laparoscopy, interventional radiology, possibilities for temporising techniques, and open abdomen options.

Severely injured patients are often under resuscitation, thus, coagulopathic, hypothermic and acidotic. No extensive laboratory indices can typically be achieved upon admission, especially in a mass casualty event. All this makes appropriate forward care to the wounded an act of confidence and courage, and this is especially relevant to abdominal injuries, which – if missed or inappropriately treated – can easily lead to death.

> Know what you have and be prepared for the worst possible scenario.
>
> Frontline surgery offers the 'opportunity' of damage control surgery for 'tactical indications' – trauma surgery in limited resources.

BRIEF REVIEW OF MATERIAL

Abdominal injuries are becoming less common in modern warfare as compared to extremity injuries, usually caused by improvised explosive devices. However, NCTH remains one of the leading causes of death in the battlefield, and until now there is no proven pre-hospital method to control this haemorrhage, with surgery being the only treatment modality to save lives.

Regardless of the mechanism of injury – penetrating or blunt – a careful physical examination is mandatory, and ultrasound exam (FAST) is a main adjacent diagnostic tool. In most cases, no computerised tomography (CT) scan is available at this echelon of care. Patients with a gunshot wound between the axilla and perineum must be suspected of having an abdominal injury. The whole-body surface must be carefully examined for a second wound, including *per rectum* and *per vaginal* examinations. There are only two absolute signs of the peritoneal injury which mandate laparotomy:

1. Organ/viscera/omentum eventration; and
2. Wound leakage of faeces, urine, bile.

The remaining signs (pain, tenderness, absence of bowel sounds, etc.) are relative and a decision about surgery should be made based on haemodynamic and physiological status. In a resource-limited environment, a diagnostic peritoneal lavage, or aspirations (DPL/DPA), may be used if ultrasound is unavailable.

Prior to any procedure, a nasogastric tube and urinary catheter are inserted.

1. A 2–3 cm longitudinal incision in the infraumbilical area is made after infiltration with local anaesthesia (in case of associated pelvic fractures, a supraumbilical approach is preferred to avoid a false-positive result due to an enlarged pelvic haematoma) (Figure 10.1). Several techniques are described. The initial steps are the same for DPL and DPA.
2. *Linea alba* is lifted by a towel clamp and a trocar is inserted into the peritoneal cavity followed by plastic tube insertion for inspection. It is the fastest, but also a relatively dangerous, technique if severe adhesions exist.
3. Consistent dissection of the periumbilical region until the peritoneum, which is taken by clamps and divided for inspection.
4. In case of a skin scar in the periumbilical region, another 'virgin' site is chosen. A left hypogastric area is preferred to avoid misinterpreting of this skin incision in the future (can be missed with a scar after appendectomy).

Once the peritoneum is opened, in DPL, a one-litre bag of crystalloid is connected to a giving set and 500 mL of fluid is allowed to pass into the abdominal cavity. The bag is then placed on the floor and the peritoneal cavity drained into the bag. It is deemed grossly positive if the contents are frank blood (unable to read text through the bag) or are the same colour as the urinary catheter of nasogastric tube. A DPA is performed with a needle and syringe prior. If frank blood is aspirated, then the DPA is deemed positive.

The approach to abdominal surgery at Role 2 is absolutely the same as the whole damage control strategy; physiology does not change because of geographical location – stop the bleeding, prevent

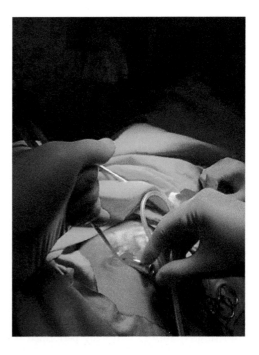

Figure 10.1 DPL. A plastic tube is inserted via a trocar placed under the umbo.

contamination, and provide the necessary 'bridge' to next level surgery for at least 12–24 hours. The surgery at Role 2 is usually provided by young well-motivated persons, who, however, lack experience with 'big, bad cases'.

A decision for laparotomy at this echelon of care depends on the current circumstances: resources, mass casualty admission, possibility of rapid transportation, duration of the evacuation. In an ideal scenario with air transport immediately available and close location of a rear-deployed hospital (a Role 3 MTF), a stable patient may be safely evacuated. In a less-than-ideal scenario (darkness, a sandstorm, hostile activity), a more aggressive approach must be undertaken. There is a significant risk of patient deterioration during transport; a stable patient with penetrating abdominal injury or with blunt injury and a significant amount of blood in the abdomen has to undergo surgical exploration. It may turn out to be non-therapeutic intervention, but it helps mitigate life-threatening intra-abdominal injuries. Patients with haemodynamic compromise and suspected abdominal injuries undergo immediate laparotomy.

FAST is good, but DPL and DPA are also useful diagnostic adjuncts at the frontline – remember and know how to do them!

Have a low threshold for laparotomy – if in doubt, do it!

HOW TO DO IT?

Aortic Control

Once trauma laparotomy is initiated (Chapter 8) – a pool of blood with uncontrolled massive bleeding – one of the following methods of temporary haemorrhage control can be performed:

1. Left anterolateral thoracotomy and aortic clamping (intrathoracic aortic clamping, IT-AC).
2. Supracoeliac aortic clamping via a smaller sac (intra-abdominal aortic clamping, IA-AC).
3. Resuscitative endovascular balloon occlusion of the aorta (REBOA).

Procedure	Difficult	Traumatic	Learning curve
IT-AC	+	+++	+
IA-AC	+++	++	+++
REBOA	+	+	+++

Abbreviations: IT-AC, intrathoracic aortic clamping; IA-AC, intraabdominal aortic clamping; REBOA, resuscitative endovascular balloon occlusion of the aorta.

The IT-AC and REBOA can be performed before laparotomy has been initiated. The former might be indicated when a patient is severely hypotensive and has a main source of bleeding (typically, a gunshot wound) in the abdomen. However, in most cases, surgeons go straight to the abdomen and try to fix the problem. REBOA is a modern technique of controlling severe intra-abdominal haemorrhage consisting of a few steps:

1. Femoral artery access and sheath placement
2. Balloon insertion and positioning (external landmarks are used – the balloon should be placed between the sternum notch and the xiphoid process)
3. Balloon inflation
4. Surgical control of bleeders: temporary (clamping, ligation, packing, etc.) or definitive (splenectomy, nephrectomy, etc.)
5. Balloon deflation and removal (a sheath can be flushed and left in place until reaching the next echelon of care)

REBOA was determined to be safe and effective in combat environments (Figure 10.2). Possibilities of early on-the-scene or en-route balloon insertion manoeuvres are also in the focus of investigators. REBOA, particularly partial REBOA (pREBOA) if placed at Role 2, can also be an option for back-up haemodynamic support during the following evacuation to Role 3. Special workshops and additional training must be undertaken to perform this manoeuvre safely.

Supracoeliac open aortic control is not as easy as it appears! It is even more difficult in haemodynamically compromised patients. It requires a clear understanding of anatomy, good technical skills, and experience. Doing the manoeuvre, you may think that you have compressed the aorta by

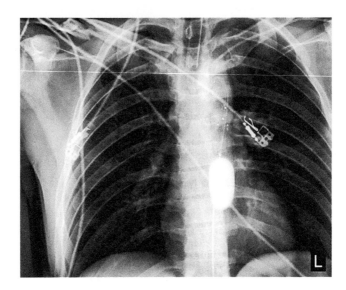

Figure 10.2 Role 2 REBOA for a patient with blunt abdominal and pelvic trauma admitted with undetectable blood pressure. An immediate rise of systolic blood pressure by 110 mmHg was noted after balloon inflation. Laparotomy and pelvic packing were successfully performed for 16 minutes aortic occlusion.

your fist or fingers, but you may not be at the correct location. This part of the aorta requires appropriate mobilisation, and the left and right walls should be clearly identified for Satinsky (or another vascular) clamp application. **There is a special instrument for aortic compression, but you will never find it in a field mobile hospital when it is needed.**

When the aorta has been temporarily occluded, it is time to fix the problem as soon as possible. Remember, a clock is ticking and ischaemic burden is accumulated, making reperfusion injury worse. Remove all the blood from the abdomen, find and address the main sources of bleeding and once controlled, start deflating the balloon/declamping the aorta. Optimal occlusion time is still unknown, but 30–40 minutes for thoracic aorta is relatively safe, but this can be greatly decreased depending on the physiological burden of injury. The stronger recommendation is to declamp (to start slow balloon deflation) the aorta as soon as feasible. pREBOA is hardly possible as it requires additional hands, monitoring, and expertise. Intermittent REBOA (15–20 minutes intervals of inflations/deflations) may be used if the patient hardly tolerates deflations.

> In a disastrous bleeding, start with aortic control. Always try to get control outside the haematoma!
>
> REBOA is a proven alternative for temporary aortic control during frontline surgery.

Abdominal Compartments

Severe bleeding can occur in two major abdominal compartments: intraperitoneal and retroperitoneal. The former is easily recognised, and usually haemorrhage from intra-abdominal organs is primarily addressed and managed. Explore them systematically, preferably in a clockwise manner starting at the liver. When the blood is removed and no continuous bleeding is seen, then keep searching – there should certainly be an injury – somewhere in mesentery or retroperitoneally.

The main sources of devastating bleeding in the abdominal region are the following:

- Intra-abdominal organs (liver, spleen).
- Mesentery.
- Retroperitoneal organs and vessels.

Liver

The most challenging damage control surgery involves the liver. It takes much of the time during damage control laparotomy. A lot is written about multiple approaches to liver surgery, using different techniques, manoeuvres, and devices. The latter will not be available, so several basic concepts and techniques must be kept in mind.

First, the understanding to do as minimal, but lifesaving, as possible is the priority. Second, there is no time to flail. A correct tactical decision and technical implementation should be made as soon as possible. Finally, some things work differently in resource-limited settings.

The well-known '**4 P**' approach **(Press, Pringle, Packing, Pictures of angiography)** has some serious limitations in resource-limited environments. Compression of the liver requires an additional pair of hands that can simply be unavailable. Moreover, it reduces the space around the patient and the zone of interest, making it difficult for an operator to manipulate intra-abdominal organs and structures. Liver packing may be the only procedure undertaken to stall to aid transport to a higher level of treatment facility or to restore physiology as part of damage control resuscitation. There is a potential that subsequent patient movements and long transportation with packs on the liver might result in bleeding to re-occur en route. Pictures of angiography are unavailable at this echelon of care.

The best manoeuvre to begin with is temporary liver packing. Abdominal pads or swabs should be applied in a regular fashion without liver mobilisation: anteriorly, inferiorly, laterally and behind the liver. The idea is to achieve effective anterior-posterior counter-compression. Sometimes, additional pads placed between a dome of the liver and the diaphragm, may be helpful in bleeding from the anterior liver surface (Figure 10.3). Packing of only the left lobe is ineffective. Cutting the ligaments of the liver makes effective packing of the liver difficult. Do it when you are ready and have a plan of action. Direct vessel ligation, finger fracture techniques, hepatic tractotomy, liver clamps or liver tourniquets, liver resections, and others are not recommended during frontline surgery because these manoeuvres invariably cause blood loss and can be used only if you know exactly what you are doing. **Now is not the time for firsts!**

The only effective and reliable manoeuvre for initial haemorrhage control in difficult cases is the Pringle manoeuvre. The Pringle manoeuvre controls the hepatic vascular inflow – the portal vein and the hepatic artery – which can be found within the substance of the free edge of the lesser omentum (the gastro-hepatic ligament) in addition to the common bile duct (CBD): portal vein posterior and CBD and hepatic artery in front. This is manually palpated by sliding the left index finger into the *foramen of Winslow* (just below the liver), which is the opening to the lesser sac (Figure 10.4). The free edge may be initially pinched between the left index finger and

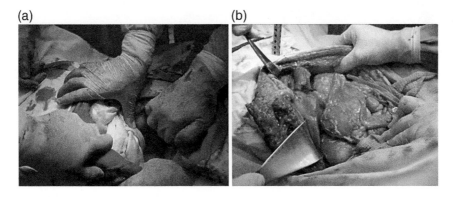

(a)   (b)

Figure 10.3 Grade IV liver injury. Massive bleeding was controlled by effective tight perihepatic packing (a). A view of the abdomen on post-operative day 5 during a staged re-laparotomy (b).

thumb, or a small window may be opened in the lesser omentum (medial to the structures to avoid damaging them), and a Foley catheter/vessel loop/ any soft silicone tube double-looped around them for control. The Pringle manoeuvre may be kept *in situ* for about 10–20 minutes (without pre-conditioning) in severe trauma (assuming normal liver function) before severe hepatic ischaemia occurs. But as with the aorta, declamp it as soon as feasible.

If the Pringle Manoeuvre Controls Bleeding, then This Is a Good Sign. If Not, Then You Have a Hepatic Vein or Retro-Hepatic IVC Injury!

While simple suture hepatorrhaphy and local haemostatic agents are techniques of choice for minor (1–3 cm in depth) hepatic lacerations; for major lacerations, one of the following reliable options must be finally applied before leaving the abdomen.

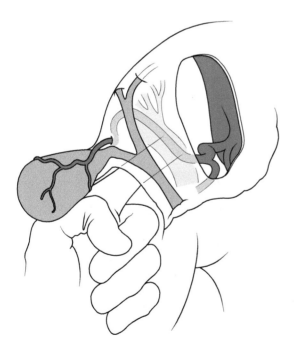

Figure 10.4 The Pringle manoeuvre to control liver bleeding.

LIVER SUTURING (DEEP SUTURE REPAIR)

A large curved needle on a Vicryl (braided) suture is a material of choice when a deep liver laceration is seen. A suture has to involve both edges (at least 1–2 cm) of the opposite sides of the ruptured capsule and must not be too superficial (otherwise, the bleeding is at elevated risk to recur). PTFE (or pieces of the peritoneum) pledgets can be used to reinforce sutures if the capsule is torn (Figure 10.5). Depending on the size and shape of the rupture, a few interrupted or horizontal mattress sutures should be applied with appropriate depth of the suture – not too superficial. A critical point here is tying the knot, so it does not cheese wire through the tissue, exacerbating the injury. In textbooks, you can find different sophisticated techniques of liver suturing, but in a difficult situation, the simplest bail-out technique is the best choice.

OMENTAL PLUGGING (PACKING)

If haemostasis is not achieved with simple suturing, or in case of a big stellate defect, an omental plug might be an alternative. An approximately 20-cm vascularised (typically on the right gastroepiploic artery) pedicle of the omentum is mobilised and put inside the liver defect as a plug (Figure 10.6). To fix this plug in place, a deep suture is applied as described. If a defect is too large, the suture may start at the liver and end at the omentum pedicle – just to fix it in place – but liver-to-liver suture anchoring the omentum carries more haemostatic effect, prevents migration, and reduces the risk of bile leakage.

LOCAL HAEMOSTATIC AGENTS

There are several commercially available haemostatic agents in the market. Not all of them are allowed for intracavitary haemostasis, but you can gently pack the wound with what you have readily available. A pair of deep suture bites over the packed wound channel will reinforce haemostatic effect if not primarily achieved. In case of a large deep laceration with a diffuse bleeding surface, off-label use of granular zeolite- or chitosan-based local haemostatic agents can be justified (Figure 10.7). It may be also used as a last resort. Scrupulous granula removal is not necessarily required.

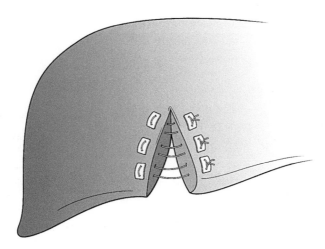

Figure 10.5 Pledget repair of liver laceration.

HEPATIC BALLOON TAMPONADE

This technique has been described for deeper through-and-through penetrating injuries to the liver (e.g., gunshot wound) that are too deep to reach with liver suturing (Figure 10.8). This will tamponade bleeding within the trajectory tract. Insert a Foley catheter into a finger of a sterile glove and tie the proximal end closed to prevent leakage. Gently insert the tip into the hepatic track as far as it will comfortably go. Once inside, infuse the Foley catheter (not its balloon) with sterile saline to inflate the finger of the glove like a balloon. The same can be done when the Foley balloon is punctured, and a Penrose drain is fixed to a Foley catheter proximally and distally. The Blackmore-Sengstaken catheter is good, but it is unlikely to be readily available.

Manual compression of the bleeding liver is your first step.

Temporary packing is your best friend. If working, do not touch the liver.

Perform only manoeuvres you are comfortable with.

(a) (b)

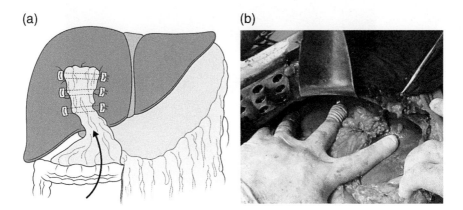

Figure 10.6 Omental packing of a deep liver injury.

(a) (b)

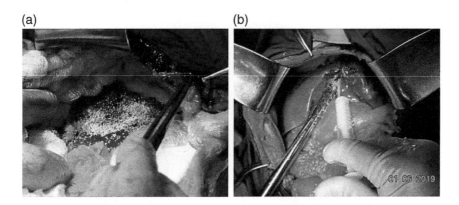

Figure 10.7 Application of a local haemostatic agent (a – zeolite-based, b – bioabsorbable liquid substance) to stop haemorrhage from a grade IV liver injury. Additional deep sutures were applied.

SPLEEN

A splenic rupture of any grade necessitates spleen removal during trauma laparotomy at a forward MTF (Figure 10.9). Any organ-sparing techniques may result in re-bleeding, unnecessary exsanguination – which would be devastating during transportation to the next echelon of care. As it was said, **the best way to preserve a spleen in trauma, is in formaldehyde**. Keep it simple!

It is known that the spleen can be 'stuck' or mobile. The former, if damaged, must be converted to mobile. Splenophrenic and splenorenal ligaments are divided, and the spleen is elevated by gentle forefinger dissection of the left hand, advancing in the retropancreatic plain, bringing the spleen into the midline. A couple of clamps are applied over the splenic hilum and the gastrosplenic ligament containing the short gastric vessels. The spleen is then removed, ligaments are ligated and/or sutured.

Use temporary liver "P" haemostatic techniques to get ready for a more reliable option.

An injured spleen is an enemy: if you do not kill it, it will kill you.

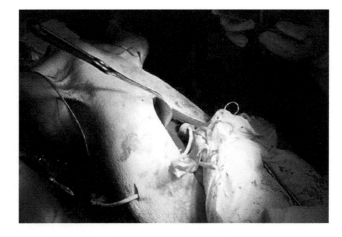

Figure 10.8 Liver balloon tamponade on an experimental porcine model. Training of military surgeons during a SMART trauma surgery workshop (Saint-Petersburg, Russia).

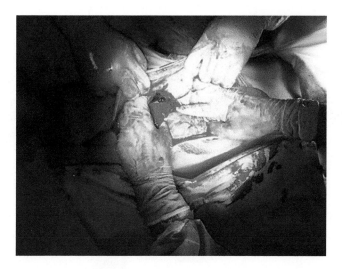

Figure 10.9 A grade III splenic rupture led to severe blood loss and hypotension (systolic blood pressure 50 mmHg). Laparotomy was undertaken at Role 2 after REBOA in a thoracic segment.

MESENTERY

Small bowel mesentery can be a source of significant bleeding which can spontaneously stop. It should be suspected if significant haemoperitoneum is found and no obvious injury is seen. The mesentery has to be inspected for possible superior (SMV) or inferior (IMV) mesenteric vein injury or their tributaries – which can be easily ligated. Arterial injuries typically manifest with a contained retroperitoneal Zone I haematoma which must be managed as described below.

All mesenteric tears even with no visible bleeding should be closed with running haemostatic sutures. It has the potential to become a significant source of haemorrhage later when blood pressure comes up.

RETROPERITONEAL HAEMORRHAGE

The retroperitoneal compartment lies behind the relatively thin wall of the parietal peritoneum and mesentery. While non-contained haemorrhage is typical for intra-abdominal trauma, retroperitoneal haemorrhage tends to stop spontaneously if the peritoneum resists in the retroperitoneum. Retroperitoneal haemorrhage usually recurs during exploration which releases the compartment pressure. Therefore, we need to be ready before opening the following retroperitoneal zones:

- **Zone I**: Central retroperitoneal compartment contains large vascular structures – aorta and inferior vena cava (IVC), their branches/tributaries, and the pancreas in the upper segment.
- **Zone II**: Lateral retroperitoneal compartment contains the flanks, kidneys, ureters and muscles of the posterior abdominal wall, and the ascending and descending colon.
- **Zone III**: The pelvic compartment contains vascular structures (Iliac arteries and accompanying veins) and pelvic organs (rectum, urinary bladder, reproductive organs) (Figure 10.10).

A Zone I haematoma mandates surgical exploration, regardless of mechanism of injury. Zone II and III haematoma should be explored only in penetrating injuries or expanding and/or pulsating haematoma. Zone III haematoma are usually associated with severe pelvic fractures. To aid haemostasis, pre-peritoneal pelvic packing should be performed via a separate incision above the pubis (Chapter 9). Zone II haematomas should also be explored in a haemodynamically compromised patient, as a shattered kidney does not haemorrhage much whilst low, but

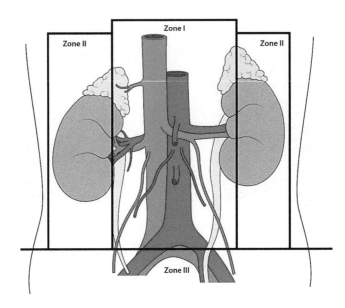

Figure 10.10 The three zones of the retroperitoneum. Zone I is the central area at the back of the abdomen, behind the parietal peritoneum and contains the major vessels including the aorta, IVC, and their branches. Zone II is the lateral RP, consisting of the kidneys and ureters. Zone III is the extraperitoneal pelvic cavity (below the iliac crests).

the bleeding has a high likelihood of recurring when the patient is back to being relatively normotensive.

MAJOR ABDOMINAL VASCULAR INJURIES

The injuries of named abdominal vessels are often fatal. Vascular injuries require prompt and reliable proximal and distal control. Major vessels injuries usually cause Zone I haematoma. An expanding/pulsating haematoma indicates main trunk of aorta or major branches of injury (Figure 10.11). Proximal control should be achieved by one of the previously mentioned techniques in virgin territory. Distal control is achieved according to the site of bleeding/haematoma by compression, temporary ligation, or clamping. Once achieved, exploration of the haematoma may be done by a direct approach (usually to the infra-renal aorta) or the classical left medial visceral rotation (especially for the supra-renal aorta). The latter is a complete mobilisation of the left flank (via the Toldt line), with the spleen (if still intact!) and with/without the left kidney. Blunt dissection is preferred as the haematoma has already done most of the

dissection required. Remember that the abdominal aorta lies on the vertebral column; therefore, do not go too deep. It allows complete visualisation of origins of all aortic visceral branches except the right renal artery.

The defect in the artery should be assessed to define the best damage control option:

- Ligation
- Shunting
- Primary repair (Prolene 3/0–5/0) or a patch (when a large defect has the potential to cause too much tension or significantly narrow the lumen)

For a large vessel injury, any plastic tube (a chest drain or a tube from a urine container) can be inserted and secured (Figure 10.12). Focus on shunt patency and make sure that it is reliably secured.

For the right renal artery and for IVC exploration, the Cattell-Braasch three-step manoeuvre is performed (Figure 10.13). It starts at the CBD, going down around the duodenum (Kocher manoeuvre – first step); then the line of Toldt is dissected to thoroughly mobilise the right flank (second step). A complete visceral rotation can be performed by dissecting all the mesentery on the Superior Mesenteric Artery (SMA)

(a)   (b)

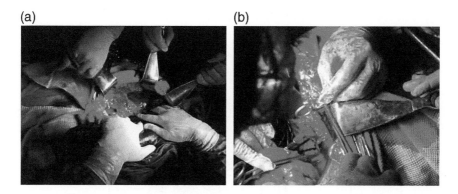

Figure 10.11 An unstable patient stabbed into the back at the left side. (a) A large expanding Zone I haematoma is seen during a laparotomy (FAST was negative). Proximal control was primarily achieved by REBOA. Distal control was achieved by manual compression. (b) A semi transection of the aorta (clamped) is revealed and sutured after the Mattox manoeuvre.

pedicle until the Treitz ligament is reached (third step) – this has the added benefit of fully visualising the third or fourth part of the duodenum as well as the proximal jejunum. However, in less experienced hands, it can lead to additional trauma; thus, it needs to be done for clear indications (i.e. full exploration of the third and fourth portions of the duodenum, extended approach to the IVC, aorta, etc.). For IVC injuries, there are numerous techniques described; the ones that work the best are usually the simplest. The soft pads of your fingers are particularly good for compression around an IVC defect; swabs on sticks can also be used for temporary proximal and distal control (Figure 10.14). No haemostats are usually applied as lumbar veins can be suddenly injured during dissection. Once a zone of injury is isolated, dry the operation field, assess the

injury pattern, and choose one of the previously mentioned options. Do not forget to look at a back wall of the IVC to rule out a through-and-through injury. If the back wall is damaged, it can be sutured by increasing the size of the anterior defect first and exposing the posterior wall defect, allowing for repair from the inside, or the IVC can be shunted with appropriately sized plastic tube (Figure 10.12b).

Ligation of the following structures has high morbidity and potential mortality:

- Aorta
- First part of the superior mesenteric artery (before at least one branch comes off)
- Supra-renal IVC (invariably fatal)
- Portal vein

(a)   (b)

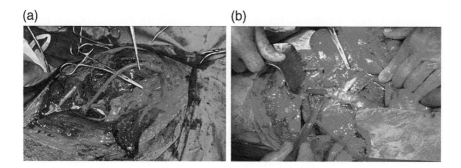

Figure 10.12 Temporary shunting for major abdominal vascular injuries: (a) hepatic artery, (b) supra-renal inferior vena cava.

(a)

(b)

Line of dissection

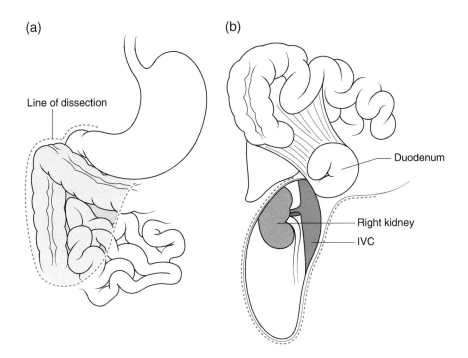

Duodenum

Right kidney

IVC

Figure 10.13 Right medial visceral rotation.

Total transection or thrombosis of the proximal SMA can be easily recognised by the 'black bowel' sign due to severe small bowel ischaemia. Surgical approach to the SMA is challenging. The options of gastric and pancreatic transections seem to be dangerous, but the left medial visceral rotation can help control the origin of the SMA, followed by exploration and shunting (have a small-calibre temporary shunt available for such vessels). Ligation of the rest of the SMA, the coeliac trunk, and the common hepatic artery is also not recommended but may be done as a last resort.

The nightmare of a military and civilian trauma surgeon is injury to the retrohepatic IVC or hepatic vein injury (so-called Zone 4 injury), which is difficult to recognise and even more difficult to manage when packing does not work effectively (remember that hepatic veins are not compressible). An additional right-sided thoracotomy with partial lower sternotomy may help visualise the injury or at least achieve total hepatic vascular isolation by clamping intra-thoracic IVC (IT-IVC), in addition to infra-hepatic IVC clamping and the Pringle manoeuvre (Figure 10.15). Another

possibility is to dissect a midline of the central tendon of the diaphragm, palpate the IT-IVC, and blindly but gently put a Satinsky clamp on it via the hole in the diaphragm.

Before the clamping, effective communication with the anaesthetist is mandatory, as they must be ready to increase volume replacement if a patient does not tolerate full IVC occlusion due to a sudden drop of cardiac preload. There are only a few minutes available to fix the IVC and/or hepatic vein injuries. **Atrio-caval shunting is not an option in this environment.** Mobilise the right lobe completely, pull it to the midline, and three/two hepatic veins can be found at the back where they enter the IVC close to each other and immediately under the diaphragm. Lateral Prolene suture of the IVC or suturing of the parenchyma at a zone of the injured hepatic vein (remember, they are not self-compressible!) or its dividing by a vascular stapler according to the injury pattern might be a method to bail out. If the achieved haemostasis is not reliably stable, add some pads for adjunct compression. This is invariably a fatal injury, with a mortality rate exceeding 80% in fully equipped

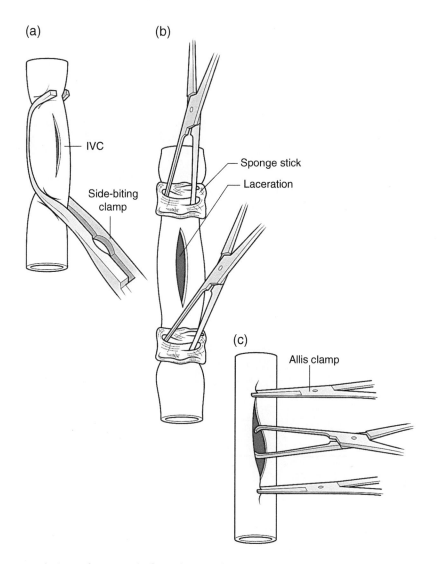

Figure 10.14 Techniques for control of IVC haemorrhage.

civilian centres, never mind a resource-limited environment.

KIDNEY

A severe kidney injury usually causes a large Zone 2 haematoma that necessitates exploration via the right or left medial visceral rotation. Surgical approach is via Gerota's fascia, which is dissected; an injured kidney is easily found inside a self-dissected haematoma; it can then be mobilised upwards and examined. In the case of compromised haemodynamics, a kidney is relatively simple to remove, the same way as the spleen, with the only exception being confirmation that another kidney exists. Superficial lacerations can be sutured, but no focus on the collecting system must be taken at this echelon of care.

Achieve proximal and distal control before entering the retroperitoneal haematoma.

Repair the vessel if permitted. Shunt, if necessary; ligate, if no other choice.

(a) (b)

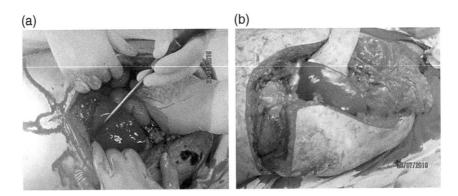

Figure 10.15 Grade V liver injury. (a) Re-bleeding after liver packing. Re-laparotomy is done 30 minutes after temporary abdominal closure. (b) Right anterolateral thoracotomy with partial median sternotomy is done to get access to the retrohepatic IVC.

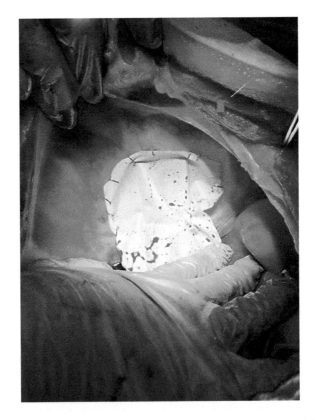

Figure 10.16 A quick damage control option for closure of the large diaphragmatic defect. A piece of plastic bag is fixed to the edges of the diaphragm by stapling.

Once life-threatening haemorrhage is controlled, other organs should be addressed to complete the damage control laparotomy.

DIAPHRAGM

The variety of diaphragmatic injuries ranges from the small holes to very big defects, sometimes very difficult for repair, especially in their posterior parts. Usually, a diaphragmatic hole may be rapidly closed using two-layer non-absorbable suturing without any tension. Again, application of two long Babcocks/Allis clamps or alternatively simple sutures that push down the diaphragm may simplify the repair. In the context of forward surgery, if the physiology of the patient allows, then the repair should be undertaken. If not, temporary abdominal closure must be undertaken, and this can be addressed at the next echelon of care.

Left-side diaphragmatic injuries which are easily suitable for primary repair, should be closed. In cases of the big defect which are not possible for simple suturing, there are two possible surgical options. The best is the closure using a piece of mesh (when no additional mobilisation of diaphragm is needed and no significant regional haematoma). Another option is a temporary (even partial) closure of the defect with a temporary bag, much like the Bogota bag, to prevent re-protrusion of abdominal contents into the chest. A piece of plastic or fabric material is simply fixed to edges of the ruptured diaphragm by silk sutures or stapler (Figure 10.16).

Always close the diaphragm when possible!

PANCREAS

Pancreatic injuries are among the most challenging and complicated to deal with. However, there are some practical issues in the context of forward surgery. First, the diagnosis of the pancreatic injury is very difficult, especially with no CT scanner. It should be suspected when peri-pancreatic haematoma is seen and confirmed after opening of the lesser sac. If the patient is operated a few hours after the injury, the signs of steatonecrosis (white patches) might appear around the pancreas, on omentum, or on the root of mesentery – indicative of pancreatic injury. Most injuries to the pancreas with no main pancreatic duct involvement may be successfully treated by adequate drainage alone and supportive therapy, including somatostatin and total parenteral nutrition. Only when the *Virsung duct* is transected are more complex and sophisticated surgical intervention is required – but this does not require definitive primary surgery! The best solution to define the extent of the pancreatic injury is not to perform aggressive pancreatic exploration. Minor damage may be easily converted to the big problem! Simply looking at the pancreatic surface and minimal haematoma evacuation may provide the necessary information about the next steps (Figure 10.17). If the pancreatic head is destroyed, drain it! If there is complete transection of the neck of pancreas is diagnosed, close both pancreatic sides using a stapling device, or multiple U-stitches. Neither Whipple's procedure nor distal pancreatectomy is recommended!

HOLLOW VISCUS INJURIES

All hollow viscus perforations and ruptures can be stratified into two groups: those suitable for simple suturing and those non-suitable for primary closure. The basic issue at Role 2 is to prevent leakage, but there are some specifications for certain organs.

OESOPHAGUS

These injuries are rare, mostly resulting from a penetrating mechanism. To evaluate the injury, the gastrohepatic ligament is opened, and the stomach is pushed caudad and centrally. The posterior wall of the oesophagus must be inspected. This may be achieved by gentle digital separation of the oesophagus from the aorta and spinal column. The oesophagus is mobilised and taken for countertraction on the large Penrose drain or the Foley catheter. In case of a small perforation of the anterior and posterior walls, the primary repair can be accomplished using Vicryl 2/0, two-layer sutures. In case of a large defect not suitable for primary repair, we recommend temporary insertion of an appropriately large-sized T-tube/chest tube into the perforation and closure of the remained defect with sutures. The chest tube can

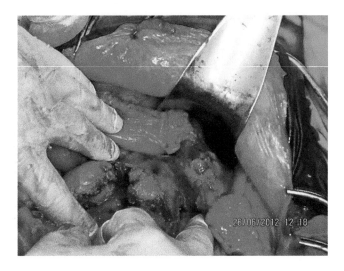

Figure 10.17 A complete transection of a body of the pancreas caused by a blunt injury. As long as no continuous bleeding is seen, a zone of injury can be simply drained in austere environments.

then be pulled through a hole in the abdominal wall and connected to a collecting bag. In case of a major defect or near/complete transection, simple closure of both sides using a GIA 60/90 stapler helps prevent contamination. Reconstruction can take place in higher echelons of care.

GASTRIC INJURIES

Gastric injuries are usually straightforward to diagnose. The posterior wall of the stomach is always to be inspected during a trauma laparotomy by opening a lesser sac, especially in penetrating injuries. Every small perigastric hematoma should be inspected. Most gastric defects may be simply sutured with or without debridement utilising two-layers Vicryl 2/0 stitches. The quickest way of temporary closure of major defects (in some cases, it may be even definitive care) is to lift both edges by long Babcocks/Allis clamps and to apply one or two TA-90 stapling devices. In a rare situation of complete transection or severe devastating gastric injury, rapid debridement and closure of the both sides with large TA-90 application might be required. Any reconstructive surgery should be avoided at Role 2. Gastric decompression must be performed with a nasogastric tube, which should be vigorously secured and left on free drainage with regular aspirations.

DUODENUM

Duodenal injuries are relatively rare, but inappropriate management may result in high morbidity and mortality. The Kocher manoeuvre should be performed for duodenal exploration (Figure 10.18). To achieve a complete duodenal examination (check for a through-and-through injury), digital dissection pushing up the peritoneal attachments from the duodenal wall is performed up to the head of the pancreas. The Ligament of Treitz must also be dissected (undertaken as described previously by a full right medial visceral rotation).

All perforations which are suitable for primary closure should be sutured using two-layer techniques. In a tricky situation, the insertion and gentle inflation of a Foley catheter prevents contamination. Leave the Foley catheter in the abdomen because all 'out-of-the-belly' tubes may be easily extracted during evacuation. Pyloric exclusion cannot be recommended as a primary procedure. In cases of massive duodenal disruptions which require multiple reconstructions, simple injury closure and drainage can be performed.

SMALL BOWEL

Some bowel injuries are suitable for primary closure, and some are not. Primary two layers suturing of the

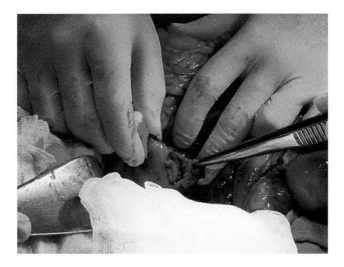

Figure 10.18 A blunt rupture of the vertical part of the duodenum. The duodenum is mobilised via the Kocher manoeuvre.

intestine is a basic surgical procedure, and a few defects may be rapidly closed. However, in the context of military injury, there are frequent situations when many holes are diagnosed, usually resulting from shrapnel or blast fragment damage. Just use as many stapling TA-30 devices to close the holes as needed and leave the abdomen open (Figure 10.19). Any primary anastomosis should be avoided.

COLON AND RECTUM

Small colonic perforations may be primarily sutured using a two-layer technique. If blast mechanism of injury is suspected, the entire colon should be totally explored, including complete mobilisation of hepatic and splenic flexures, even if no significant pericolic haematoma or spillage is seen. If the primary closure is unsuitable, the colostomy and exteriorisation are the options. In a damage control scenario, after debridement, simple closure of both colonic sides with TA 60–90 devices are performed, leaving both ends in the abdomen. In case of significant colonic dilatation, the bowel loop may be pulled out, secured via a window in the Bogota bag, and then safely opened. An injured segment of the colon may be rapidly exteriorised via the lateral abdominal wall in a critical situation.

Rectal injuries are usually because of a blast mechanism. If the patient is diagnosed with any type of perineal or perianal injury, in absence of clear indications for immediate laparotomy, the repair of such injuries should be delayed and only an end colostomy is required if patient is stable. If a rectal perforation is accidentally found during trauma laparotomy, the attempt to close such perforation should be performed by simple closure or GIA stapling of both edges. Extensive injuries would likely require externalisation as an end colostomy with delayed reconstruction.

Enteric intra-abdominal spillage prevention is mandated.

Simple closure in any fashion is the best solution when is possible. Avoid immediate reconstructions.

URINARY TRACT INJURIES

An intraperitoneal urinary bladder injury easily identified during laparotomy is repaired in two layers using an absorbable suture, and both the bladder and the pelvic cavity should be drained by a large urinary catheter and a large drain, respectively. Ureteric injuries

(a)

(b)

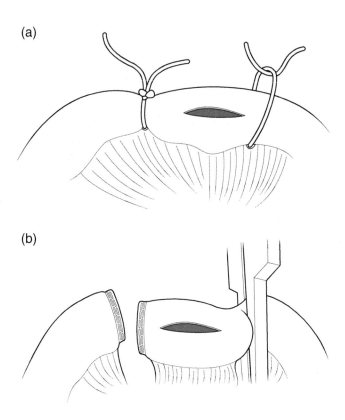

Figure 10.19 Bowel injury damage control.

can be subtle; however, there is no need to explore ureters for possible injuries detection at Role 2. If the injury is accidentally found, then simple ligation can be done with long sutures left in place for easy identification during the second surgery. Reconstructive surgery is quite sophisticated and thus not indicated. If the injury is suspected, then simple draining of a zone of injury is an appropriate choice.

Stapling devices and drains are the best adjuncts in hollow viscus and urinary tract injury management.

No reconstructions and sophisticated procedures are needed at Role 2. Just bridging techniques to prevent contamination.

TEN KEY POINTS

1. Priority is to stop haemorrhage.

2. The simpler and more reliable technique you choose, the better the chance for patient survival.
3. Plan ahead (tactical/strategical evacuation, surgery at the next echelon of care, timeline, etc.).
4. Forward surgery mandates an aggressive surgical approach.
5. A ruptured spleen has is best kept in a bucket.
6. If in doubt, be brave and aggressive.
7. No blind clamping of a hypothetical vessel.
8. Three damage control options for abdominal vascular injuries – ligation, shunting, simple repair.
9. GI Staplers work. They make damage control timeline feasible; therefore, bring them to a mission.
10. Opening the abdomen in tents make things simple and reliable: clamp, ligate, staple, drain, leave open, and inform the next echelon surgeon what has been done.

FURTHER READING

1. Bulger EM, Perina DG, Qasim Z, Beldowicz B, Brenner M, Guyette F, et al. Clinical use of resuscitative endovascular balloon occlusion of the aorta (REBOA) in civilian trauma systems in the USA, 2019: a joint statement from the American College of Surgeons Committee on Trauma, the American College of Emergency Physicians, the National Association of Emergency Medical Services Physicians and the National Association of Emergency Medical Technicians. *Trauma Surg Acute Care Open*. 2019; **4(1)**:e000376.

2. Remick KN. The surgical resuscitation team: surgical trauma support for U.S. Army Special Operations Forces. *J Spec Oper Med*. 2009;**9(4)**:20–25.

3. Fisher AD, Teeter WA, Cordova CB, Brenner ML, Szczepanski MP, Miles EA, et al. The role I resuscitation team and resuscitative endovascular balloon occlusion of the aorta. *J Spec Oper Med*. 2017 Summer; **17(2)**:65–73.

4. D'Angelo M, Losch J, Smith B, Geslak M, Compton S, Wofford K, et al. Expeditionary resuscitation surgical team: the US Army's Initiative to provide damage control resuscitation and surgery to forces in austere settings. *J Spec Oper Med*. 2017 Winter;**17(4)**:76–79.

5. Greaves I, editor. *Military medicine in Iraq and Afghanistan: A comprehensive review*. CRC Press, 2018.

6. Feliciano DV, Mattox KL, Jordan GL, Burch JM, Bitondo CG, Cruse PA. Management of 1000 consecutive cases of hepatic trauma (1979–1984). *Ann Surg*. 1986 Oct;**204(4)**:438–445.

7. Schein M, Rogers, PN, Leppäniemi, A, Rosin, D, eds. *Schein's common sense prevention and management of surgical complications: for surgeons, residents, lawyers, and even those who never have any complications*. TFM Publishing Limited, 2013.

8. Benz D, Balogh ZJ. Damage control surgery: current state and future directions. *Curr Opin Crit Care*. 2017;**23(6)**:491–497.

9. Imran JB, Tsai S, Timaran CH, Valentine RJ, Modrall JG. Damage control endografting for the unstable or unfit patient. *Ann Vasc Surg*. 2017;**42**:150–155.

10. Roberts DJ, Zygun DA, Faris PD, Ball CG, Kirkpatrick AW, Stelfox HT; Indications for trauma damage control surgery international study group. Opinions of practicing surgeons on the appropriateness of published indications for use of damage control surgery in trauma patients: an international cross-sectional survey. *J Am Coll Surg*. 2016;**223(3)**:515–529.

11. Krige JE, Kotze UK, Setshedi M, Nicol AJ, Navsaria PH. Surgical management and outcomes of combined pancreaticoduodenal injuries: analysis of 75 consecutive cases. *J Am Coll Surg*. 2016;**222(5)**:737–749.

12. Coleman JJ, Zarzaur BL. Surgical management of abdominal trauma: hollow viscus injury. *Surg Clin North Am*. 2017;**97(5)**:1107–1117.

13. Aiolfi A, Matsushima K, Chang G, Bardes J, Strumwasser A, Lam L, Inaba K, Demetriades D. Surgical trends in the management of duodenal injury. *J Gastrointest Surg*. 2019;**23(2)**:264–269.

14. Ordoñez C, García A, Parra MW, Scavo D, Pino LF, Millán M, Badiel M, Sanjuán J, Rodriguez F, Ferrada R, Puyana JC. Complex penetrating duodenal injuries: less is better. *J Trauma Acute Care Surg*. 2014;**76(5)**:1177–1183.

15. Faulconer ER, Branco BC, Loja MN, Grayson K, Sampson J, Fabian TC, Holcomb JB, Scalea T, Skarupa D, Inaba K, Poulin N, Rasmussen TE, Dubose JJ. Use of open and endovascular surgical techniques to manage vascular injuries in the trauma setting: a review of the American Association for the Surgery of Trauma PROspective Observational Vascular Injury Trial registry. *J Trauma Acute Care Surg*. 2018;**84(3)**:411–417.

16. Galili O, Hebron D, Dubose J, Horer T, Heidelberg E, Gefen S, Kessel B. Use of endovascular balloons may simplify the proximal and distal control in complicated vascular trauma. *J Endovas Resuscit Trauma Manag* 2017;**1(1)**:39–41.

17. McDonald AA, Robinson BRH, Alarcon L, Bosarge PL, Dorion H, Haut ER, Juern J, Madbak F, Reddy S, Weiss P, Como JJ. Evaluation and management of traumatic diaphragmatic injuries: a Practice Management Guideline from the Eastern Association for the Surgery of Trauma. *J Trauma Acute Care Surg*. 2018;**85(1)**:198–207.

18. Ward J, Alarcon L, Peitzman AB. Management of blunt liver injury: what is new? *Eur J Trauma Emerg Surg*. 2015;**41(3)**:229–237.

19. Choron RL, Hazelton JP, Hunter K, Capano-Wehrle L, Gaughan J, Chovanes J, Seamon MJ. Intra-abdominal packing with laparotomy pads and QuikClot™ during damage control laparotomy: a safety analysis. *Injury*. 2017;**48(1)**:158–164.

20. Roberts DJ, Ball CG, Feliciano DV, Moore EE, Ivatury RR, Lucas CE, Fabian TC, Zygun DA, Kirkpatrick AW, Stelfox HT. History of the innovation of damage

control for management of trauma patients: 1902-2016. *Ann Surg.* 2017;**265(5)**:1034–1044.

21. Doklestić K, Stefanović B, Gregorić P, Ivančević N, Lončar Z, Jovanović B, Bumbaširević V, Jeremić V, Vujadinović ST, Stefanović B, Milić N, Karamarković A. Surgical management of AAST grades III-V hepatic trauma by damage control surgery with perihepatic packing and definitive hepatic repair-single centre experience. *World J Emerg Surg.* 2015 **1(10)**:34.

22. DuBose JJ, Inaba K, Teixeira PG, Shiflett A, Putty B, Green DJ, Plurad D, Demetriades D. Pyloric exclusion in the treatment of severe duodenal injuries: results from the National Trauma Data Bank. *Am Surg.* 2008;**74(10)**:925–929.

23. Walker NM, Eardley W, Clasper JC. UK combat-related pelvic junctional vascular injuries 2008-2011: implications for future intervention. *Injury.* 2014;**45(10)**:1585–1589.

24. Patel JA, White JM, White PW, Rich NM, Rasmussen TE. A contemporary, 7-year analysis of vascular injury from the war in Afghanistan. *J Vasc Surg.* 2018;**68(6)**:1872–1879.

25. Smith IM, Beech ZK, Lundy JB, Bowley DM. A prospective observational study of abdominal injury management in contemporary military operations: damage control laparotomy is associated with high survivability and low rates of fecal diversion. *Ann Surg.* 2015;**261(4)**:765–773.

26. MacFarlane C, Vaizey CJ, Benn CA. Battle injuries of the rectum: options for the field surgeon. *J R Army Med Corps.* 2002;**148(1)**:27–31.

27. Asensio JA, Chahwan S, Hanpeter D, Demetriades D, Forno W, Gambaro E, Murray J, Velmahos G, Marengo J, Shoemaker WC, Berne TV. Operative management and outcome of 302 abdominal vascular injuries. *Am J Surg.* 2000;**180(6)**:528–533.

28. Blackbourne LH. *Defining combat damage control surgery. US Army Med Dep J.* 2008:67–73.

29. Martin MJ, Beekley A, editors. *Front line surgery: a practical approach.* 1st ed. New York: Springer; 2011.

30. Martin MJ, Brown CVR. (2014) Colon and rectal trauma. In: Steele SR, Maykel JA, Champagne BJ, Orangio GR (eds) *Complexities in colorectal surgery.* Springer, New York, NY.

31. Hirshberg A, Mattox KL. Top Knife: Art and Craft in Trauma Surgery.

32. Eastridge BJ, Mabry RL, Seguin P, Cantrell J, Tops T, Uribe P, et al. Death on the battlefield (2001-2011): implications for the future of combat casualty care. *J Trauma Acute Care Surg.* 2012 Dec;**73(6 Suppl 5)**: S431–S437.

33. Stockinger ZT, Turner CA, Gurney JM. Abdominal trauma surgery during recent US combat operations from 2002 to 2016. *J Trauma Acute Care Surg.* 2018;**85(1S Suppl 2)**: S122–S128.

34. Hathaway E, Glaser J, Cardarelli C, Dunne J, Elster E, Safford S, et al. Exploratory laparotomy for proximal vascular control in combat-related injuries. *Mil Med.* 2016;**181(5 Suppl)**:247–252.

35. Smith IM, Beech ZK, Lundy JB, Bowley DM. A prospective observational study of abdominal injury management in contemporary military operations: damage control laparotomy is associated with high survivability and low rates of fecal diversion. *Ann Surg* 2015;**261(4)**:765–773.

36. Smith JW, Matheson PJ, Franklin GA, Harbrecht BG, Richardson JD, Garrison RN. Randomized controlled trial evaluating the efficacy of peritoneal resuscitation in the management of trauma patients undergoing damage control surgery. *J Am Coll Surg* 2017;**224(4)**: 396–404.

37. Sorrentino TA, Moore EE, Wohlauer MV et al. Effect of damage control surgery on major abdominal vascular trauma. *J Surg Res* 2012;**177(2)**:320–325.

38. Rotondo MF, Schwab CW, McGonigal MD et al. 'Damage control': an approach for improved survival in exsanguinating penetrating abdominal injury. *J Trauma* 1993;**35(3)**:375–382; discussion 382–383.

39. Morrison JJ. Noncompressible torso hemorrhage. *Crit Care Clin* 2017;**33(1)**:37–54.

40. Moore EE, Burch JM, Franciose RJ, Offner PJ, Biffl WL. Staged physiologic restoration and damage control surgery. *World J Surg* 1998;**22(12)**:1184–1190; discussion 1190–1191.

Acute Care Emergency Surgery 11

Marcelo A. F. Ribeiro and Mansoor Khan

RESOURCE LIMITATION CONCERNS

Limitation of resources is a major challenge for medical staff, especially in the face of dubious diagnoses. Often, a lack of resources such as laboratory and imaging tests can lead to errors and inadequate therapeutic planning.

From a laboratory standpoint, remote healthcare units can often be said to have equipment that enables staff to perform basic tests such as blood gas analysis, haematocrit and haemoglobin levels, blood counts, electrolyte dosing, blood glucose, and lactate, among others. It should be noted that a blood count, a lactate dosage – as well as a blood gas analysis – can provide the teams with valuable data to predict the severity of the patient.

As for imaging studies, examinations such as X-ray and ultrasound are now readily available and increasingly portable. They provide important information such as the presence or absence of pneumoperitoneum, radiological signs of intestinal obstruction, presence of free fluid in the cavity, and with the growing mastery of point-of-care ultrasound techniques, the trained surgeon can refine their capabilities in extreme situations for diagnoses such as appendicitis or acute cholecystitis.

Importantly, in extreme situations, a good history, as well as a thorough physical examination, will often be the most important tools in formulating diagnostic hypotheses and subsequent surgical therapeutic planning.

ACUTE APPENDICITIS

Acute appendicitis represents the most commonly performed urgent abdominal surgery worldwide, with a lifetime risk of 8.6% in men and 6.9% in women in developing the disease.

Clinical diagnosis using objective parameters such as the Alvaro Score evaluates the presence of migratory pain to the right iliac fossa (one point), nausea and vomiting (one point), anorexia (one point), right iliac fossa defence (two points), painful decompression in the right iliac fossa (one point), fever >37.2 °C (one point), leucocytosis (two points), and left shift of the leukocytes (one point).

With a score between 7–10, there is a 93% chance that the patient will have acute appendicitis. It has been shown to be an important tool in resource-limited settings and has been corroborated with computerised tomographical findings.

Nowadays, the gold standard in treatment continues to be the appendicectomy, preferably by laparoscopic approach. In certain circumstances, the treatment will be performed by an open surgical procedure and, in selected cases, treated by antibiotic therapy with or without interval appendicectomy. The treatment of non-perforated acute appendicitis remains surgical, preferably within the first 12 hours after diagnosis. However, this approach can change in a resource-limited environment. The patients can have delayed presentation and surgery in this environment should only be undertaken if absolutely necessary.

Patients presenting with complicated appendicitis, haemodynamic compromise, sepsis, and free cavity perforation require emergency treatment with appendix removal, irrigation, drainage, and sometimes even right hemicolectomy.

Non-operative treatment is currently reserved for patients with uncomplicated acute appendicitis, with intravenous antibiotics being used for 1 to 3 days, followed by oral antibiotics until 10 days after treatment. The patient should be advised that the rate of treatment failure and recurrence is typically between 15–25%. Regarding morbidity, the most common complication after appendectomy is surgical site infection, from simple wound infections to the appearance of intra-abdominal abscesses.

Procedure

Open appendicectomy in adults was first described by McBurney in 1891. Since then, the technique has remained largely unchanged.

Antibiotics: the flora of the appendix is composed of gram-negative aerobes and anaerobes. We may suggest Intravenous Cephalosporins and Metronidazole. If the patient is allergic to penicillin and cephalosporins, then they should be administered clindamycin plus ciprofloxacin, or other suitable locally authorised antibiotic therapy.

Surgical steps:

- After anaesthesia, the patient is re-examined. If a palpable mass is identified, the incision can be located over the mass.
- Classical incisions are McBurney (one-third of the distance from the anterior superior iliac spine to umbilicus – curvilinear incision) or Rockey-Davis. In cases where there is an elevated risk of a complicated appendix (long evolution time), a middle line incision may be advisable (Figure 11.1a).
- After skin incision identifies the external oblique fascia, make a sharp lateral incision lateral to the rectus sheath.
- Proceed using a muscle-splitting technique, separating the fibres from the external and internal oblique muscles as well as the tranversus abdominis.
- Peritoneum is sharply entered (Figure 11.1b).
- Sweep your finger laterally to medially in the right paracolic gutter. If the appendix cannot be identified by palpation, it can be located by

following the taeniae coli to its origin at the caecal base.

- After identification of the appendix, deliver the appendix through the incision and proceed with the ligation of the vascular structures of the mesoappendix until you find the appendiceal artery. Divide the artery between haemostatic clips, tied with 3-0 absorbable sutures (Figure 11.1c).
- After crushing the appendiceal base with a Kelly clamp, the appendix is double sutured with 2-0 absorbable sutures. The appendix is excised with a scalpel and the remaining stump is cauterised to prevent a mucocele (Figure 11.1d). You may invert the stump into the caecum although the usefulness of stump inversion is debatable.
- The surgical bed is then irrigated with saline carefully. First, clean the purulent collection (if present) and then apply irrigation judiciously. The goal is to dilute and remove infected material without spreading the infection to the rest of the abdomen.
- Closure in layers with 2-0 running absorbable suture beginning with the peritoneum, followed by muscular plane and the Scarpa's fascia. Remember to irrigate each layer. You may inject the external oblique fascia with local anaesthetic (Figure 11.1e). Skin can be closed by simple monofilament 4-0 sutures or staples. In perforated appendicitis, the skin may be left open to avoid surgical site infection.

Patients with a phlegmon on the right lower quadrant should be treated with intravenous antibiotics. **The authors do not recommend immediate appendicectomy in patients with phlegmon associated with perforated appendicitis.**

There is no evidence of benefits for abdominal cavity drainage, either to avoid intra-peritoneal abscess or wound infection.

Key Concepts

- For adults with nonperforated appendicitis, we suggest appendectomy rather than nonoperative management with antibiotics.
- Surgery must be performed within 12 hours of diagnosis.
- Always provide a single prophylactic

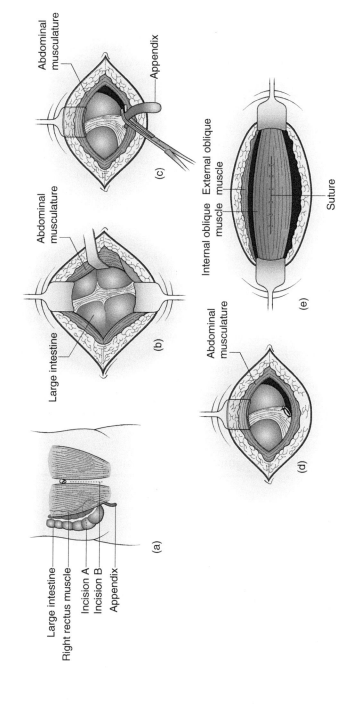

Figure 11.1 Examples for redraw.

antibiotic within 60-minute window before incision.

- In severe cases, you may need to perform a right hemicolectomy.
- Immediate appendicectomy is an alternative option for patients who present with an appendiceal abscess, especially if the abscess is not amenable to percutaneous drainage or you don't have the appropriate tools.

HERNIA

Umbilical and Paraumbilical Hernia Repair

An umbilical hernia is classified as ventral hernia occurring anteriorly at the abdominal wall. They can be congenital (most common during childhood) or acquired (para-umbilical) when the defect develops because of weakening or disruption of the fibromuscular tissues of the abdominal wall.

Para-umbilical hernias are common and have been found in 2–50% of individuals screened by physical exam or ultrasound. They occur more commonly in females than in males, with a 3:1 ratio and can present incarcerated with omentum or preperitoneal fat within the hernial sac.

Most small defects are asymptomatic. As the size increases, the symptoms become more frequent and can vary from different degrees of pain and discomfort as the hernia contents protrude through the defect. Majority of the time, the patient will complain of a bulge somewhere in the abdominal wall.

A physical exam will be enough to provide a correct diagnosis. The patient should be examined both standing and lying down. In nonobese patients, the hernia is typically easy to identify, and the edges of the fascial defect can often be palpated. The entire abdominal wall, particularly along the length of any incision, should be palpated carefully to identify other coexistent hernia sites. In large defects, due to increased pressure in the hernial sac, the surrounding skin may have its vascularity compromised resulting in erythema, ischaemia, or ulcerations. This is notably more pronounced when the contents of the hernia become ischaemic. Ultrasound, when available, can help in some cases, but it is not the most appropriate study, requiring a good expertise to provide support to your clinical suspicions. The treatment of symptomatic para-umbilical hernias is operative repair.

Operative Repair:

In a situation of limitation of resources, the best approach to umbilical hernia repair is as follows:

- After anaesthesia, the patient is re-examined. If a palpable mass is identified, the incision can be located over the mass.
- Classical incision is a vertical or curvilinear incision adjacent to the hernia sac (Figure 11.2a).
- Identification and dissection of the sac to its fascial attachments (Figure 11.2b).
- Once the fascia has been cleared, the hernia sac can either be inverted or excised, then the fascia can be closed with a nonabsorbable suture (Figure 11.2c).
- In the cases where the fascial defect is too big and cannot be closed without tension, the surgeon may consider the use of a mesh (Sublay; Figure 11.2d).
- Whenever possible, a suture to tack the skin of the umbilicus to the fascia to recreate a cosmetically appealing umbilicus should be done (Figure 11.2e).

Recurrence rates range from 0–3% after a mesh repair and up to 14% after sutured repair.

Inguinal Hernia Repair

Inguinal hernia repair is among the most common procedures performed by the general surgeon. There are two types: indirect and direct. Indirect hernias develop at the internal ring, where the spermatic cord or the round ligament enter the inguinal canal. They originate lateral to the inferior epigastric vessels – in contrast to the direct hernias which protrude through Hesselbach's triangle (rectus abdominis muscle medially, the inguinal ligament inferiorly, and the inferior epigastric vessels laterally) medial to the inferior epigastric vessels.

The definitive treatment of all hernias regardless of their origin or type is surgical repair. In a situation of limited resources, the surgeon will need to perform an open repair and, if available, utilise a mesh. If no mesh is at hand, the Shouldice repair (more

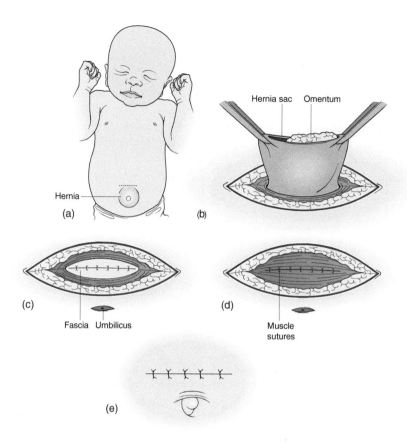

Figure 11.2 Umbilical and para-umbilical hernia repair.

complex and time-demanding) or a Bassini repair with a McVay relaxing incision are alternatives. In cases of femoral hernias – which count for less than 10% of all the groin hernias but represent 40% of hernia emergencies – the Lichtenstein repair cannot be used since it does not address the femoral ring. In these cases, the McVay technique is still considered the most appropriate.

In a situation of limitation of resources, the best approach to inguinal hernia repair is as follows:

- After anaesthesia, the patient is re-examined to try to identify the presence of direct or indirect defect.
- A short transverse incision over the region of the internal ring is performed, the incision continues down by planes. Sharply dissect the subcutaneous tissue and ligate the superficial epigastric vein (Figure 11.3a).

- When the surgeon reaches the aponeurosis of the external oblique muscle, the aponeurosis is open in the direction of the fibres. Once the incision has been made, the groin is explored. If exploration of the internal inguinal ring and Hesselbach's triangle fails to identify an inguinal hernia, the preperitoneal space must be explored to inspect the femoral canal. This can be accomplished by incising the transversalis fascia over the Hesselbach's triangle (Figure 11.3b).
- Mobilisation of the hernia sac (Figure 11.3c):

  - Indirect hernias: The sac is normally mobilised from the adjacent cord structures. The excess sac is then excised, and the case of the sac is transfixed with a suture (Figure 11.3d,e). In the case of a large sac, the distal elements of the sac can be left in place to avoid ischaemic orchitis due to excessive dissection.
  - Direct hernias: Usually have a broader base. The

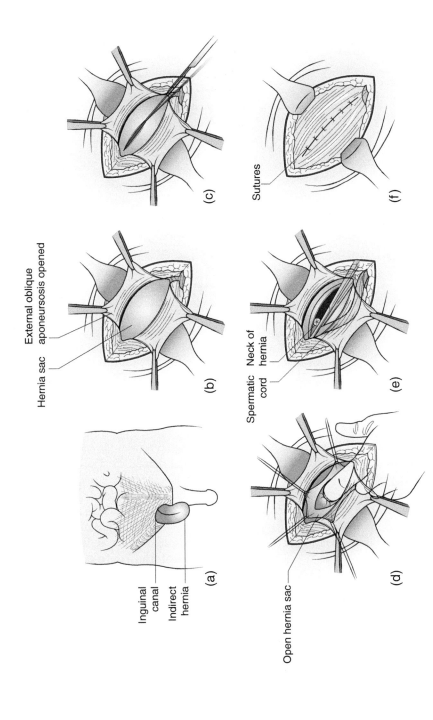

Figure 11.3 Inguinal hernia repair (a–f).

attenuated fascia associated with these cases may be mistaken for peritoneal sac.

- Plication of the posterior wall is done using a continuous suture to aid placement of the mesh, if available. The external oblique aponeurosis is repaired using an absorbable suture material (Figure 11.3f).
- Mesh for open hernia repair: Macroporous polypropylene meshes are preferred over other prosthetic materials. Microporous meshes do not promote a sufficient inflammatory response and do not provide sufficient tissue incorporation.
- Mesh fixation (Figure 11.4) is performed, suturing it to the aponeurotic tissue over the pubic bone and continuing over the lower edge, attaching the mesh to the shelving portion of the Poupart ligament to a point just lateral to the internal ring with a running suture using a non-absorbable suture. A slit is made at the lateral end of the mesh and the cord stays between the two tails, creating a 'neo-internal inguinal' ring. The upper edge is sutured to the internal oblique aponeurosis using a few sutures to leave the mesh in place. Some new self-fixing meshes as well as tissue glue have been described to reduce the incidence of chronic pain with interesting results.

Some tips:

- Sutures must not entrap the ilioinguinal, iliohypogastric, or genital branch of the genitofemoral nerves
- The tails of the mesh should be sutured together, lateral to the spermatic cord, to avoid recurrence.

- There must be no tension on the mesh.
  Bassini repair:
- Primary tissue approximation approach, in which the weakened inguinal floor is strengthened by suturing the conjoined tendon to the inguinal ligament from the pubic tubercle medially to the area of the internal ring laterally.
  McVay repair:
- The only open, non-mesh repair for femoral hernias.
- The procedure starts by incising the traversalis fascia in the region of the Hasselbach's triangle to enter the preperitoneal space and expose the pectineal ligament (Cooper's Ligament).
- The conjoined ligament is then sutured to Cooper's ligament from the pubic tubercle laterally.
- The inguinal floor is then repaired by approximating the conjoined tendon to the inguinal ligament, extending laterally to the area of the internal ring.
- The anterior rectus sheath behind the external oblique aponeurosis should be exposed from the pubic tubercle cephalad for approximately 6 cm along the external oblique aponeurosis.

Key Concepts

- Physical exam is still very accurate for diagnosis.
- Surgical treatment remains as the only definitive option for hernias.
- In most cases, the surgical repair includes the use of non-absorbable meshes.

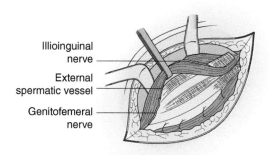

Illioinguinal nerve

External spermatic vessel

Genitofemeral nerve

Figure 11.4 Mesh repair of inguinal hernia.

> • In strangulated hernias, always be sure about intestinal viability; ischaemia and perforations can be present and are usually devastating for the patient.

RIGHT HEMICOLECTOMY

For Acute Care Surgery in resource-limited environments, the reasons for a right hemicolectomy would likely be infective, inflammatory, or obstructing neoplasm. Given the potential heterogeneity of the workforce (i.e. military, humanitarian, displaced persons, refugees, etc.). All pathologies must be considered, therefore the most common reasons for this procedure in resource-limited or austere environments would be necrotising appendicitis involving the caecum, complication of infectious diseases (i.e. Tuberculosis), obstructing neoplasm, or caecal volvulus.

Surgical Considerations

The resection for benign disease involves the resection of the terminal ileum, right colon, and proximal transverse colon, followed by ileocolic anastomosis. The extension required for malignant lesions depends on the tumour margin and the need for oncologic lymphadenectomy as defined by the blood supply. Depending on local resources and the evacuation chain, it is preferable to send the specimen for histological analysis; however, the infrastructure of the environment may deem this impossible.

• A midline incision in the emergency setting is the most appropriate.
• For oncological cases, the location of the lesion will determine the line of resection. If the tumour is in the caecum, a 10 cm segment of terminal ileum must be resected; however, if the tumour is in the ascending colon, only a few centimetres of the ileum is required as margin. The line of resection should extend to the right side of the transverse colon at level with the right branch of the middle colic vessels.
• The surgeon must preserve the main branch of the middle colic vessels. To ensure proper lymph node

harvesting, the right colic and ileocolic vessels are taken at their origin.
• Mobilisation of the colon: The right colon is mobilised by incising the line of Toldt and rotating the caecum anteriorly and medially (Figure 11.5). During mobilisation, proper care must be taken to identify and posteriorly displace the gonadal vessels and ureter.
• Resection can be undertaken at the determined area in between soft bowel clamps or by using a gastrointestinal stapling device.
• Creation of anastomosis: This step can be performed either with a stapler or by the use of handsewn technique.

LEFT HEMICOLECTOMY

The indications for operative intervention on the left hemicolon and sigmoid colon are the same for the right side: infective, inflammatory, and consequences of neoplasm.

• A midline incision in the emergency setting is the most appropriate.
• The principles for surgical margins and lymph node resection are the same for the right colon when the procedure is performed for oncological purposes.
• The mobilisation is the same for the left medial visceral rotation (Figure 11.6). The surgeon opens the line of Toldt from the splenic flexure down to the level of the pelvic brim.
• At this point, the surgeon must identify the left ureter crossing the gonadal vessels.
• In the medial aspect, the mesentery is lifted from the retroperitoneal attachments, helping identify the inferior mesenteric artery (IMA) and vein (IMV). They are then ligated and divided. If the lesion remains at the splenic flexure, it may be necessary to ligate the left branch of the middle colic artery.
• Once the segment is mobilised, the ends of the colon are divided, and the two ends are prepared for anastomosis using a stapler or by handsewn technique.
• If the entire sigmoid is removed, the colorectal anastomosis is usually performed using a handsewn parachuting technique.

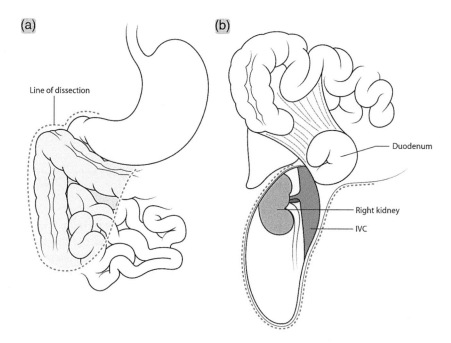

Figure 11.5 The Cattell-Braasch manoeuvre (right medial visceral rotation): (a) illustrates the avascular plane for division of the peritoneum lateral to the ascending colon (akin to the dissection for a right hemi-colectomy). (b) After division of this peritoneal 'white line' of reflection, the ascending colon and hepatic flexure are rotated upwards and medially. Continue the dissection plane to also elevate the small bowel down to the root of the mesentery and lift it out of the surgical field, thus exposing the right kidney (kept down and covered in Gerota's fascia) and IVC.

Handsewn anastomosis:

- After placing crushing bowel clamps across the colon, the rectum, and subsequent resection, place non-crushing clamps straight across the colon and the rectum to divide them. There are three types of anastomosis that can be created: end-to-end, end-to-side, or side-to-side.
- To aid approximation, place 3–0 single-layer in the corners of the bowel. Make a single layer continuous 3–0 suture, beginning with the posterior row and making sure not to strangle them. Then, remove the occluding clamps to allow blood flow to return to the ends of the bowel.
- After the anastomosis is done, it can be tested for any leaks by placing the patient in the reverse Trendelenburg position and filling the pelvis with saline. Using a 60 mL syringe after clamping the colon proximal to the air, and, the surgeon inflates the colon with air, and the area is checked for adequate distention and the presence of bubbling.

If gross contamination is found (e.g., faecal spilling due to diverticulitis), it is acceptable to leave the cavity open (damage control for a second look in severely ill patients with septic shock).

STOMA FORMATION

Stomas are constructed to connect a body cavity to the outside and are named according to their anatomical location (i.e. colostomy, ileostomy, etc.). Before formation of a stoma, many factors need to be considered, such as the type of injury, the physiology of the casualty, the evacuation timelines, and the ultimate destination of a casualty.

When treating the local population in a resource-limited setting, it is better to discontinue medical care and resume when the casualty's physiology allows, rather than forming a stoma as medical infrastructure in the country may not facilitate care of a casualty with one.

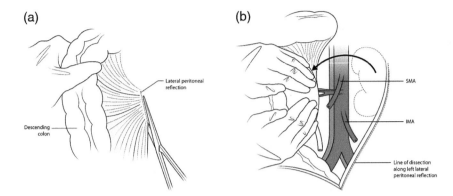

Figure 11.6 Mattox manoeuvre. (a) Division of the peritoneum along the line of Toldt. The lateral white line of Toltz is a relatively avascular plane (often the haematoma has performed most of this dissection already). The descending colon and sigmoid are stretched towards the midline, exposing the lateral peritoneal reflection, which in turn is excised in a longitudinal fashion which allows the bowel to be mobilized further to the midline exposing the retroperitoneum. (b) The left lateral avascular peritoneal reflection plane has been divided and the left colon reflected from left to right. The lateral dissection plane is continued lateral to and behind the left kidney (and Gerota's fascia) to elevate the left kidney forward and towards the midline. Often the haematoma has performed much of the dissection already. Once performed, this allows massive exposure of the aorta from the common iliac arteries and up to the visceral aorta (i.e., segment containing the renal vessels, superior mesenteric artery and coeliac artery). Remember, the left renal artery will now be anterior to the aorta (and not left lateral) due to the elevation of the left kidney.

There are two main forms of stomata: loop or end. Loop stoma is usually formed to relieve a distal obstruction or divert enteric contents away from a new anastomotic site. As mentioned earlier, in a damage control situation, no stomata should be formed, and the bowel should be left in discontinuity. In a forward surgical environment, this is the preferred option, with restoration of intestinal continuity or formation of a stoma taking place at higher echelons of care. In low/middle-income countries where humanitarian operations are being undertaken, if possible, then intestinal continuity should be restored, even if it requires temporary abdominal closure – restore physiology; then return to theatre.

Loop stoma formation:

- Define the location of the stoma preoperatively.
- Middle line incision is usually required for bigger patients; in slim patients, a small transverse incision in the right (ileostomy) or left (colonic) lower quadrant over the rectus muscle. Remember to split the muscle in the direction of its fibres.

- The bowel is mobilised sharply from its attachments.
- A mesenteric window is created between the marginal artery and the mesenteric border of the bowel. The loop of bowel is pulled through the incision carefully to ensure that no tension is placed. The fascial opening should be wide enough to accommodate the bowel and one finger.
- If the middle line was opened, it should be closed before the stoma matured.
- A transverse incision along the length of the loop of bowel is performed. It should be long enough to allow visualisation of the posterior wall of the colon.
- Full thickness 3-0 polyglactin sutures are placed from the bowel wall to the dermis.
- Ileostomies are everted by placing 'triplicate' sutures. First, suture is placed through the dermis, followed by a seromuscular bite 4–5 cm from the proximal to the distal end of the ileum. The final bite is passed full thickness through the cut end of the bowel. Gaps can be closed with standard sutures between the triplicate sutures (usually, three are enough).

- If a supporting bridge was used, it can be removed in 4–5 days.

For an end stoma, deliver the previously divided bowel through the abdominal wall without twisting it **(Make sure the right limb of the bowel is brought out!)**. Confirm that the bowel is not twisted.

PERFORATION OF GASTRIC AND DUODENAL ULCERS

Peptic ulcer disease (PUD) affects four million people worldwide annually. In the presence of risk factors (NSAIDs, *H. pylori*, smoking, etc.), recurrence of ulcer is common despite initial successful treatment. The pillars of treatment are prompt resuscitation, intravenous antibiotics, analgesia, proton pump inhibitory medications (PP), nasogastric tube, urinary catheter, and surgical source control.

Operative Versus Non-operative Management

A major decision when treating patients with ulcer perforation is whether and when to operate. After resuscitation, emergent operation and closure with a piece of omentum is the standard of care for patients with acute perforation and a rigid abdomen with free intraperitoneal air. If the patient is stable or improving, especially if spontaneous sealing of the perforation has been demonstrated, nonoperative management with close monitoring is a reasonable option. With any free perforation, regardless of the presence or size of the leak, if the patient's status is deteriorating, urgent surgery is indicated. Prolonged efforts to establish a diagnosis or pursue nonoperative care despite worsening status can be counterproductive, since a needed operation will be delayed. In addition, surgery is suggested in circumstances where the cause of an acute abdomen has not been established or the patient's status cannot be closely monitored.

Simple patch closure of the perforation should be considered in ongoing shock, delayed presentation, significant medical comorbidities, or significant peritoneal contamination. Patch closure may also be appropriate for patients who have never been treated for peptic ulcer disease and are candidates for proton pump inhibitors and antibiotic therapy for *H. pylori*.

For gastric perforations, the choice of procedure is usually made during the operation. The preferred approach is partial gastrectomy to include ulcer because of the risk of gastric malignancy, especially in large ulcers – unless the patient is at an unacceptably considerable risk because of advanced age, comorbid disease, intraoperative instability, or severe peritoneal soilage.

Key Concepts

- It can be treated in selective cases with medications instead of elective surgery.
- X-ray may not establish the diagnosis, and a high index of suspicion is essential.
- Early diagnosis, prompt resuscitation, and urgent surgical intervention are essential.
- Exploratory laparotomy and omental patch remain the gold standard.
- Partial gastrectomy is recommended in patients with large or malignant ulcer to enhance outcomes.

Key points

1. Patient physiology dictates the requirement and expediency of operative intervention.
2. If possible, consider non-operative intervention.
3. Surgical treatment remains as the only definitive option for hernias.
4. In most cases, surgical repair includes the use of non-absorbable meshes.
5. In strangulated hernias, always guarantee intestinal viability. Ischaemia or perforations can be present and are usually devastating for the patient.
6. You can leave a patient in discontinuity until the next echelon of care or re-look when physiology allows.
7. Avoid formation of stomas on local populace if there is inadequate post-formation established to care for such patients.

8. Perforated duodenal ulcer, if sealed, can be managed non-operatively.
9. Partial gastrectomy is recommended in patients with large or malignant ulcer to enhance outcomes.
10. If in doubt about patient stability en route, keep hold of the patient!

FURTHER READING

Alvarado A. A practical score for the early diagnosis of acute appendicitis. *Ann Emerg Med* 1986;**15**:557.

Chung KT, Shelat VG, Perforated peptic ulcer – an update. *World J Gastrointest Surg* 2017;**9(1)**:1–12.

Di Saverio S, Sibilio A, Giorgini E. et al. The NOTA Study (Non Operative Treatment for Acute Appendicitis): prospective study on the efficacy and safety of antibiotics (amoxacilin and clavulanic acid) for treating patients with right lower quadrant abdominal pain and long-term follow-up of conservatively treated suspected appendicitis. *Ann Surg* 2014;**260**:109.

Di Saverio S, Bassi M, Smerieri N et al. Diagnosis and treatment of perforated or bleeding peptic ulcers: 2013 WSES position paper. *World J Emerg Surg* 2014;**9**:45.

Earle AE, McLellan J. A Repair of umbilical and epigastric hernias. *Surg Clin North Am* 2013;**93**:1057.

Halm JA, Heisterkamp J, Veen HF, Weidema WF. Long-term follow-up after umbilical hernia repair: are there risk factors for recurrence after simple and mesh repair. *Hernia* 2005;**9**:334.

Hentati H, Dougaz W, Dziri C. Mesh repair versus non-mesh repair for strangulated inguinal hernia: systematic review with meta-analysis. *World J Surg* 2014;**38**:2784.

The HerniaSurge Group. International guidelines for groin hernia management. *Hernia* 2018;**22**:1–165.

Korner H, Sondenaa K, Soreide J A et al. Incidence of acute nonperforated and perforated appendicitis: age-specific and sex-specific analysis. *World J Surg* 1997;**21**:313.

Lau JY, Sung J, Hill C et al. Systematic review of the epidemiology of complicated peptic ulcer disease: incidence, recurrence, risk factors and mortality. *Digestion* 2011;**84**:102–113.

Lee EC, Garrett K. Left colectomy: open and laparoscopic. Evans SRT, ed. *Surgical pitfalls: prevention and management.* Philadelphia: Saunderns Elsevier; 2009. 265–272.

Lockhart K, Dunn D, Teo S et al. Mesh versus non-mesh for inguinal and femoral hernia repair. *Cochrane Database Syst Rev* 2018;**9**:CD011517.

Lofgren J, Beard J, Ashley T. Groin hernia surgery in low-resource setting – a problem still unsolved. *N Engl J Med* 2018;**378**:1357.

Mahmoud NN, Bleier JIS, Aarons CB et al. Colon and rectum. Townsend CM Jr, Beauchamp RD, Evers BM, Mattox KL, eds. *Sabiston textbook of surgery: the biological basis of modern surgical practice.* 20th ed. Philadelphia: Elsivier; 2017. 1312–1393.

Malik T, Lee MJ, Harikrishnan AB. The incidence of stoma related morbidity – a systematic review of randomized controlled trials. *Ann R Coll Surg Engl* 2018;**100(7)**:501–508.

Park AE, Roth JS, Kavic SM. Abdominal wall hernia. *Curr Probl Surg* 2006;**43**:326.

Ribeiro Jr MAF, Barros EA, Carvalho SM. Open abdomen in gastrointestinal surgery: which technique is best for temporary closure during damage control? *World J Gastrointest Surg* 2016;**8**:590.

Sartelli M, Baiocchi GL, Di Saverio S et al. Prospective observational study on acute appendicitis worldwide (POSAW). *World J Emerg Surg* 2018;**13**:19.

Smith AJ, Driman DK, Spithoff K et al. Guideline for optimization of colorectal cancer surgery and pathology. *J Surg Oncol* 2010;**101(1)**: 5–12.

Spina C, Marconi AP, Ribeiro Jr MA F et al. Alvarado score in the diagnosis of acute appendicitis: correlation with the tomographic and intra-operative findings. *Int J Radiol Radiat Ther* 2018;**5**:00135.

Street D, Bodai BI, Owens LJ et al. Simple ligation vs stump inversion in appendectomy. *Arch Surg* 1988;**123**: 689.

Whitehead A, Cataldo PA. Technical considerations in stoma creation. *Clin Colon Rectal Surg* 2017;**30**:162–171.

Frontline Consideration for Paediatric Emergency and Trauma Surgery

Nicholas Alexander

INTRODUCTION

Paediatric surgery emergencies comprise around 5–15% of admissions to frontline hospitals in austere environments. The aetiology of admissions ranges from combat (burns, blast, penetrating) to non-combat-related trauma (burns, falls, blunt injury). As a group, their all-comer mortality remains independently higher than adult patients. The skill set required to carry out the operative procedures in the emergency setting is not demonstrably different from the adult patient, but the differences lie in assessment and delivery of resuscitation to infants and children, which are the most challenging. The physiological reserve of a child is considerably less than that of an adult, and this is amplified in prepubescent. With extended timelines and resource-limited settings, many severely injured children do not survive to admission at an appropriate medical facility.

ANATOMICAL CONSIDERATIONS

Paediatric patients are not just 'small adults', and there are certain anatomical differences which create unique challenges for their care.

Infants and children have a significantly increased surface area to body ratio compared to adults – therefore, they lose heat quickly. For infants (<1 year of age), the head is the major source of heat loss and simple measures (such as hats) to mitigate these losses should be employed.

A large surface area–to–body ratio and relative lack of body fat results in much higher rates of insensible fluid losses in infants and children. This is of importance not only in the acute presentation, but also in the operating room where an inadequately warmed environment can cause significant fluid shifts through increased water loss.

The suture lines in the skull do not fuse until around 18–24 months. Infants' skulls can, therefore, expand and accommodate significant increases in pressure, masking initial clinical signs. Although the plasticity of the skull at this age may dissipate some of the force of direct trauma compared to the fused skull, the transfer of energy leads to increased shearing forces on the vessels and increased risk of subdural haemorrhage.

Infants and younger children have comparatively shorter necks, making assessment for tracheal deviation or signs of raised jugular venous pressure difficult.

Infants and children have significantly higher proportions of ligamentous cervical injuries due to their larger head and increased mobility of the cervical spine. Almost half of children with spinal injuries have no radiological signs (SCIOWRA) due to the ligamentous laxity.

The chest wall and, particularly, the ribs are not yet ossified in younger children. Rib fractures are much less common in adults; as a result, the traumatic force is transferred to the lungs, which exhibit higher rates of contusion.

The abdominal solid organs are proportionately larger sized – especially the liver, which is the size of a preterm baby – and may extend well below the umbilicus. A combination of size and relatively less well-developed abdominal musculature results in relatively benign blunt trauma commonly injuring organs.

PHYSIOLOGICAL CONSIDERATIONS

Evaluation of the child at initial presentation can be challenging, but the initial assessment is often simply focussed on the impression of the patient, with an abnormal general appearance being associated with a seriously unwell child. Children compensate very well but then rapidly deteriorate; therefore, it is essential to assess every child with scepticism and assume they are unwell (Figure 12.1).

The expected vital signs used vary according to age (Table 12.1). Whilst tachycardia and tachypnea are almost universally seen in both trauma and non-trauma admissions, the presence of bradycardia and bradypnea is sinister and are signs of impending cardiorespiratory arrest. Unlike adults, infants and small children are unable to increase their stroke volume and are, therefore, dependent on elevated heart rate exclusively to meet cardiac output demands.

Temperature: hypothermia is often a concern due to increased surface area–weight ratio and causes increased oxygen demand, leading to bradycardia and apnoeas. In neonates (<28 days), hypothermia will inactivate surfactant function, leading to respiratory distress.

Hypoventilation often drives worsening acidosis in the trauma patient and is the typical cause of cardiac arrest in children. Delayed capillary refill, cool peripheries, and weak pulses are reliable early signs of hypovolaemia in paediatric patients. Hypotension is an extremely late sign of hypovolaemia in children, often occurring after more than 40% of circulating volume is lost.

THE INITIAL ASSESSMENT

Resuscitation of paediatric surgical patients presenting to the department should be carried out in a systematic fashion as laid out in the Paediatric Advanced Life Support and Advanced Trauma Life Support guidelines. As described above, there are discrete differences and potential pitfalls in managing infants and children. Resuscitation adjuncts such as the Broselow Tape system will allow clinicians to effectively estimate weight and age from the length of the presenting patient.

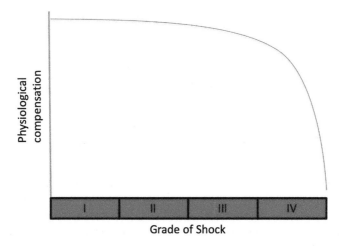

Figure 12.1 Compensatory mechanism in children.

Table 12.1 Normal vital signs

Age	Weight (kg)	Respiratory rate (breaths min⁻¹)	Heart rate (beats min⁻¹)	Systolic blood pressure (mm Hg)
Premature	<3	40–60	130–170	45–60
Neonate (0–28 days)	3	35–60	120–160	60–70
Infant (1 month–1 year)	4–10	25–50	110–150	70–100
Toddler (1–2 years)	10–13	20–30	90–130	75–110
Young child (3–5 years)	13–18	20–30	80–120	80–110
Older child (6–12 years)	18–40	15–25	70–110	90–120
Adolescent (13–18)	>40	12–20	55–100	100–120

Airway

Ensuring airway patency is vital in the initial assessment. Children have a relatively large tongue and a prominent occiput, which has a tendency to flex the neck forward. Simple manoeuvres such as a jaw thrust is often all that is required to clear the airway. Airway adjuncts should be considered early if the airway remains compromised.

Breathing

Respiratory rate should be compared to age-appropriate norms. Tachypnoea – more than 60 breaths per minute – is always abnormal. A respiratory rate which falls towards the expected normal is reassuring only if the patient's clinical appearance is also improving – bradypnea is often indicative of impending respiratory arrest.

Signs of respiratory distress in infants and children include tracheal tug, drawing in of the costal margin, and sternal recession. The presence of grunting (expiratory noise) is found in infants with alveolar or airways collapse, and is an attempt to increase intrathoracic pressure. High-flow oxygen should always be administered.

Circulation

Initial assessment of response and reaction of the child is often a good guide to the state of perfusion. Cerebral obtundation is reflective of poor cerebral perfusion – a quiet or sleepy child is worrying in the acute setting.

Capillary refill time should be assessed centrally and peripherally and should be less than 2 seconds. Tachycardia not only is the earliest and most reliable sign of hypotension but can also accompany anxiety and pain.

Vascular Access

Large-bore cannulae should be inserted to deliver fluid resuscitation. In younger children and infants, early intraosseous access should be used in the anterior tibial plateau 1–2 cm below the tibial tuberosity (picture showing IO needle insertion).

Fluid Resuscitation

A 20 mL/kg⁻¹ initial fluid bolus with crystalloid should be given. This can be repeated up to 60 mL/kg⁻¹ before considering the use of inotropic support. In acutely ill paediatric patients, excessive crystalloid administration is independently associated with higher mortality, worse ventilation outcomes, and cerebral oedema (Feast Study). This finding is mirrored in the context of paediatric trauma patients who received large volumes of crystalloid.

In the context of haemorrhage, PRC transfusion should be considered early. Although the evidence for balanced blood component transfusion (1:1:1 PRC:FFP:Plts) is strong in adults, similar protocols have been introduced in paediatrics with little evidence to support them.

Resuscitation response should be assessed by measuring haemodynamic parameters as well as clinical assessment. Determining level of distal limb perfusion (capillary refill time, skin warmth) is of paramount importance as this enables quantification of a child's repose to instigated resuscitation.

Disability

The AVPU assessment – **A**lert, responds to **V**erbal stimulus, response to **P**ainful stimulus, **U**nresponsive – is most appropriate for the initial neurological survey, along with pupillary testing for size, equality, and reaction to light. The Modified Glasgow Coma Scale (Table 12.2) is best employed after the initial resuscitative efforts.

Exposure

Careful examination to ensure that no injuries are missed while keeping the patient warm.

Imaging

FAST scans are readily available and whilst they are accurate in identifying cardiac tamponade, haemothorax, and haemoperitoneumin adults, they are not accurate in assessing organ damage and will miss a significant proportion of injuries in paediatric patients. The gold standard imaging in children remains the computerised tomography scan. Unfortunately, this may not be possible in a resource-limited environment.

ASSUME EVERY CHILD IS SICK

Adult Adjuncts for Paediatric Trauma.

Tranexamic Acid (TXA)

The CRASH-2 study showed clear and obvious benefit for TXA, reducing morbidity and mortality in adult trauma-related haemorrhage. Such data do not exist for paediatric trauma because of the relative infrequency. However, there are some retrospective

Table 12.2 Paediatric GCS evaluation

Eye-opening	Spontaneous	Spontaneous	4
	To speech	To speech	3
	To pain only	To pain only	2
	No response	No response	1
Verbal	Coos and babbles	Orientated and appropriate	5
	Irritable cries	Confused	4
	Cries to pain	Inappropriate words	3
	Moans to pain	Incomprehensible sounds	2
	No response	No response	1
Motor	Moves spontaneously and with purpose	Obeys commands	6
	Withdraws to touch	Localises to painful stimulus	5
	Withdraws to pain	Withdraws to pain	4
	Abnormal flexion posture to pain	Flexion in response to pain	3
	Abnormal extension posture to pain	Extension in response to pain	2
	No response	No response	1

series demonstrating a reduction in mortality and ventilator-associated morbidity for paediatric combat trauma patients receiving TXA. In these series, there were no prothrombotic complications seen such as thromboembolic events.

Although there is little firm evidence for TXA administration criteria, dosing, and so on, the potential benefits for early TXA in paediatric major trauma would suggest that it should be considered part of normal trauma care.

Massive Transfusion

The definition of massive transfusion in paediatric patients has been arbitrarily defined as requirement of blood products of more than 50% circulating volume. This is not a validated measure and comparison between retrospective series to investigate balance transfusions is complicated. A retrospective series suggested more than 40 mL/kg^{-1} of blood products is associated with excess mortality, which may represent a more appropriate definition.

There have been no prospective large studies to assess the benefits of balanced transfusions, but in the interim, most paediatric trauma units have adopted adult practices. A large retrospective case series with conflict injuries has suggested that in paediatric patients requiring massive transfusion, those that received balanced blood components had an independently higher mortality.

In the Operating Room

As stated previously, hypothermia in infants and children is one of the biggest challenges – it will worsen acidosis and coagulopathy rapidly. Once a body cavity is open, the insensible fluid and heat losses accelerate. Emphasis should be placed on having a prewarmed theatre, forced heaters, and the use of warmed intravenous fluids intraoperatively. If the bowel is exposed, it should be covered with warm, wet gauze to minimise fluid, and thermal losses and should be returned to the peritoneal cavity early.

All attempts should be made to keep the child from lying in pooled fluids during the operation. The use of adhesive clear drapes applied before the

sterile surgical ones can divert fluid away from the patient.

Shared space working particularly in polytrauma is an important consideration for infants and small children. Attention should be paid in securing IV lines and tubing away from the operating field, so they are not displaced or kinked during procedure.

Placement of incision is important, particularly in infants and younger children. Although a midline laparotomy is appropriate for older children, transverse lower abdominal incisions, particularly in infants, is recommended due to a relatively large liver which can extend down to the umbilicus. A transverse incision in these patients permits access to all four quadrants necessary for Damage Control Surgery.

When dealing with vascular trauma in children, a high proportion of injuries are amenable to primary repair. Vascular injury can be difficult to manage in children; the vessels are small and are prone to intense vasoconstriction which makes shunting difficult. However, if possible, shunting remains the optimal option for maintaining oxygenation in damaged limbs. Another damage control surgery option for severely injured limbs with vascular compromise is early amputation. Though it can be a difficult decision to make, it is often well tolerated because of children's capacity to adapt and learn new skills. In addition, long-term reconstruction with multiple operations and prolonged hospitalisation can sometimes be more detrimental to the child's development than early amputation and rehabilitation.

When closing the abdomen, carefully use an absorbable suture and not a non-absorbable one, as the child will grow, and the non-absorbable suture will not!

FURTHER READING

Gray, J, et al. *Pediatric trauma: management from an austere prospective. J Spec Oper Med.* **17(1)**:p. 46–53.

Spinella, PC, M.A Borgman, and K.S Azarow, *Pediatric trauma in an austere combat environment. Crit Care Med*, 2008; **36(7 Suppl)**:p. S293–S296.

McKechnie SP, et al. Pediatric surgery skill sets in role 3: the Afghanistan experience. *Military Med*, 2014; **179(7)**: p. 762–765.

RLE Orthopaedic Injury Management 13

Jowan Penn-Barwell and Daniel Christopher Allison

DAMAGE CONTROL PRINCIPLES

The concept of damage control arose from the US Navy, to immediately address critical areas of loss while maintaining the ship's and the mission's integrity. In the early 1990s, this same concept of damage control was applied to emergency treatment of severe human bodily trauma. The concept in this setting involves postponing definitive surgical repair of injury until optimal host physiologic status has been achieved. In the orthopaedic realm of massive systemic trauma as often seen in combat – especially in the setting of limited resources – the principles of damage control involve addressing only the factors necessary to sustain life and expeditiously initiate provisional stabilisation that promotes early restoration of normal physiology and optimises future definitive repair.

The principles of approaching these injuries aim to prevent loss of life, restore normal host hemodynamic and physiologic status, and prevent loss of limb while maximising future potential function and rehabilitation. The key damage control principles as they relate to conflict orthopaedics are the following:

1. **Control of haemorrhage.** Haemorrhage is the most common cause of combat death, and approximately 20% of these deaths can be prevented through appropriate compression and initial response. Bleeding from major vessels needs surgical treatment, which requires proximal and distal vascular control, as described in Chapter 8, followed by vascular ligation, repair, or shunting.

2. **Immediate compartment decompression.** A rise in pressure in a myofascial compartment due to haemorrhage or tissue swelling after trauma or reperfusion can lead to soft tissue ischemia and is commonly seen in high energy injuries and can be limb-threatening. Prompt recognition of the clinical presentation and rapid surgical treatment, and prophylaxis in high-risk cases, prevent development of this potentially limb-threatening complication.

3. **Expeditious fracture stabilisation.** Unstable long bone fractures cause pain, perpetuate haemorrhage, increase local soft tissue injury, and exacerbate the systemic inflammatory response. Early restoration of anatomic length, alignment, and rotation of the limb with associated provisional mechanical stabilisation promote physiologic stabilisation of the patient in the short term and maximises the potential for optimal recovery in the long term.

4. **Prevention or treatment of infection.** Appropriate early debridement of all foreign material and contaminated, devitalised, or infected soft tissue or bone, in addition to optimising the soft tissue envelope, ensuring optimal mechanical stability of the area, and delivering the appropriate antibiotic locally and systemically prevents life or limb-threatening sepsis.

5. **Local wound care.** The promotion of the appropriate healing of wounds – through optimal soft tissue management and incorporation of primary, secondary, graft, or flap modalities – minimises further complications and optimises long-term limb function.

RESOURCE LIMITATION CONCERNS

Orthopaedic trauma surgery often requires a significant amount of equipment, extensive personnel, meticulous sterile technique, and prolonged time – none of which are available in austere environment.

Surgical equipment and implants in combat setting, even the most basic fragment fixation set, are likely to be unavailable, un-replenishable, un-sterilisable, or all three. Fractures and injuries that could be easily managed in civilian setting will often need to be temporised to facilitate transport for definitive care in a more equipped location.

The multiple surgical assistants and operating room personnel required to fix complex periarticular and long bone fractures are frequently unavailable in conflict medical settings. Therefore, the initial treatment of these cases must have these personnel restrictions in mind, and only basic provisional stabilisation and treatment of such injuries should be performed.

In wartime, the ability to maintain sterility in the surgical theatre and cleanliness postoperatively is often challenging. The implantation of internal hardware in austere environment often imposes an unacceptable risk of contamination and infection. Definitive wound closure may also be contraindicated in gross contamination.

A further potential limitation that constrains management options in wartime setting includes significant restrictions in time and early follow-up of these injured patients. Patients are often transferred through to increasingly higher levels of care. The timing of these transfers is often unpredictable, and obstacles such as weather, equipment malfunction, lack of personnel, or hostile activity may interrupt the transfer for hours or days. Under these circumstances, surgeons may consider more definitive early management of high-risk wounds, though it may limit future reconstructive options. For example, a surgeon may opt to perform a more proximal amputation for a devasting limb injury that permits immediate direct primary closure outside of the zone of injury. In a less constrained environment, the same case could often be managed with serial surgical inspections, which could preserve bone and soft tissue, resulting in a distal amputation or even limb salvage.

Given these significant limitations in equipment, personnel, sterility, and time, the frontline surgeon should assume that the mainstay of treatment

options available for management of combat limb injuries will include the following:

1. Basic debridement or amputation instrumentation (scalpel, scissor, rongeur, bone saw)
2. Splinting or casting equipment (plaster, fibreglass)
3. Skeletal or soft tissue traction modalities (traction pin, Hare splint)
4. External fixation devices (Synthes large external fixator, Stryker military field kit)

PROCEDURES

The orthopaedic procedures that a surgeon may have to perform in a conflict zone are as diverse as the injuries themselves but can be simplified and categorised according to the basic principles described. Prior to deployment, a surgeon should have mastery of these important principles as well as the procedures and techniques to address them. In addition to the techniques described in this chapter, pelvic stabilisation and packing is further described in Chapter 9, vascular control in Chapter 7, and plastic surgical soft tissue techniques in Chapter 17.

Wound Incision

If wounds require exploration (gross open contamination, vascular compromise, compartment syndrome), the wound should be extended proximally and distally to the areas of un-injured tissue as shown in Figure 13.1. below. Neurovascular structures and tissue planes identified, and *the zone of injury explored from anatomic, uninjured tissue.* Consider that the zone of injury in high-energy combat wounds often evolves and may not be fully evident for days or even weeks, which is why repeat surgical explorations are often required.

Anytime compartment syndrome is even considered (high-energy blunt trauma, proximal tibial fracture, significant deep swelling, pain out of proportion to the injury both at rest and with passive toe or finger range of motion, and evolving neurologic symptoms), then decompression of *all* regional muscle compartments through *complete* longitudinal incisional fasciotomy is essential and a potential

(a)

(b)

(c)

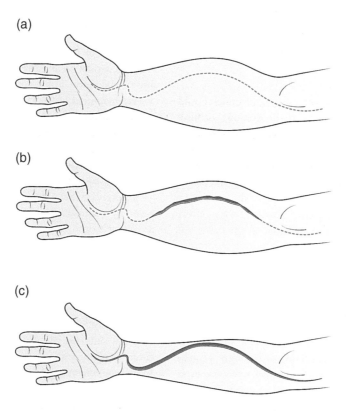

Figure 13.1 Surgeons faced with a traumatic wound (a) can be tempted to excise necrotic or heavily contaminated tissue from within the wound. This risks inadvertently damaging neurovascular structures within the zone of injury. A superior strategy is to extend the wound in line of the potential fasciotomy incisions (b) and then dissect back from normal anatomy, having identified neurovascular structures and tracing them back into the zone of injury (c).

limb-saving procedure. Compartment fasciotomy is described in greater detail in Chapter 17.

In the case of open fractures, the incision should be extended proximally and distally sufficiently to allow complete visualisation of the contaminated area and to 'deliver' the ends of the fractures out of the wound for inspection, debridement, and cleaning. Commonly in the setting of severely contaminated open fractures, multiple serial debridement is required before achieving a clean fracture site.

Wound Excision

Wound excision is sometimes referred to as soft tissue 'debridement' and encompasses the removal of foreign material, gross contamination, and all marginal, devitalised, and necrotic soft tissue and bone. To assess tissue viability adequately, the wound must be extended

proximally and distally to uninjured tissue as previously described. A systematic approach should be used to ensure no areas are missed. The authors follow a 'top-down' approach of fully inspecting and addressing the injured area – starting with the skin, then progressing to the subcutaneous tissue, followed by fascia and then muscle and bone, as necessary.

The surgeon should attempt to remove all gross contamination; however, it might be impossible to remove every piece of debris driven along tissue planes by high-energy wounding mechanisms. Greater effort should be made to remove organic material like vegetation or wood compared to metallic fragments.

Muscle tissue viability should be assessed according to the '4 Cs':

- Colour (healthy red as opposed to purple or brown);

- Contractility (contraction in response to mechanical or electrical stimulation);
- Capillary bleeding; and
- Consistency (normal structure by look and feel).

Grossly devascularised soft tissue and bone should be excised. Tissue of marginal or dubious viability presents a dilemma: in a well-resourced environment, when a patient can be monitored for wound progression and sepsis and returned for further surgery as required, such tissue can be given the 'benefit of the doubt', and potentially be preserved; however, in a resource-constrained environment, every effort should be made to ensure that the all the tissue left in the wound is viable and unlikely to deteriorate.

The decision on the extent of debridement can be difficult. In high-energy wounds spanning large areas, tissue damage is likely to be extensive, and profound excision of non-viable tissue should be performed, as shown in Figure 13.2. below. Certain high-energy wounds (bilateral above-knee traumatic amputation from improvised explosive devices or landmines) can be particularly prone to invasive fungal infection, especially due to systemic immunocompromise, which can be life-threatening. In these cases, the debridement should be as aggressive as the underlying condition. Similarly, if a patient arrives at a medical treatment facility several days after injury, without prior debridement, the wound is likely to be heavily colonised or infected, requiring a more radical excision. These judgements can be challenging and will change according to the clinical context.

Amputation

In devastating limb injuries for which reconstruction is not advised or possible, a well-performed amputation can set a patient on an early path to functional recovery and rehabilitation. The decision to salvage or amputate a severely injured limb can be challenging, and several scoring systems have been developed to aid in this assessment (Mangled Extremity Severity Score [MESS], Limb Salvage Index [LSI], Predictive Salvage Index [PSI]). Unfortunately, these systems have been proved to be poor predictors of limb viability and function.

In austere combat setting, the optimal management of a severely traumatised limb involves emergent treatment according to the damage control principles previously described, while deferring or postponing definitive amputation and associated amputation level to higher echelons of care, after the zone of injury has fully demarcated, and the true extent of the injury and future function can be completely characterised. Postponing the decisions about amputation until this point significantly simplifies this judgement, increases options for future reconstruction, and may improve long-term functional outcome.

When the choice has been made to proceed with immediate amputation, the surgeon has two further important decisions to make: (1) whether to primarily close the stump or leave it open and (2) what the most appropriate length to fashion the amputation stump is. The decision to close the stump will be primarily based on the degree of underlying contamination and risk for infection. In clean wounds, even if the viability of skin flaps is in question, closing the wound will

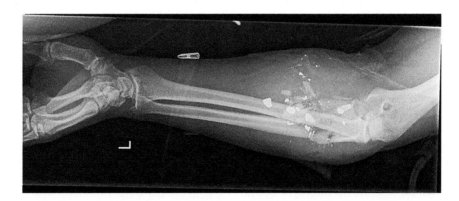

Figure 13.2 This radiograph demonstrates features of high energy transfer from a 9×19-mm low-energy handgun round, that is bone fragmentation bullet disintegration and fragment retention.

Table 13.1 Alternative strategies for determining amputation level	
Amputation from within zone of injury	**Amputation proximal to the zone of injury**
Longer residual limb – mechanical advantage	Shorter residual limb
Multiple surgeries – impact on patient physiology and hospital resources	Single surgery
Irregular 'stump' with scar tissue – potentially challenging for limb fitting	Regular 'stump' with healthy load-bearing surface

result in less deep bone contamination and will prevent soft tissue contracture, which could facilitate future wound coverage.

There are two broad strategies to determine amputation level, and the most appropriate will depend on the patient and the operational context, as summarised in Table 13.1.

In general, attempts should be made to preserve upper extremities at the most distal level possible because of their functional importance and the lack of equivalent prosthetic compensation. In a similar vein, the significantly improved function and increased prosthetic wear associated with below-knee amputation when compared with above-knee amputation should prompt the surgeon to save the knee joint when safely possible. If the patellar tendon insertion is preserved, a prosthesis can be fashioned to preserve at least some degree of knee function. Along the same lines, above-knee amputation at any level is significantly preferred over hip disarticulation, as long as it does not risk the patient's life.

Application of Splints and Casts

Splints (non-circumferential [along one, two, or three sides of the limb]) and casts (circumferential) are firm supports made of plaster or fibreglass which can confer relative stability to unstable extremity fractures and joint injuries through immobilisation. In the case of long-bone fractures, splints and casts work by immobilising the joint above and below the fracture after basic length, alignment, and rotation of the bone or joint have been restored. Application of a splint or cast to a fractured humerus or femur can be technically challenging, and these devices can even exacerbate movement at the fracture site, especially if the joint above (shoulder, hip) is not adequately included and immobilised. Casts of any material will require a mechanical saw to remove, which can be challenging in austere environments. Options for splint and cast types are summarised in Table 13.2.

Splints and casts are usually applied in two layers. First, a circumferential layer of soft padding (usually cotton-based) material is applied. Great care should be taken to pad bony prominences to minimise the risk of skin necrosis, especially if the splint or cast will be left for an indeterminate duration. After length, alignment, and rotation of the fractured bone or joint has been restored, multiple layers (~10–15) of plaster of fibreglass are applied (along one, two, or three sides in the case of a splint or circumferentially in the case of a cast) and held in position until the substance cures (usually 5–15 minutes). Cautiously immobilise the patient in the 'safe' position to minimise joint contracture, which can set in a matter of days. The main 'safe' position for common splint or cast applications are discussed in the following sections.

UPPER EXTREMITY

Elbow and forearm:

- Elbow at 90° of flexion.
- Forearm at neutral pronation/supination (thumb pointed up).

Wrist and hand:

- Wrist at 30° of extension.
- Metacarpophalangeal joints at 90° of flexion.
- Interphalangeal joints fully extended.

LOWER EXTREMITY

Knee:

- Knee between 0–30 of flexion.

Ankle and foot:

- Ankle at 90° (neutral flexion).
- Hindfoot at neutral (plantigrade foot).

Table 13.2 Options for cast type and design

Immobilisation type	Advantages	Disadvantages
Cast	More robust	Difficult to remove
	More stable	Does not allow inspection
		May cause skin pressure wounds
		May cause compartment syndrome
Splint	Allows swelling to expand	May cause skin pressure wounds
	Ease of inspection	May not be robust enough
	Ease of removal	
Materials		
Plaster (CaSO$_4$)	Inexpensive	Heavy
	Easy to mould	Vulnerable to water damage
	Easier to remove	
'Soft cast'	More comfortable	Difficult to apply
	Not affected by water	Hard to remove
Fibreglass	Most Robust	Difficult to apply
	Lighter	Very difficult to remove

These 'safe' positions are extremely important, especially in settings where delays and obstacles to definitive care exist. A poorly placed splint or cast could result in complicated ulcers or severe joint contractures that could significantly impact further care and outcome.

Both plaster and fibreglass cure in the form of an exothermic reaction, and use of hot water as the activating agent, inadequate skin padding, and external heat applied during the curing process can result in severe burns.

The decision to proceed with a splint or cast immobilisation (as opposed to no immobilisation or external fixation) can be difficult and is always based on the injury, available resources, and future care. Patients who will not have certain follow up (host nationals) should not be treated in a circumferential cast. In general, unstable injuries from the elbow to the fingers in the upper extremity and from the distal tibia to the foot in the lower extremity can be well treated with splinting or casting. If stability cannot be achieved with a splint or cast (especially in the setting of humerus or femur fractures), external fixation should be applied.

Prior to deployment, surgeons should spend time in their hospital's 'plaster room' or 'cast room' to familiarise themselves with common splint and cast configurations and techniques. It is beyond the scope of this text to provide details on immobilisation

management of all different fracture types. However, the *AO Foundation* provides an exhaustive, open-source digital manual for non-operative fracture management which is available online, and deployed surgeons should download and familiarise themselves with this resource (provide citation here).

Application of Traction

Traction involves application of a distracting force across a fracture site to restore general length, alignment, and rotation of the bone and provide stability of the fracture through soft tissue tension. Traction can be applied through the soft tissues or the bone.

Soft tissue traction techniques include Buck's traction (a weight applied to a soft ankle boot) and Hare traction (a splint that secures the soft tissues above and below a femur fracture and applies a distracting force). Problems with these methods include (1) insufficient purchase which precludes appropriate distracting force generation and (2) soft tissue ischaemia and compromise. These methods are temporary and not always amenable to treatment in combat setting.

Pelvic binding represents a non-invasive variation of soft tissue traction (compression) which deserves mention in this section. In the setting of anterior-posterior pelvic injuries (pubic symphysis diastasis, bilateral pubic rami fractures) the pelvic basin or ring can actually 'open up' and lose its ability to apply compression to retroperitoneal vascular injury. A circumferential binder around the pelvis (in the form of a bed sheet or formal pelvic binder apparatus) applied at the level of the greater trochanters and wrapped with tension can effectively 'close down' this pelvic basin and allow lifesaving compression of pelvic bleeding. Given the potential for pressure sores and skin necrosis, pelvic binders placed for these injuries should normally be replaced with external fixation within 24 hours.

Skeletal traction involves distraction forces placed through fixation of a bone distal to the fracture site. Skeletal traction is a more secure and durable technique and used almost exclusively in femoral fractures, unstable acetabular fractures, and vertical shear pelvic ring injury. Insertion of a pin for skeletal traction requires little equipment, is technically straight forward, and can be performed under local anaesthetic outside of an operating theatre.

In general, skeletal traction can be applied through a 3–5-mm stainless steel pin placed across the distal femur or the proximal tibia. The proximal tibia may be a technically easier site for pin insertion but results in traction being applied across the knee joint – it must be avoided if ligamentous injury is suspected. Both locations confer some degree of neurovascular injury during insertion.

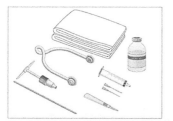

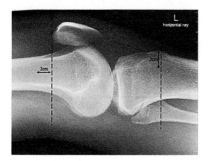

Equipment required:
- Pin-smooth or threads in centre (Denham pin)
- T-handle chuck
- Scalpel
- Stirrup
- Local Anaesthetic

Insertion Site: Distal Femur
- Medial to lateral
- Internally rotate the leg to ensure foot and patella are pointing straight up
- Aim for the centre of the femur at level 2 cm proximal to the superior pole of the patella.

Insertion Site: Proximal tibia, 2 cm posterior to the tibial tuberosity
- Lateral to medial
- Internally rotate leg to ensure point straight up 2 cm posterior to the tibial tubercle, 4 cm distal to the joint line

Traction of around 10% of a patient's body weight should be applied – weight can be adjusted depending on X-ray assessment in traction or comparing limb lengths – anterior superior iliac spine to patella. The patient's bed should be tilted head down to avoid them being dragged to the end of the bed. More complex counter-balanced traction allowing patient rehabilitation can be set up over the following weeks.

Problems with traction treatment of extremity injuries include interruption of traction forces when no proximal opposing force is applied (i.e. the patient is pulled down the bed distally and the weight touches the ground, eliminating the traction force). Traction can be especially problematic during the combat transfer process from one echelon to the next. These interruptions in traction can result in repetitive unnecessary fracture displacement, bleeding, and soft tissue injury.

Application of Extremity External Fixation

For cases where stability cannot be reliably or practicably achieved through splinting/casting or traction, external fixation represents a secure and durable technique which stabilises the fracture through skeletal fixation applied above and below the fracture site, which is in turn linked to a rigid construct (carbon fibre bars) that lies outside the body. There are two main types of external fixation: circular (multi-planar) frames and unilateral (uniplanar) fixators. Circular frames (also referred to as Ilizarov frames or fine-wire frames) are robust and used for definitive treatment, while unilateral external fixators are quicker and easier to apply but are less robust and normally will not be durable enough to support a bone to definitive union. In austere combat setting, unilateral fixators are the only practical form of external fixation.

As previously discussed, the decision to proceed with external fixation is based on the location and overall stability of the fracture, the type of injury, the status of the soft tissues, and the medical status of the patient. In austere combat setting, high energy injuries involving the middle-to-proximal tibia, femur, and humerus benefit from external fixation prior to transport for definitive care. In less common cases of severe bone comminution or loss in the distal tibia or distal radius, external fixation of the ankle or wrist joints may be required to provide stable restoration of length, alignment, and rotation. Certain pelvic injuries may also benefit from external fixation (see the next section).

Advantages of external fixation include speed of application, minimisation of soft tissue trauma, multiple degrees of alignment and rotational freedom through modularity, strength of construct, and durability of the construct. External fixators reliably stabilise the bone after restoration of basic length, alignment, and rotation, and subsequently stabilise the soft tissue envelope. There are three basic components to an external fixator set summarised in Table 13.3.

Appropriate pin insertion is instrumental to avoid complications and optimise outcomes of external fixation. Two pins in the proximal fragment and two pins in the distal fragment are usually sufficient. First, pins should be placed through healthy skin and 'safe corridors' (i.e. avoiding neurovascular structures and joints). Pins should be inserted through a longitudinal skin incision, the length of which should be twice the diameter of the pin being inserted. Clips or scissors should be used for a blunt dissection down to the near cortex. The pin should be rested against the cortex and 'swept' anterior and posterior to ensure that it is being inserted perpendicular to the broadest cross-section. Insertion can be performed by hand or under power. Insertion by hand allows the surgeon to feel the increase and decrease in resistance which accompanies passing in and out of the near cortex, followed by entry and exit of the far cortex, respectively. The far cortex should only be penetrated by <5 mm of the pin tip.

The safe corridors/locations for pin insertion in the upper and lower extremity are as discussed in the following sections.

UPPER EXTREMITY

Humerus

Proximal pins

   o Placed anterolaterally. Care must be taken to avoid the axillary and musculocutaneous nerves.

Distal pins

   o Placed directly laterally. The radial nerve is at significant risk (traversing from posterior to anterior in this location) and an open incision with direct visualisation of all bone and soft tissue should be performed.

Elbow

Proximal pins

   o Placed directly laterally or posteriorly in the distal humerus. Again, great care must be

Table 13.3 The three main components required for linear external fixation

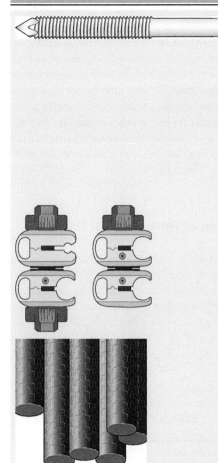

Pins are placed through the skin into the bone.

They are normally 'half-pins' (also known as *Schanz* pins) which do not go all the way through the limb.

Can use full pins (also known as *Denham* or *Steinmann* pins) which fully penetrated the limb at safe sites (i.e. the heel or distal femur).

Can be self-drilling or require pre-drilling before insertion.

Modern pins with an HA coating on the threads will last longer without infection/loosening.

Single use.

Clamps connect pins to bars, and bars to bars.

A wide variety of types are available.

Can be re-used after adequate sterilisation.

Allow a rigid construct to span skeletal instability.

Frequently made from radiolucent material, but radio-opaque material achieves the function of stability, but obscure subsequent imaging.

Can be re-used after adequate sterilisation.

taken to avoid the radial nerve. An open incision with direct visualisation of all bone and soft tissue should be performed.

Distal pins

  o Placed posteriorly along the subcutaneous border of the ulna. If one remains directly at this subcutaneous border, there is minimal risk to surrounding structures.

Forearm

Proximal and distal pins

  o Placed posteriorly along the subcutaneous border of the ulna as previously described.

Wrist

Proximal pins

  o Placed directly radially (laterally) along the subcutaneous border of the radius. Care must be taken to avoid the superficial radial nerve.

Distal pins

  o Smaller diameter pins are placed dorsally through the second metacarpal.

LOWER EXTREMITY

Femur

Proximal and distal pins

  o Placed directly laterally or anterolaterally. Important neurovascular structures are medial and posterior in the thigh, and care must be taken not to penetrate while pre-drilling or inserting the pins.

Knee

Proximal pins

o Placed laterally or anterolaterally in the distal femur as previously described.

Distal pins

o Placed directly at the centre of the broad subcutaneous tibia at the anteromedial leg and aimed perpendicularly (toward the posterolateral leg). This area is very safe, as long as the drill or pins do not penetrate too far posteriorly.

Tibia

Proximal and distal pins

o Anteromedially placed directly in the centre of the subcutaneous tibia and aimed perpendicularly.

Ankle

Proximal pins

o Anteromedially placed directly in the centre of the subcutaneous tibia and aimed perpendicularly.

Distal pins

o Usually through the entire calcaneus, starting medially 2 cm posterior and 2 cm distal to the posterior tibial artery and aimed directly laterally, with exposed pin on the medial and lateral sides of the calcaneus. A second smaller-diameter pin is usually placed through the second metatarsal or the cuneiforms medially to facilitate, maintaining the ankle and foot in neutral position.

The safe immobilisation positions for external fixators spanning joints are the same as those outlined in the splinting/casting section.

The primary goal of external fixation is to achieve rigid skeletal stability after length, alignment, and rotation of the bone have been restored while preserving the soft tissue envelope, facilitating transport, and optimising definitive treatment. The most crucial factor to improve the rigidity of the external fixation construct is anatomic apposition of the bone edges at the fracture site. Further stability can be achieved in the ways discussed in Table 13.4.

Application of Pelvic External Fixation

Grossly unstable pelvic ring injuries can result in life-threatening haemorrhage secondary to the retroperitoneal bleeding that inevitably ensues, and the body's relative inability to tamponade said bleeding secondary to loss of the pelvic basin. Therefore, external fixation of pelvic ring injuries plays an essential role in *haemorrhage control*, particularly in high energy anterior-posterior compression injuries (pubic symphysis diastasis, bilateral pubic rami fractures) and longitudinal distraction injuries (vertical shear dissociation). Reduction and stabilisation of a disrupted pelvic ring in these cases will restore the pelvic basin and allow tamponage and compression of extensive small vessel bleeding, autogenously – if open, pelvic packing is performed.

In a resource-constrained environment which precludes patient transfer to a higher echelon of care and allows for long-term follow-up, reduction and stabilisation with an external fixator might be the only potential treatment for displaced, unstable pelvic ring injuries. Given the contribution of slow-to-heal ligaments to pelvic stability, a fixator used for this purpose will need to be in place for 8–12 weeks.

Pelvic external fixator pins inserted under these circumstances and without image intensification should be placed in the iliac crest via an open technique (Table 13.5).

Table 13.4 Techniques for increasing the strength and stiffness of an external fixator construct	
Pin size	Pins should be as thick as possible – up to a third of the width of the bone into which it is being inserted.
	As a rule:
	5 or 6 mm for femur and tibia
	5 mm for the humerus
	4 mm for forearm
	3 mm for first meta-tarsal
Pin position 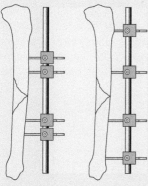	Pins should be positioned 'near and far' – that is near the fracture and far from the fracture, creating the maximum distance between the pins within the constraints of the injury and anatomy.
Bar size 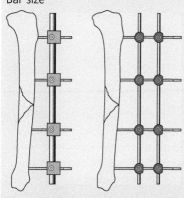	For a given material, a thicker bar will be stiffer.
	If it is not possible to use thicker bars, then increasing the number of bars will also increase stiffness.
Bar position 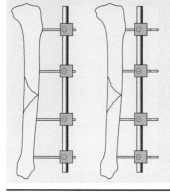	The closer the bar is to the bone, the stiffer the construct. Sufficient space must be left for swelling and care of pin sites.

Table 13.5 The stages of managing a pelvic fracture with external fixation.

Incision

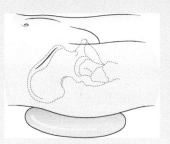

The iliac crest is sub-cutaneous and easily palpable posterior to the anterior superior iliac spine (ASIS), between the external oblique muscles of the anterior abdominal wall proximally and gluteus maximus distally.

The incision begins 1 cm posterior to ASIS and continues posteriorly for 5 cm along the crest

Deep dissection 1

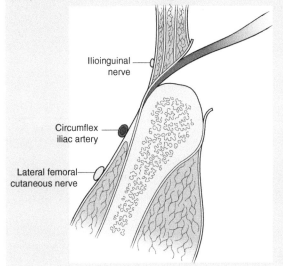

Ilioinguinal nerve

Circumflex iliac artery

Lateral femoral cutaneous nerve

The fascial interval between the external oblique and gluteus maximal is sharply incised directly onto the iliac crest.

Deep dissection 2

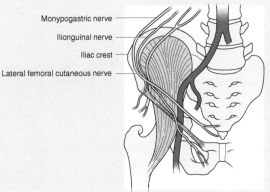

Monypogastric nerve

Ilionguinal nerve

Iliac crest

Lateral femoral cutaneous nerve

The iliac crest is exposed by lifting the gluteus maximus and iliacus muscles from the inner and outer surface of the iliac wing. This can be initiated with a periosteal elevator and continued with a gauze pack.

Table 13.5 (*continued*)

Pin insertion 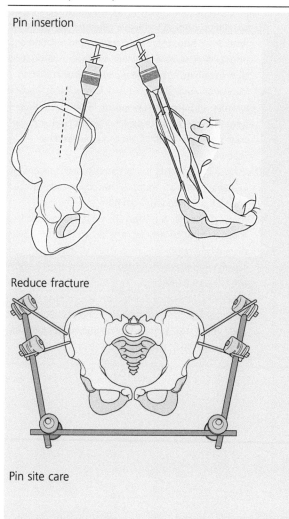	Pins should be inserted underhand or powered in through the narrow corridor between the two cortical tables of bone of the iliac wing.
	A method to visually identify this corridor is to lay a Kirschner wire or similar narrow instrument on either side of the iliac wing, as shown in the diagram.
	At least two pins need to be inserted.
Reduce fracture	The frame should be constructed with the clamps holding the pins to the bars fully tightened and the clamps between bars lose.
	The reduction manoeuvre is performed according to the fracture displacement.
	Whilst the reduction is held, the rest of the clamps should be tightened.
Pin site care	The reduction maneuverer may have resulted in skin tension against the pins – this should be released.
	The incision should be closed around the pins with sutures and dressed.

KEY POINTS

Frontline surgeons must assume that they will spend much of their time managing bone and soft tissue injuries to the upper extremity, lower extremity, and pelvis. Surgical management of traumatic wounds in these areas is the most common operation performed in conflict – your pre-deployment training should focus on this skill.

Understanding and applying damage control principles in combat medical setting is essential and involves preventing loss of life, restoring normal host hemodynamic and physiologic status, and impeding loss of limb while maximising future potential function and rehabilitation. The key orthopaedic damage control principles include termination of bleed, expeditious compartment release, provisional stabilisation of fractures and unstable limbs, decontamination of grossly contaminated wounds, and appropriate wound care.

The goals of fracture care in conflict involve restoring basic anatomic length, alignment, and rotation of the limb and providing expeditious and safe stabilisation that decreases bleeding, preserves the soft tissue envelope, decreases pain, facilitates patient transfer, and optimises definitive fixation and wound management. The stabilisation method depends on the location and degree of injury, mechanism, available resources, and patient status. Stabilisation methods range from no stabilisation at all to splinting/casting, application of traction, application of external fixation, or early amputation.

In these austere or dangerous settings, there may be one opportunity for surgical intervention. Surgeons should accept that their intervention will be aimed at saving life and limb and recognise that compromises will have to be made regarding wound debridement and limb salvage that would not be required in greater resources. The combat setting often requires establishing delicate balance between optimising long-term functional outcome and providing lifesaving immediate – though radical – care.

FURTHER READING

AO Foundation. AO handbook-nonoperative fracture treatment. Davos 2013. https://ao-alliance.org/wp-content/uploads/2015/07/ao-alliance-handbook-nono-perative-fracture-treatment-complete.pdf.

AO foundation surgical technique guide for basic external fixation. https://surgeryreference.aofoundation.org/orthopedic-trauma/adult-trauma/humeral-shaft/basic-technique/basic-technique-modular-external-fixation.

AO foundation surgical technique guide for Pelvic fracture external fixation-by Dankward Höntzsch. https://surgeryreference.aofoundation.org/orthopedic-trauma/adult-trauma/pelvic-ring/basic-technique/external-fixation.

BOA/BAPRAS. Standards for open fracture management, available online: https://www.boa.ac.uk/resources/knowledge-hub/boast-4-pdf.html.

Noblet, T., Lineham, B., Wiper, J. et al. Amputation in trauma—how to achieve a good result from lower extremity amputation irrespective of the level. Curr Trauma Rep 5, 69–78 (2019). https://doi.org/10.1007/s40719-019-0159-1.

Penn-Barwell J, Rowlands T. Infection and combat injuries-historical lessons and evolving concepts. Bone Joint 360. Vol. 2, No. 5 https://online.boneandjoint.org.uk/doi/full/10.1302/2048-0105.25.36071

Neurotrauma in the Field 14

Down Range

Kevin Tsang

CRANIAL TRAUMA

Introduction

As mentioned, traumatic brain injury (TBI) is extremely common and accounts for many trauma-related deaths. It is difficult to find accurate data relating to military trauma, but large US and European epidemiological studies on civilian trauma estimated around 15 per 100,000 population per year would die from a brain injury — that's a significant fatality rate of 11%. Military trauma is more often related to open, penetrating, or blast injuries rather than closed injuries, which would likely translate to an even higher fatality — hence, the need for frontline clinicians to be appropriately trained in dealing with these cases.

Considerations

There are many differences between casualties of a combat setting and civilian trauma. The most obvious difference is that most civilian trauma are closed head injuries due to blunt trauma, whilst the majority of military trauma are either due to blast injury (56% of all military TBI in one study) or penetrating injury (missiles either from fragments or debris created by an explosive device, or some form of ballistic such as bullets). As a result of the mechanism, they are also much more likely to be polytrauma patients with major haemorrhage, major burns, and complex skeletal injuries. These make it exceedingly difficult to accurately assess the severity of the TBI.

In addition, due to the primary blast wave, these patients are much more likely to have vascular injuries and strokes. Therefore, some form of vascular imaging upon arrival to the care facility should be considered.

All of these partly explain the severe and irreversible nature of primary brain injury, but as a result of polytrauma, secondary brain injury is extremely common in this group of patients. The severe burns and major haemorrhage can result in significant hypotension, hypothermia, and acidosis; the burns and significant facial fractures encountered in these cases may also make definitive airway insertion difficult with resultant hypoventilation, hypoxia, and hypercarbia. All of these will amount to secondary brain injury which may be very tricky to control in a combat field.

Therefore, rapid and efficient stabilisation and transfer to the definitive care facility are of utmost importance in these situations.

Common Cases and Treatment

BLAST INJURY

Various blast waves have different impacts on brain tissue. The primary wave causes significant tissue oedema. The airway compromise and cardiorespiratory compromise because of body oedema can obviously result in secondary brain injury, but the wave itself can cause significant brain oedema and the patient may require a bifrontal decompressive craniectomy to adequately control this brain swelling (see the following discussion). However, this should not be necessary in the field and should be treated like any closed brain injury with neuroprotective measures alone, including adequate sedation, ventilation to maintain normal range pCO_2 (4.5–5.0 kPa), and the use of osmotherapy.

The secondary blast injury is related to the debris and fragmentation of the explosive device and acts more like a ballistic type of penetrating injury, which is described in detail later. Due to the multiple nature of this, compared to single gunshot wounds, the need to operate is very rare. However, these ballistics tend to have a much higher velocity than normal gunshots and may result in more damage with worse prognosis.

The tertiary blast injury results from sudden acceleration and deceleration (from the body being thrown in the air) with resultant diffuse axonal injury (DAI). Compared to a closed high-velocity brain injury (e.g., road traffic accident), this has a significantly higher chance of a cerebrovascular injury (up to 27% in one study), and patients should all undergo an angiogram (in the form of a CTA) upon transfer to definitive care centre. There is a high chance of vascular dissection and resultant ischaemia and infarction but the only treatment available in the field would be adequate cerebral perfusion by maintaining a mean arterial pressure (MAP) of 90 mmHg, which may not be possible if the patient is haemorrhaging from another source.

Quaternary blast injury refers to thermal and toxic inhalation injuries and may contribute towards a secondary brain injury if not adequately treated but has no direct contribution to primary brain injury.

In the extremely unlikely event that a bifrontal decompressive craniectomy is required, here are the steps to follow:

1. Standard preparation of the patient.
2. Bicoronal incision (i.e. incision from the top of one ear across the top of the head to the other ear; Figure 14.1).
3. Raise the scalp flap forwards to the level of the supraorbital ridge, ideally preserving the pericranium and temporalis fascia to be raised as a separate layer as this can be used to cranialise the frontal air sinus.

   a. Beware of the temporal branch of the frontal nerve which runs within the temporal fat pad; one should incise the temporalis fascia just superior to the fat pad and raise this with the scalp as a single layer to protect the nerve.

4. Depending on how lateral the decompression needs to be, the temporalis muscle may need to be detached from the attachment (superior temporal line) and raised as a separate flap laterally onto the zygoma.
5. The most important structure to be aware of during the craniotomy is the midline superior sagittal sinus. One option is to create multiple burr holes on either side of the midline (Figure 14.2) to allow the dura to be stripped off the bone across the midline before connecting the holes (Figure 14.3; including ones placed laterally on the temporal bone) to remove the bone flap (Figure 14.4).

   a. A second option is to raise two separate craniotomy bone flaps (Figure 14.5), leaving a strip of bone in the midline. Once the dura has been exposed, it is much easier to strip the dura of the midline strip of bone under direct vision. This strip of bone is removed as a third bone flap.

   b. In the unfortunate event that the sinus is injured, and major haemorrhage is encountered whilst not in a hospital setting, one can just take a stitch (e.g., 3-0 Vicryl) and tie off the sinus altogether. It is safe to tie off the anterior third of the sinus, but the risk of venous infarction of the brain increases if it is done more posteriorly.

   c. The other concern, if the sinus is injured, is that of an air embolus. Therefore, one must irrigate the sinus continuously until it has been secured. Ensure the anaesthetist is informed, both for blood loss and $etCO_2$ drop monitoring, which is the first sign of an air embolus.

6. The dura can be opened bilaterally in a U-shaped fashion, with the base towards the midline to prevent injury to the sinus.

   a. If the brain is very oedematous, it may start to herniate through the durotomy. In this setting, ensure the anaesthetist maximise the neuroprotection manoeuvres whilst the surgeon closes the wound immediately; otherwise, the herniation will be so significant that the wound cannot be closed without some brain resection, which

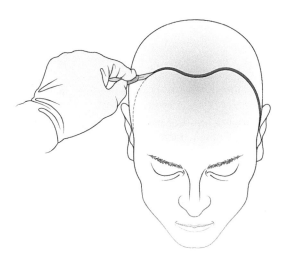

Figure 14.1 Ear to ear (bicoronal) scalp incision

obviously carries an extremely poor prognosis.

7. In a hospital setting, the frontal air sinus can be cranialised at this point, but this is unnecessary if the procedure is not done in a definitive care setting.

8. Place the pericranium over the dural surface to reduce the chances of CSF leak and close the scalp wound with 2-0 Vicryl to the galea and clips to skin.

9. Apply a head bandage (not too tight!).

BALLISTICS

When considering ballistic wounds, considerations should be given to the physics of the weapon used. This is described in detail in previous chapters of this book. A bullet fired through the skull, first, creates a soft tissue wound and a depressed skull fracture, sometimes with fragments driven into the brain tissue. Just like any other solid organs, the bullet would de-stabilise and 'wobble' upon entering the density of the brain, creating an area of primary damage that is beyond expected of a 'straight' trajectory. A temporary vacuum created will also attract hair, debris, and any other types of soiling into the brain, increasing the risk of infection (brain abscess) to around 10%.

The patient should be stabilised in terms of a primary survey, followed by the consideration given to

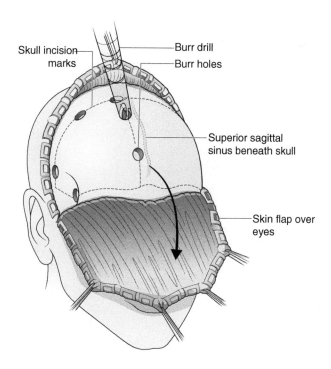

Figure 14.2

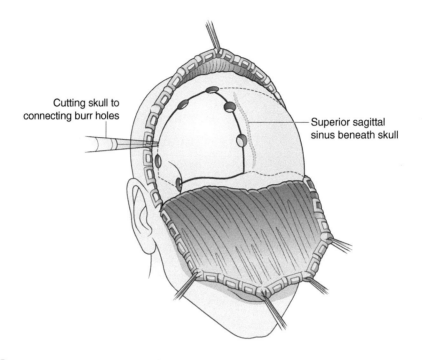

Cutting skull to
connecting burr holes

Superior sagittal
sinus beneath skull

Figure 14.3

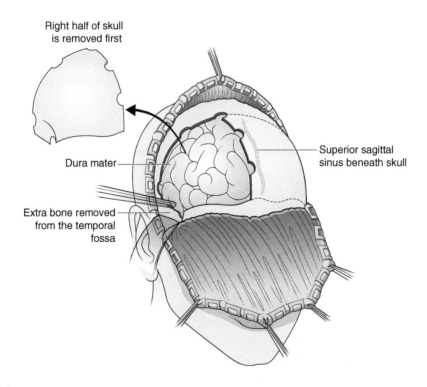

Right half of skull
is removed first

Dura mater

Extra bone removed
from the temporal
fossa

Superior sagittal
sinus beneath skull

Figure 14.4

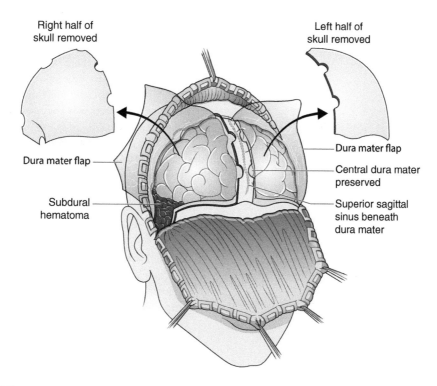

Right half of skull removed

Left half of skull removed

Dura mater flap

Subdural hematoma

Dura mater flap

Central dura mater preserved

Superior sagittal sinus beneath dura mater

Figure 14.5

the brain injury. Anyone with a penetrating brain injury and an altered level of consciousness should be intubated even if the GCS is still above 8, the traditional cut-off for airway protection. This is because the patient is likely to have a more significant brain injury than anticipated, which will deteriorate over time, and controlled ventilation to maintain normal pCO_2 would be protective for the brain. If there are signs of raised intracranial pressure (ICP), then the patient should be adequately sedated, and osmotherapy given. This can be either mannitol (although this may worsen hypotension associated with a polytrauma patient) or hypertonic saline.

The immediate surgical consideration is whether there may be a localised haematoma that can be efficiently evacuated through a simple burr hole. This is much more likely if the patient has lowered GCS and lateralising signs, such as a unilateral weakness or unilateral pupillary dilatation. The haematoma is likely to be ipsilateral to the side of the impact or wound, with further clues coming from pupil dilation or motor weakness. However, it is possible to have false lateralising signs. Kernohan's notch — which describes significant subfalcine herniation resulting in compression

of the contralateral cerebral peduncle causing weakness that is ipsilateral to the weakness — may make the diagnosis difficult. See the later discussion for the actual procedure for burr-hole creation.

It is extremely rare to need to perform a craniotomy in the field. Two recent studies, DECRA and RescueICP, both showed that decompressive craniectomy can improve survival but significantly increase the disability of living patients (i.e. converting GOS 6 patients to GOS 5), and therefore, it still controversial as to whether this is the correct treatment. Certainly, there should be no reason to perform such a procedure before adequate imaging in a definitive centre. Similarly, there is no reason to elevate any depressed skull fractures or try to remove any bullets from the brain in the field. If there is some form of soft tissue cover to prevent cerebrospinal fluid (CSF) leak, thereby reducing the risk of meningitis, then the patient is ready for transfer. This can be done by simple irrigation of the wound and primary closure — in the case of significant soft tissue loss, a simple washout and water-tight dressing (such as a head bandage) — and then transfer (Figures 14.6–14.11).

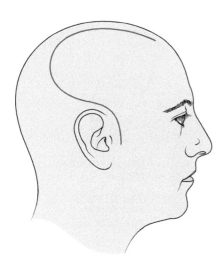

Figure 14.6 Use of burr hole to allow turning of craniotomy flap using either a power-driven craniotome or the Gigli saw.

CLOSED HEAD INJURIES

This is much less common in a combat situation but may be important in a humanitarian crisis zone. If it is necessary to perform exploratory burr-holes due to lowered GCS and inability to arrive in definitive care centre rapidly, then it should be made on the side that is most likely to be injured (see the earlier discussion). In a closed head injury, where there is suspicion of incranial haemorrhage (Figure 14.12) where there is no wound to be found, a temporal burr hole just anterior and superior to the ear (near the pterion) would be the best place to start as this is the most likely site of haematoma formation (due to injury to the middle meningeal artery). Failing this, a frontal burr hole in the mid-pupillary line 10–15 cm from the eye is the second possible site of injury, followed by parietal or occipital sites, which are less common.

To create the burr hole follow these simple steps:

1. Simple linear incision should be made after adequate cleaning in the area of interest (Figure 14.13).
2. Strip the pericranium off the bone using a periosteal elevator to prevent the drill from sliding.
3. The burr hole is created using either a Hudson brace (Figure 14.14) or a pneumatic perforator. The inner cortex of the skull is hard, and the operating surgeon should feel stiffening of the brace — a sign to slow down the drilling to prevent injuring the brain.
4. The haematoma should be visible or, in most

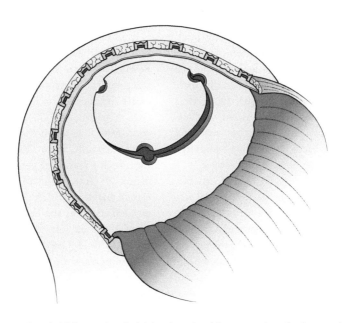

Figure 14.7 A very tense dura (which may be dark blue in colour) is suggestive of a large subdural haematoma.

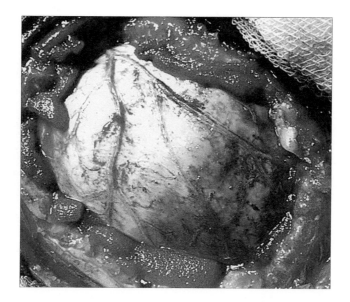

Figure 14.8 If there are doubts about brain herniation which may worsen operative outcome, make multiple slits to allow evacuation of the haematoma without allowing the brain to herniate out.

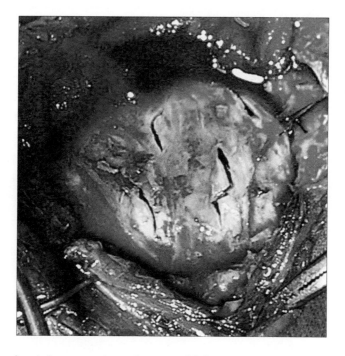

Figure 14.9 Once the dura is less tense, it can be opened fully.

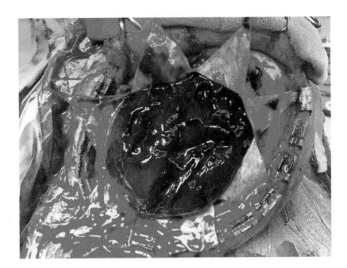

Figure 14.10 Clot present.

cases, will start to self-evacuate due to high pressure. If this is not the case, the dura may have to be opened using a scalpel (Figure 14.15) in a cruciate manner.

5. Washout the haematoma as much as possible through the burr-hole. This is an immediate life-saving procedure to reduce ICP and not designed to achieve complete evacuation of the haematoma or haemostasis. A craniotomy is required to achieve these goals.

6. The scalp is then closed using 2-0 Vicryl to galea and clips to skin.

SPINAL TRAUMA

Introduction

As with traumatic brain injuries, military spinal injuries are more severe and complex than those of

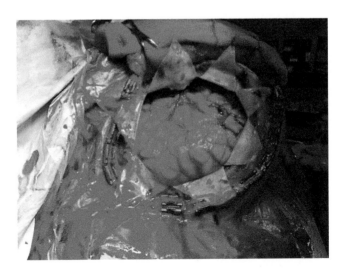

Figure 14.11 After-clot evacuation.

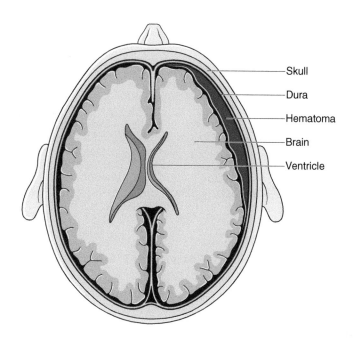

Figure 14.12 Pre-operative condition. Cut-away view from above.

civilians. Most of these are in the thoracolumbar region (up to 65% and 60%, respectively) and mainly relate to blast and gunshot injuries, like in brain injuries. Many of these patients are ASIA A (American Spinal Injury Association), which means they have complete cord injury. Interestingly, spinal cord injuries (SCI) tend to be more common in marine service (incidence up to $5.3/100,000$ year^{-1}).

Military Versus Civilian

Military spine injuries tend to be related to blast injuries, which area mainly blunt (81.6%) rather than penetrating (18.4%) in nature, according to a study of the Iraq and Afghanistan veterans. These military patients have high injury severity score (ISS) due to the polytrauma nature, with a considerable proportion having concomitant brain injury. These blast and gunshot injuries result in significant comminution of the vertebrae, rather than the simpler compression wedge fractures, which are much more common in civilian trauma. This means that the spine is much less likely to be stable and full spinal precautions must be taken. Similarly, the high incidence of spinal cord injury means that the field medics need to be more aware of the potential impact of neurogenic shock.

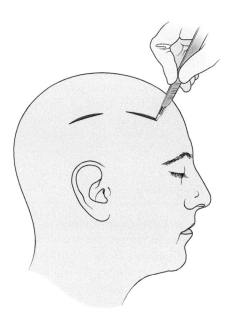

Figure 14.13 Incisions are made into the right side of the head.

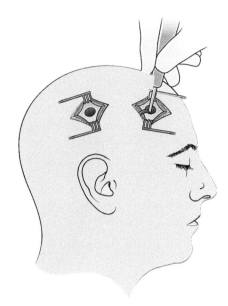

Figure 14.15 The dura is entered, and the blood is evacuated from the surface of the brain.

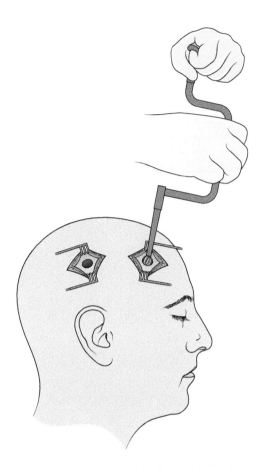

Figure 14.14 A hole is drilled through the skull at each incision site.

Spinal Column Injury

It is not recommended to place a collar on any patients with a penetrating injury as this will compromise the assessment of the wound and may contribute towards airway obstruction. Similarly, in a patient involved in a blast injury, the high likelihood of airway obstruction and lung injury from barotrauma is a contraindication to the use of a collar. Therefore, as a general rule, military patients with suspected spinal injuries should be immobilised either manually or with blocks and tapes alone. A spine board is helpful in transferring the patient efficiently whilst maintaining alignment, but there is an elevated risk of pressure sores even if only used for a brief period, and the spine board will contribute significantly to hypothermia in a polytrauma patient. These need to be considered when immobilising such patients.

There is no reason to perform any spinal fixation surgery in the field. Even with comminuted fractures and retropulsed fragments in the spinal canal, studies suggest that surgery within 24 hours provide better outcome than those performed beyond 24 hours, but there is no evidence that earlier surgery would further improve the outcome. Therefore, these patients just need to be transferred carefully with consideration given to the spinal column. Similarly, a presumed epidural haematoma in the spine (e.g., progressive paraplegia) need urgent attention at the definitive care centre but not in the field.

Spinal Cord Injury

Neurogenic shock may play a crucial role in these patients due to higher rates of spinal cord injury. This is an interruption to the sympathetic nervous system with resultant bradycardia and hypotension. Any patient not responding to normal fluid resuscitation should be started on inotropes as early as possible. Studies have shown that maintaining a good perfusion pressure to the spinal cord (current

British Association of Spine Surgeons guidelines suggest MAP of more than 90 mmHg) will result in better neurological outcome.

More important, if possible, these patients should be catheterised at the earliest opportunity after stabilisation of the vitals. This is because any patient with a cord injury (above T6 level) is at risk of autonomic dysreflexia, and this is mainly triggered by a significant stimulus within the pelvic region (e.g., very full bladder or sudden emptying of a very full bladder). The patient develops a sympathetic overdrive with tachycardia, hypertension, flushing, and sweating and may progress to seizures, coma, and death. The mortality is over 80%, and only supportive treatment in ICU is possible. The best treatment is, therefore, prevention by catheterising the patient early (and then ensuring the bowels open regularly, but this is irrelevant in the field).

KEY POINTS

1. In a combat zone, blast and ballistic injuries are much more common than closed injuries.
2. Immediate treatment is stabilisation of the patient with irrigation and covering of the wound.
3. Spinal immobilisation is all that is required in those with suspected spinal column injury, with no reason for any surgical intervention prior to arrival at definitive care.
4. Maintain adequate perfusion to the nervous system in suspected head and spinal injuries.
5. Safe and efficient transfer to definitive care is of utmost importance.

FURTHER READING

1. Tagliaferri F, Compagnone C, Korsie M et al. A systematic review of brain injury epidemiology in Europe. *Acta Neurochir* 2006; **148**:255–268.
2. Division of Injury Response. *Traumatic brain injury in the United States. Emergency department visits, hospitalizations, and death. National Center for Injury Prevention and Control,* 2006.
3. Wilberger J, Harris M, Diamond D. Acute subdural haematoma: morbidity, mortality and operative timing. *J Neurosurg* 1991; **74**:212–218.
4. Bell R, Vo A, Neal C, Tingo J, Roberts R, Mossop C. Military traumatic brain and spinal column injury: a 5-year study of the impact blast and other military grade weaponry on the Central Nervous System. *J Trauma Acute Care Surg* 2009; **66(4)**:S104–S111.
5. The CRASH-3 collaborators. Effects of tranexamic acid on death, disability, vascular occlusive events and other morbidities in patients with acute traumatic brain injury (CRASH-3): a randomised, placebo-controlled trial. *Lancet* 2019; **394(10210):1713–1723.**
6. Cooper D, Resenfeld J, Murray L, Arabi Y, Davies A, D'Urso P et al. Decompressive craniectomy in diffuse traumatic brain injury. *NEJM* 2011; **364**:1493–1502.
7. Hutchinson P, Kolias A, Tomofeev T, Corteen E, Czosnyk M, Timothy J et al. Trail of decompressive craniectomy for traumatic intracranial hypertension. *NEJM* 2016; **375**:1119–1130.
8. Furlan J, Gulasingam S, Craven B. Epidemiology of war-related spinal cord injury among combatants: a systematic review. *Global Spine J* 2019; **9(5)**: 545–558.
9. Szuflita N, Neal C, Rosner M, Frankowski R, Grossman R. Spine injuries sustained by US military personnel in combat are different from non-combat spine injuries. *Military Med* 2016; **181(10)**:1314–1323.

Management of Ballistic Face and Neck Trauma in an Austere Setting

15

Johno Breeze

RESOURCE LIMITATION CONCERNS

- Computerised tomography (CT) is essential for correct management of penetrating face and neck trauma.
- Surgical intervention should be delayed until CT is available, unless casualties are haemodynamically unstable.
- Interventional radiology for penetrating neck injury (PNI) unlikely to be available – meaning that conventional access to vascular damage may be required.
- Such surgery for PNI has potential morbidity and the need for early exploration should balance the risks.
- Endoscopy is essential for PNI in a resource-limited environment, even when CT is available.
- Equipment for temporarily stabilising facial fractures for evacuation is cheap but requires practice to be performed correctly.

STEP-BY-STEP PROCEDURES

1. Surgical cricothyroidotomy.
2. Arresting facial bleeding by nasal and oral packing.
3. Access to the common carotid artery in neck Zone 2.
4. Maxillary–mandibular stabilisation with IMF screws.

EXSANGUINATING HAEMORRHAGE

Immediate management of penetrating face and neck injury is based on the modified Advanced Trauma Life Support principles used by most common militaries, in which catastrophic haemorrhage precedes the airway. Multiple types of haemostatic agents are available to first responders and are highly effective for neck wounds, especially if pressure is maintained by pressing on the dressing. In this author's opinion, combat gauze type dressings are the most recommended for open neck wounds, as it not only can be packed without causing further damage but also easily removed at the time of surgery. Facial bleeding in comparison can be catastrophic, and most sources of facial bleeding are often inaccessible anyway without surgery.

AIRWAY PROVISION

In experienced hands, endotracheal intubation should be performed even with suspected laryngotracheal injury. In less-experienced hands – particularly in the pre-hospital setting – surgical cricothyroidotomy is recommended instead of endotracheal intubation (Figure 15.1). Intubation can be complicated by the associated expanding neck hematoma, laryngotracheal injury, and suspicion of an associated cervical spine injury. Specialist kits are available for performing surgical cricothyroidotomy with a greater lumen diameter than

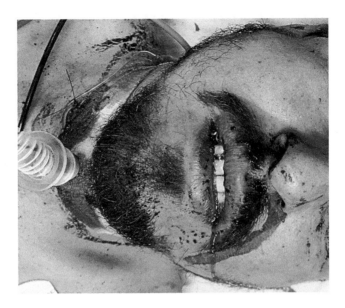

Figure 15.1 Clinical image of a pre-hospital placed surgical cricothyroidotomy in situ while in the Emergency Department.

using a wide bore needle cannula alone. There is no role for either surgical or percutaneous tracheostomy in truly acute setting. Should delays in evacuation be anticipated, or if treatment of PNI or facial fractures is performed, a surgical tracheostomy may be indicated.

STEP-BY-STEP PROCEDURE 1: SURGICAL CRICOTHYROIDOTOMY

- Identify landmarks (Figure 15.2).
- Infiltrate both the skin and through the cricothyroid membrane with lidocaine and epinephrine.
- Horizontal puncture through a cricothyroid membrane with a scalpel – make sure you do not to hit the posterior wall of the larynx.
- Insert a small lumen endotracheal tube.
- Inflate the cuff and check pressure.

CERVICAL SPINE IMMOBILISATION

The probability of cervical spine instability from a facial injury from either a GSW or a blast in a patient who is conscious – neurologically intact and moving all limbs – is low. Immobilisation is recommended unless it would place the clinician at risk. There is no consensus, however, for penetrating cervical wounds, and most casualties will arrive in a collar, which must be carefully removed; immobilisation is maintained during the primary survey.

MANAGEMENT OF FACIAL HAEMORRHAGE

The face is rarely the site of torrential haemorrhage sufficient to be the sole contributor to hypovolaemic shock. Bleeding from the nose may represent oral (such as a mandible fracture) or nasal injury. Similarly, oral bleeding can represent injuries at both sites. All conscious patients should be sat up and, in extremis, rolled onto their front. Cauterisation of severe nasal haemorrhage is usually challenging unless a clinician is well trained, has good light, and ideal magnification. Instead, nasal bleeding should be managed first by insertion of a haemostat into each nostril such as Merocel® or Rapid Rhino®. Should this fail, anterior packing of each nostril should be performed with a ribbon-type haemostatic dressing; if this fails, then additional posterior packing should be performed.

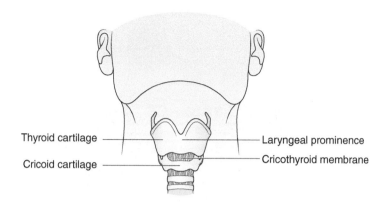

Figure 15.2 Surface landmarks in performing a surgical cricothyroidotomy.

Oral bleeding is far more challenging and may require intubation. Although bite props can be used to impact the maxilla, this can displace fractures and should be performed by an experienced clinician. Oropharyngeal bleeding that cannot be arrested requires careful packing that cannot be properly performed without a definitive airway. Blind clamping of external areas of facial bleeding should be avoided because critical structures, such as the facial nerve or parotid duct, are susceptible to injury. Ligation of the external carotid artery to stop facial bleeding is rarely successful due to collateral circulation and is not recommended.

STEP-BY-STEP PROCEDURE 2: ARRESTING FACIAL BLEEDING BY NASAL AND ORAL PACKING

- Identify the source of bleeding.
- If likely nasal bleeding, insert a nasal epistatic into both nostrils.
- Should bleeding continue, remove both epistats and pack each nostril with a ribbon-type haemostatic dressing (Figure 15.3).
- Should bleeding continue, insert a 10–14 French urinary catheter into each nostril, inflate with 5 mL of air, and pull back until it lodges in the nasopharynx.
- Although a CT to rule out a base of skull fracture is taught, in reality, such fractures are far too small to allow a urinary catheter to pass through them.

- Repack the anterior nose.
- Any further bleeding is likely to be from nasopharynx running into the mouth and can only be addressed by packing the oropharynx.
- This, in turn, requires the patient to be orally intubated, or through a surgical airway.

DAMAGE CONTROL SURGERY FOR PENETRATING NECK INJURY

Damage Control Surgery (DCS) is a principle where early identification of life-threatening injuries is made and the decision to avoid complicated, sometimes lengthy, definitive repairs in an unstable patient. Patients with 'hard signs' of PNI should be taken to the operating room for surgical exploration prior to CT (Table 15.1). Soft signs include hematemesis, haemoptysis, hoarseness or change in voice, dysphagia, or odynophagia. In a stable patient, these signs mandate further evaluation and exclusion of vascular and aero-digestive injury. Transcervical gunshot wounds, in particular, have a high probability of underlying damage and, in the lack of availability of CT, would generally indicate a need for surgical exploration.

The use of serial physical examinations alone to guide management decisions in PNI from ballistic injury is highly debatable and depends on the experience of the clinicians looking after them. For example, asymptomatic military patients injured by fragmentation were found to have vascular damage

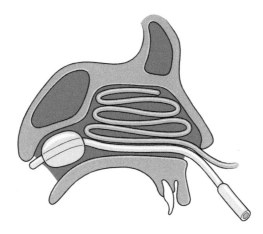

Figure 15.3 A Foley catheter (yellow) is inflated within the posterior nasopharynx and haemostatic gauze packed against it into both nasal cavities.

Table 15.1 Clinical 'hard signs' of penetrating neck injury warranting immediate surgical exploration
Vascular: ongoing bleeding from the neck region that is not amenable to pressure, an expanding haematoma, and a bruit or thrill in the neck.
Aerodigestive injury: crepitus or subcutaneous emphysema, dyspnoea or stridor, air bubbling from the wound, tenderness or pain over the trachea, hoarse or abnormal voice, hematemesis, or haemoptysis.

in 25% of cases, even when no wound tract seem to involve vessel and fragment in close proximity.

Damage to the hypopharynx and oesophagus may be clinically silent and escape serial physical examinations. Missed oesophageal injuries are the cause of the majority of delayed complications seen with penetrating neck injuries. Early signs of oesophageal injury include subcutaneous air, crepitus, dysphagia, odynophagia, drooling, and hematemesis. When an oesophageal leak progresses to mediastinitis, morbidity and mortality are significant.

INVESTIGATIONS OF PENETRATING NECK INJURY

Unstable patients and those with hard signs should proceed straight to DCS. Otherwise, if available, CT Angiography (CTA) using contrast is recommended for all but most innocuous injuries, with a Positive

Predictive Value (PPV) of up to 100% for diagnosis of carotid arterial injuries in experienced units (Múnera et al. 2000). In ballistic injury, CTA can be non-diagnostic in up to 20% of cases due to metallic artefact and, therefore, a lower threshold for exploration will occur. CT is less sensitive for the diagnosis of injuries to the larynx and trachea. Flexible laryngoscopy can be performed in intubated patients either pre- or intra-operatively and can visualise damage up to and past the carina.

The diagnosis of oesophageal injury in neck injuries is the most difficult, with CT of 40–79% and NPV of 82–100% (Conradie and Gebremariam 2015; Kazi et al. 2013; Teixeira et al. 2016). Intra-operative direct oesophagoscopy (preferably both flexible and rigid) provide the highest sensitivity for diagnosis of oesophageal injury but requires experience to perform, especially in a patient with an immobilised cervical spine. A Gastrografin® contrast swallow imaging study can be performed but require a stable, cooperative patient. When combined, oesophagoscopy with oesophagography has a sensitivity of up to 90%.

THE USE OF NECK ZONES

In the civilian environment where CT scanning and interventional radiology is readily available, the use of neck zones to guide management has decreased. However, in austere settings, particularly when CT is not available, dividing the neck into three zones still has a key role. Zone I is classed from suprasternal notch to cricoid cartilage, Zone II from the cricoid cartilage to mandibular angle, and Zone III from mandibular angle to base of the skull. Exercise caution as the neck entry zone may not reflect the trajectory of projectiles once in tissues.

ZONE 1 INJURIES

This zone contains the origin of the common carotid artery, the subclavian vessels and the vertebral artery, the brachial plexus, the trachea, the oesophagus (Figure 15.4), the apex of the lung, and the thoracic duct. Acute assessment is analogous to chest injury; a chest radiograph should be taken to exclude haemo- or pneumothorax. Stable patients with Zone 1 injuries should be first assessed by CT to guide management. Since up to one-third of patients with a clinically significant Zone 1 injury may have no symptoms at their initial presentation, many centres advocate vascular evaluation of the aortic arch and great vessels, with an oesophageal evaluation. In a haemodynamically unstable patient, particularly if polytrauma is present, clinicians should be sure that the neck is the source of instability before proceeding to surgery. In the prescribe of instability or hard signs, an incision parallel to sternocleidomastoid is generally utilised (Figure 15.5(a)) and can be extended into a midline sternotomy (Figure 15.5(b)). A surgical tracheostomy is recommended in most cases.

ZONE 2 INJURIES

The following structures are located here: the carotid and vertebral arteries, the internal jugular veins, trachea, and the oesophagus. This zone has comparatively easy access for clinical examination and surgical exploration. It is the largest zone and the most injured in the neck. Even in austere setting, stable casualties with Zone II injuries and no hard signs can be managed conservatively without surgical exploration until CTA is available. This is, however, dependent on the mechanism of injury, with authors describing underlying damage in 78% of asymptomatic ballistic military neck wounds. Damage to vascular and airway structures in Zone II should be repaired, with delayed repair of oesophageal injuries generally recommended. Most cases do not, in fact, require a surgical tracheostomy unless severe disruption of the larynx or trachea is found requiring delayed or secondary repair. An incision parallel to SCM can be used, but should coexisting facial fractures be present, a low collar incision is recommended (Figure 15.5(c)); this is analogous to an incision performed for a neck dissection and enables a mandible fracture to be fixed externally.

ZONE 3 INJURIES

Zone III is the most challenging to manage, due to its anatomy and the lack of familiarity of many surgeons in this era of increasing sub-specialisation. Zone III contains the distal carotid and vertebral arteries, oro- and nasopharynx. The anatomy is challenging to assess clinically and access surgically, due to being close to the base of the skull and medial to the mandible (most Zone III injuries are in fact facial injuries). Casualties with Zone III injuries without hard signs should have frequent intraoral examination to observe for oedema or expanding haematoma within the parapharyngeal or retropharyngeal spaces. Cranial nerves exiting the skull base such as the glossopharyngeal and hypoglossal are near the great vessels, with neurological deficits, therefore suggestive of associated injury. Surgical access to Zone III injuries has been classically described by extending the sternocleidomastoid (SCM) incision superiorly behind the ear. However, those injuries medial to the mandible often require a mandibulotomy to access them. In the author's experience, surgical access is better managed through a unilateral collar incision extended into a lip split to one side of the midline (Figure 15.5(d)). The mandible is divided using a saw, which may require tooth extraction. For this reason, even if damage in Zone II is found on CT, exploration in a stable patient is best delayed until performed by a surgeon used to dealing with such injuries. Such injuries in a civilian setting are generally managed through percutaneous

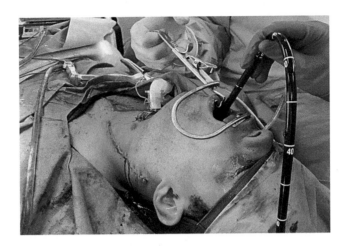

Figure 15.4 Intra-operative oesophagoscopy used to rule out cervical oesophageal injury. No damage was seen on pre-operative CT.

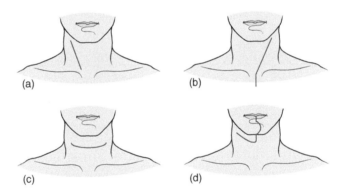

Figure 15.5 Operative approaches to the neck include (a) sternocleidomastoid incision, (b) sternocleido-mastoid incision with sternotomy extension, (c) collar incision, and (d) unilateral collar incision extended into midline lip split.

angiography, and evacuation of the casualty from austere setting to a medical treatment facility is highly recommended.

SURGICAL TREATMENT OF PENETRATING CERVICAL VASCULAR INJURY

The primary objective during operative management is to preserve antegrade flow to the carotid and vertebral arteries to optimise neurological function, if possible. Common and internal carotid artery injuries should be repaired unless there is truly uncontrollable haemorrhage or devastating vessel injury. A temporary vascular shunt with a short piece of plastic can be used while an autogenous graft is harvested to reduce the need for cross-clamping (Figure 15.6). Ligation of the external carotid and internal jugular is generally well tolerated unless performed bilaterally. Defects larger than 2 cm in diameter will often require either a patch or graft; such grafts can come from an adjacent damaged internal jugular vein, reversed

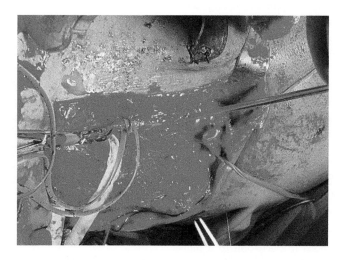

Figure 15.6 Surgical repair of a common carotid artery wound using temporary stent bypass and subsequent vein graft, as the internal jugular was too damaged to be used.

long saphenous vein or an alloplastic material such as polytetrafluoroethylene (PTFE). The latter may save ischaemic time if the artery is temporarily clamped during repair but has an increased risk of infection.

Damage to a vertebral artery that is actively bleeding in an austere environment without access to endovascular angiographic embolisation requires surgical exploration. The proximal portion of the vertebral artery enters the spinal transverse process at the level of C6. It is usually impossible to get access distal to that point. The most practical method is to ligate the vertebral artery at its origin on the second part of the subclavian and then occlude the vertebral foramen with bone wax.

STEP-BY-STEP PROCEDURE 3: ACCESS TO THE COMMON CAROTID ARTERY IN NECK ZONE II

- Mark an 8–10-cm skin incision along the anterior border of the SCM.
- Dissect through skin and platysma to identify the SCM.
- SCM should be retracted posteriorly to identify the carotid sheath below, containing the common carotid artery, internal jugular vein (IJV), and vagus nerve.

- The IJV is generally superficial to the artery and should be retracted to one side, or clamped, if time is critical.
- The key is to obtain proximal and distal control of the bleeding vessel prior to dissecting the area of damage.
- The proximal end of the artery should be clamped, and the area of damage inspected.
- Small holes can be repaired, but larger holes require a patch or graft.
- Utilise the IJV if required or, if potentially damaged, harvest a saphenous vein or superficial femoral vein graft.
- If harvesting a graft, consider a stent to ensure temporary perfusion is maintained.

SURGICAL TREATMENT OF LARYNGOTRACHEAL INJURIES

Patients presenting with such injuries can be approached using either an anterior SCM or collar incision, although the latter provides greater access. Most laryngeal defects from penetrating trauma can be repaired primarily. Although repair is often performed with sutures, small titanium plates used for midface maxillofacial fractures are often better. Small defects noted on endoscopy can be managed non-operatively. If the cartilaginous framework has been disrupted beyond management with a primary repair, delayed repair is recommended, and an endotracheal tube kept in situ. The role of tracheostomy in these patients remains controversial, with some authors recommending one is placed distal to large repair. If performed, surgical tracheostomy should be avoided in the area of injury. The use of temporary stents is, again, controversial and is not recommended in austere setting.

SURGICAL TREATMENT OF OESOPHAGEAL INJURIES

Surgical repair of oesophageal injuries in austere setting is not recommended if evacuation to a higher level of care is possible. Unless grossly disrupted, a nasogastric tube can be passed under endoscopic guidance to enable feeding. Should repair of a cervical oesophageal injury be performed, it is best approached through an anterior SCM incision. Should there be an associated laryngotracheal injury, however, these combination injuries are best approached through a collar incision. Maximal exposure of the oesophagus is achieved through retraction of the trachea, the thyroid medially and the carotid sheath laterally. An indwelling nasogastric tube can facilitate not only the localisation of the oesophagus, but also the identification of the oesophageal injury through the instillation of air or methylene blue. Primary repair is nearly always possible through either a single- or two-layered approach. The main complication from such injuries is the risks of tracheo-oesophageal fistula, although most of such fistulas will heal without surgical intervention. Their risk of occurrence can be minimised by using a tissue flap such as dividing the clavicular head of the SCM muscle and mobilising it to separate the trachea and oesophagus. All patients should remain fed by nasogastric tube only until a contrast swallow performed at 5–7 days postoperatively has excluded a leak.

SOFT TISSUE FACIAL TRAUMA

Early and aggressive debridement of high-energy facial wounds from ballistic trauma is required to prevent infection and tattooing of the skin. This is best undertaken with a surgical scrubbing brush with an antiseptic solution. Most facial wounds can be closed within 36 hours after injury, and delayed closure is rarely necessary. Closed tissues must be tension free, and if distortion of the tissues is seen, sutures should be started again. Although local flaps can be used in the early setting, these are rarely required, and any residual defects should be packed with an impregnated dressing. Removal of most explosive fragments is actually futile, surprisingly difficult in reality, and of no proven clinical benefit. If severed branches of the facial nerve or a damaged parotid duct are encountered, they should be tagged with a non-absorbable suture for later anastomosis, unless a clinician with those skills are present. There is added importance in achieving multiple-layer primary closure in the face, as any leakage of saliva around a wound will slow healing.

IMAGING OF FACIAL FRACTURES

Plain radiographs, with some limitations, can be used to diagnose most mandible (lateral obliques and posteroanterior films) and midface fractures (occipito-mental films). These are usually supplemented by tomographic radiographs in civilian environment but are unlikely to be available in austere setting. Therefore, if possible, management should be delayed following CT imaging and subsequent three-dimensional bone reconstructions, especially if comminution or high-energy transfer has occurred. Missing teeth should be meticulously accounted for as they represent an airway hazard.

STABILISATION OF FACIAL FRACTURES WITH MAXILLARY–MANDIBULAR FIXATION

DCS of facial fractures comprises temporary reduction and immobilisation of mobile mandible and maxilla fractures; this can be highly effective in reducing both bleeding and pain (Figure 15.7). Ballistic facial fractures are often comminuted and open to both the cutaneous and mucosal surfaces.

Mobile fractures are most effectively stabilised using upper and lower Erich arch bars (Figure 15.8). However, such they are time-consuming to place (an

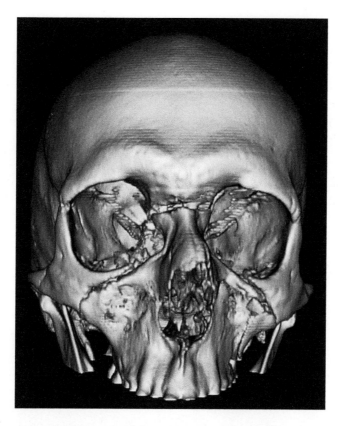

Figure 15.7 A LeFort 2 midface fracture visualised with computed tomography including three-dimensional reconstruction. The whole midface was mobile but was temporarily stabilised using IMF screws and elastic bands.

hour of operating time), require experience to perform correctly, and run the risk of a sharps injury as they require stainless steel wires. Intermaxillary fixation (IMF) screws are rapid but, again, require practice and there is a risk of damaging tooth roots if performed incorrectly (Figure 15.9; Jones, 1999). Once placed, either method should use tight elastic bands to hold the mandibular teeth to the maxillary teeth so they can be cut with scissors should vomiting occur (see Step-by-Step Procedure 4).

STEP-BY-STEP PROCEDURE 4: MAXILLARY–MANDIBULAR STABILISATION WITH IMF SCREWS

- Inject local anaesthesia into the vestibule in all four quadrants: this makes fracture manipulation and insertion of screws more comfortable.

- Identify the optimal entry position of the screws: most commonly, this is between the roots of the first and second premolar teeth in each quadrant.
- Load an 8-mm IMF screw into the specially designed screwdriver: it is extremely hard to do this with a conventional screwdriver used for plating.
- Start to insert the screw – there should be initial resistance as it threads through cortical bone but should become easier as soon as cancellous bone is encountered.
- Careful tactile feedback is essential to ensure that the screw does not go into a tooth root: this is felt with increased resistance, and the screw should be withdrawn completely and reinserted from the beginning.
- The screw should not be torqued, or it may snap: should this occur, it is best to leave it for attempted removal by a specialist later.

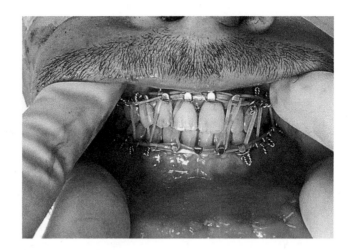

Figure 15.8 Upper and lower Erich arch bars placed for closed reduction with elastic intermaxillary fixation of a comminuted right angle of mandible fracture.

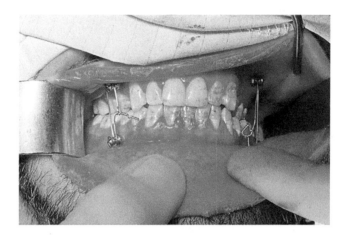

Figure 15.9 IMF screws with wires being used to provide temporary stabilisation for a left mandible fracture.

- Attempt to reduce the fracture and ensure maximum interdigitation of teeth.
- At this point, place elastic bands tightly between the screws, modifying the alignment of bands to ensure the position of the jaws.
- Ensure that the tongue is not caught between the teeth.
- Additional screws with elastic bands between them can be placed on either side of the fracture line but this is generally recommended only for displaced fractures.

- The bands should produce good reduction of the fracture

INTERNAL FIXATION OF FACIAL FRACTURES

No evidence exists that most facial fractures result in greater morbidity if they are not fixed early. On the contrary, military evidence gained from Iraq and Afghanistan has reiterated lessons from earlier conflicts that inappropriate use of internal fixation reduces vascularity and predisposes towards infection. Internal fixation should only be considered in the first 48 hours in non-comminuted clean fractures representative of those seen in civilian practice and should be performed by a clinician used to managing such injuries. If in doubt, temporary stabilisation with MMF as described in the previous section is recommended.

EXTERNAL FIXATION OF FACIAL FRACTURES

Although an external fixator can provide temporary anatomical reduction and fragment stability, their use is challenging to those unfamiliar to treating facial fractures and, again, is not recommended (Figure 15.10). Clinicians should attempt to learn their use if possible, particularly when there is a delay in evacuation of casualties to higher echelons of care. Unlike IMF, there is no compromise to the airway, and no special precautions for the release of fixation are required during patient evacuation as they are attached to the mandible or midface alone.

Any soft tissue or bony defects may continue to be debrided with the fixation device in situ. As the mouth can be opened during fracture healing, oral hygiene and patient nutrition are improved, and trismus due to fibrosis and scarring is reduced.

TEN KEY POINTS

1. Penetrating neck Injury can be a source of exsanguinating haemorrhage, but facial bleeding of that magnitude is rare.
2. Airway compromise can occur both from direct injury to the larynx or trenches or from bleeding into them.
3. Standard intubation should be performed if possible, but should there be any doubt or difficulty, surgical cricothyroidotomy is recommended.
4. There is no rule for either surgical or percutaneous tracheostomy in acute setting.
5. Haemorrhage from the mouth and nose should be arrested by packing, in conjunction with nasal epistats, optimally following intubation.
6. Neck haemorrhage should be packed with pressure applied to haemostatic dressings but may require damage control surgery.
7. Surgical options for cervical vascular damage include repair, which in turn may require temporary shunting and ligation.
8. Aero-digestive injury is best identified by direct endoscopy in conjunction with CT, if available.
9. Facial fractures may be stabilised for airway and pain control through simple techniques, but these require practice to be performed correctly.
10. Facial fractures should not be fixed until clinicians with the appropriate equipment and level of training are available.

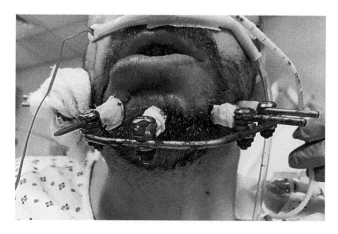

Figure 15.10 An external fixator is used to treat a comminuted mandible fracture; the patient was evacuated by aeroplane awake.

FURTHER READING

Conradie, Wilhelmus Jacobus, and Fekade Admassu Gebremariam. "Can Computed Tomography Esophagography Reliably Diagnose Traumatic Penetrating Upper Digestive Tract Injuries?" *Clinical Imaging*, **36(6)**, Elsevier Inc., Nov. 2015, pp. 1039–1045, doi:10.1016/j.clinimag.2015.07.021.

Jones D. "The Intermaxillary Screw: A Dedicated Bicortical Bone Screw for Temporary Intermaxillary Fixation." *British Journal of Oral and Maxillofacial Surgery*, 1999;**37(3)**:pp. 115–116, doi:http://dx.doi.org/10.1054/bjom.2001.0771.

Kazi, Maliha, et al. "Utility of Clinical Examination and CT Scan in Assessment of Penetrating Neck Trauma." *Journal of the College of Physicians and Surgeons Pakistan*, 2013;**23(4)**

Múnera, Felipe, et al. "Diagnosis of Arterial Injuries Caused by Penetrating Trauma to the Neck: Comparison of Helical CT Angiography and Conventional Angiography 1." *Radiology*, 2000;**216(2)**:pp. 356–362.

Teixeira, Frederico, et al. "Safety in Selective Surgical Exploration in Penetrating Neck Trauma." *World Journal of Emergency Surgery*, **11(1)**, BioMed Central Ltd., July 2016, doi:10.1186/s13017-016-0091-4.

Management of Ophthalmic Injuries by the Forward Surgical Team

16

Richard J. Blanch, Johno Breeze, and William G. Gensheimer

INTRODUCTION

Ocular trauma is a common civilian injury, affecting up to 20% of the population at some point in their life. Ocular trauma also affects military patients, frequently dependent on the use of combat eye protection, at 10–15% of combat-related injuries during Operation Enduring Freedom (OEF) and Operation Iraqi Freedom (OIF).

NATO joint medical doctrine is to undertake damage control surgery not involving the eye within two hours of wounding (Allied Joint Doctrine). Although time to specialist treatment of ocular injuries has not been defined, multi-disciplinary consensus states that this should be done within 24 hours. In a theatre of conflict, this level of medical support requires both the deployment of ophthalmologists and overall air superiority. Future conflicts are likely to have delays in evacuation and are likely to require local, Role 2 or 3, management for up to five days post-injury.

Prolonged Field Care (PFC) is described within US doctrine as 'field medical care, applied beyond doctrinal planning timelines', and culminates in evacuation to a higher-level medical treatment facility (MTFs). For trauma, PFC may be thought of as an extension or follow-on treatment to Tactical Combat Casualty Care (TCCC), when evacuation is delayed, and providers are forced to address the patient's needs beyond the initial resuscitation and preparation for transport. The principles of PFC are to reduce morbidity and should include only the most serious and critical casualties. Although analogous in concept, the UK utilises the NATO doctrinal term 'prolonged hospital care' instead of PFC to describe 'in-theatre surgery' that is required when evacuation timelines are protracted, termed 'in-theatre surgery' in NATO doctrine and 'prolonged field care' in US joint doctrine.

The aim of this chapter is to support the development of the following knowledge, skills, and abilities in practitioners who may be required to conduct initial as well as prolonged field or hospital care of eye injuries:

1. Recognise that ocular pathology is present.
2. Assess whether that pathology requires time-critical management.

3. Understand how to safely temporise and package serious ocular pathology.
4. Understand some of the issues around prolonged care of eye injuries, including the effect of delay and the risk of endophthalmitis and sympathetic ophthalmia.

RECOGNISE THAT OCULAR PATHOLOGY IS PRESENT

Diagnosing eye injury or other pathology requires an understanding of it, a thorough history, and examination and pattern recognition. The key pathology to recognise after ocular trauma are chemical injury, open globe injury, orbital compartment syndrome, hyphaemia and retinal detachment or dialysis.

History

If the patient can give a history of the key features to pick out are as follows:

- Awareness of an eye injury.
- Maintain a high index of suspicion based on the mechanism of injury.
- Altered or reduced visual acuity and its extent and constancy. Blurry vision that clears with blinking suggests a tear film problem, intermittent or sudden total loss of vision in one eye may be

caused by carotid dissection, and transient visual loss of any severity (but rarely exceeding 30 seconds) may be associated with elevated intracranial pressure and papilledema, when transient visual loss may be unilateral or bilateral.
- Visual field defect, if this was preceded by flashing lights or floaters in one eye, may be associated with retinal detachment.
- Eye pain. Foreign body sensation localises to the cornea, photophobia usually localises to the front half of the eye.
- Double vision presents with one eye open suggests an opacity in the optical media; with both eyes open it suggests neurological or bony damage causing misalignment of the eyes.
- Symptom onset and duration, particularly in respect of the injury.
- Substance applied if chemical injury.

Examination

The critical feature of an eye examination is an assessment of function, which includes best-corrected visual acuity (BCVA) and testing of pupils with the swinging flashlight test.

INSPECT THE EYES

Open globe injuries may cause obvious distortion in eye shape (Figure 16.1).

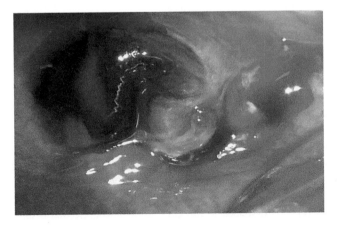

Figure 16.1 A severe open globe injury with loss of volume and distortion of shape, suggesting extrusion of ocular contents.

Open globe injuries may also be hidden by sub-conjunctival haemorrhage (Figure 16.2a,b).

Prolapsed ocular contents also indicate an open globe injury (Figure 16.3).

The presence of total hyphaemia (space behind the cornea completely obscured by blood), or an eye that looks soft and easily deformed, should also raise suspicion of open globe injury (Figure 16.4).

Closed Globe Injury

Once open globe injury has been excluded, the main closed globe injury to recognise on inspection is hyphaemia (Figure 16.5). The height of the blood level from the bottom of the cornea should be measured in millimetres and estimated in terms of the proportion of the anterior chamber (the space between the cornea and the iris) as <⅓, ⅓–½, >½ but less than complete or completely full of blood.

Orbital Compartment Syndrome

Orbital compartment syndrome is a diagnosis made after assessment, but suspicion should be raised if the lids are severely bruised and/or swollen and difficult to open.

VISUAL ACUITY IS TESTED AS FOLLOWS

- Preservative-free topical anaesthetic may aid testing if the patient is in pain.

(a)

(b)

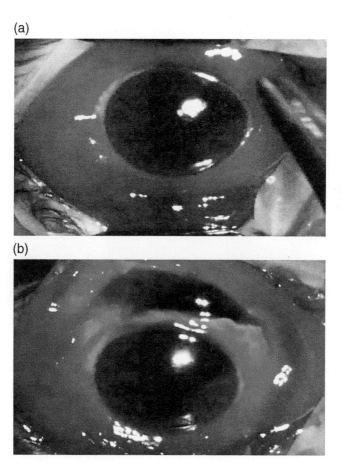

Figure 16.2 (a) Extensive subconjunctival haemorrhage obscuring a superior rupture. Note that the pupil is dragged superiorly into the rupture. (b) When the conjunctiva and Tenon's capsule are dissected off, the rupture is obvious.

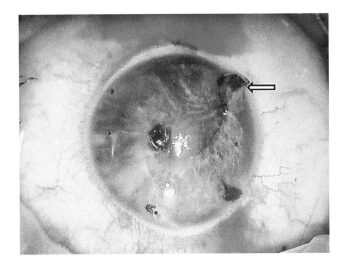

Figure 16.3 The iris is prolapsed out of the eye superonasal (arrow) indicating penetration of the cornea by a foreign body that has traversed the lens and lodged in the vitreous. The pupil is also dragged towards the penetration. Large metallic foreign bodies are also deeply embedded in the cornea centrally and inferonasal.

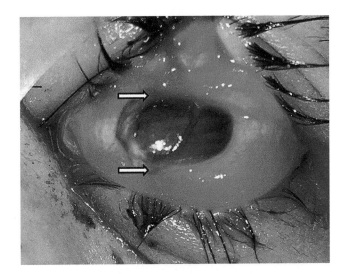

Figure 16.4 There is diffuse conjunctival swelling (chemosis); no iris details are visible because the anterior chamber is full of blood (hyphaemia) and the eye looks soft and mildly deformed. A circumferential limbal rupture is present nasally between the two arrows but also extends posteriorly through the medial rectus insertion.

- Always test with the patient's own refractive correction if available (and near correction where relevant).
- Always occlude the other eye to prevent visual clues from the other eye, but do NOT put pressure on eye with suspected open globe injury.

- If a chart is available and the patient can cooperate, place the patient at the chart's designated testing distance. This is 6 m for most Snellen charts, but if the patient cannot read the top of the chart, it should be moved closer.

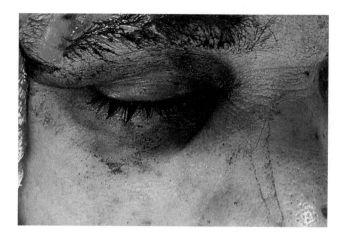

Figure 16.5 Orbital compartment syndrome – note the bruising and swelling of eyelids.

- Improvised letters can give a rough idea: a standard uniform name stripe at 3 ft is roughly equivalent to 6/60, whilst standard newspaper print is font size eight at 40 cm is roughly equivalent to 6/15.
- If the patient is unable to see letters, test as follows:

  o Count fingers: ask the patient to count the number of fingers on one hand and record the greatest distance at which counting fingers is done accurately.
  o Hand motion: Is the patient able to detect a hand waving in front of the eye?
  o Light perception: Use the brightest light available and shine in the eye. Record the patient's response as light perception (LP) can detect the light. Ensure the other eye is thoroughly occluded, for example, with double folded tissues and the palm of your hand.
  o Record the patient's response as no light perception (NLP) if unable to detect the light. Record the light source used for testing (e.g., penlight or flashlight).

- Record the acuity measurement as a notation (example 6/6) in which the numerator represents the testing distance and the denominator represents the numeric designation for the smallest line read.
- Test both eyes.

PUPILS ARE TESTED AS FOLLOWS

- Ask the patient to fixate on a distant target to prevent accommodation and pupil constriction.
- Examine the size of both pupils in bright and dim conditions. They should be the same size. Pupil size differences may indicate ocular trauma (with iris sphincter damage); neurological damage (third nerve palsy is a false localising of elevated intracranial pressure and is accompanied by ptosis and eye movement abnormalities) or prior unilateral application of a mydriatic agent.
- Lower the ambient lighting as much as possible and use the brightest light source available to test pupil reflexes.
- Shine the light on each eye. Both pupils should react to light and there should be a symmetric consensual response in the other eye.
- Perform the swinging flashlight test by shining the light onto the first pupil for 2 seconds, and then moving to the other pupil, taking less than one second to swing across. The light is then moved back to the first pupil after 2 seconds. This is repeated several times and the pupil reactions observed, which should be equal. If either pupil appears to dilate when the light is shone on it, that indicates either very poor retinal function or reduced optic nerve function compared to the other side (a relative afferent pupillary defect, RAPD).
- If one pupil is immobile when testing direct and consensual reflexes, the swinging flashlight test

should still be performed. Because direct and consensual pupil reactions are symmetrical, the swinging flashlight test may be performed whilst examining the pupil size of only the eye with the mobile pupil but still swinging the light between both eyes.

ASSESS WHETHER THE PATHOLOGY REQUIRES TIME-CRITICAL MANAGEMENT

The time-critical eye injuries are orbital compartment syndrome, open globe injury, closed globe injury with hyphaemia, retinal detachment and dialysis, and closed globe injuries after refractive surgery.

Chemical Injury

Ocular chemical injury is an emergency requiring immediate action and may be caused by contact with either acid, such as sulphuric acid (e.g., battery acid), or alkali such as calcium hydroxide, (e.g., in cement or other caustic compounds such as volatile organic compounds). Begin irrigation of the eye immediately if there is a chemical injury. pH can be tested immediately and rapidly (using pH strips) and topical anaesthetic applied if they are available before irrigation, but treatment should not be delayed for any reason. Remove any visible foreign bodies from the eye and irrigate and sweep the conjunctival fornices. Alkaline injuries are often the most severe because alkali saponifies corneal cell membranes and increases its corneal penetration, with pH change detectable in the aqueous humour of rabbits one minute after alkaline injury, indicating severe damage has occurred [9].

Orbital Compartment Syndrome

Orbital haematomas are usually mild, diagnosed on CT, and should be managed conservatively. However, if the orbit is very tense, especially if associated with limitation of eye movements or reduced vision, this indicates an orbital compartment syndrome – which requires emergency management. A CT scan is not appropriate

until after initial decompression, as it causes delay to appropriate management.

A haematoma in the orbit or (often) in the subperiosteal space may increase intraorbital pressure sufficiently to impair blood supply to the eye and optic nerve. This may or may not be associated with orbital fractures.

Orbital tension is assessed by gently palpating over the swelling through the upper lid ONLY AFTER ensuring that an open globe injury is not present by direct inspection of the globe. It may be necessary to use a speculum to retract the eyelids after the application of preservative-free topical anaesthetic. It is important to never press on a penetrated eye as the pressure rise may cause the intraocular contents to extrude. If the globe is closed and the orbit feels tense, this should cause suspicion for an orbital compartment syndrome.

The features of orbital compartment syndrome are:

- Pain and often nausea
- Proptosis (eyeball moved forwards out of the orbit and into the eyelids)
- Tense orbit and tight eyelids over the globe
- Reduced or absent eye movements
- Reduced visual acuity
- RAPD

Management of an orbital compartment syndrome is time-critical, and decompression should be undertaken immediately as permanent visual loss occurs within 2–4 hours.

Open Globe Injury

Open globe injuries are classified using the Birmingham Eye Trauma Terminology system into penetrating injuries, where a sharp object has entered the eye; intraocular foreign bodies when the object remains in the eye; perforating injuries when the object has traversed the eye (entry and exit wound); and ruptures when blunt trauma has caused the eye to burst. Perforating and rupture injuries are the most severe and, in the context of military injuries, have extremely poor prognosis.

Open globe injuries have a substantial risk of devastating intraocular infection that increases with delays to primary repair (surgical closure of the eye). In addition, final visual acuity declines with delays to primary repair even in the absence of infection. The recommended time window for closure of an open globe injury is 12–24 hours. Visual acuity, the presence of a RAPD, or infection and injury type all have prognostic value.

Hyphaemia

When a closed globe injury has blood in the anterior chamber, there is a risk of elevated intraocular pressure, which increases with the size of the hyphaemia from 13.5% when less than half the anterior chamber is full of blood, to more than 50% when the whole anterior chamber is full of red cells. High intraocular pressure (>40 mmHg) is an ophthalmic emergency, as it can compromise blood supply to the retina and requires urgent treatment. For this reason, ophthalmic assessment should be arranged within 24 hours of injury. Treatment is usually medical with systemic and topical ocular anti-hypertensives, but up to 5% of patients with hyphaemia require surgery to wash out the blood. The other complication of hyphaemia is rebleeding (increase in size or recurrence of hyphaemia), which also increases the risk of increased pressure and is also more common when assessment by ophthalmology occurs more than 24 hours after injury.

In the context of closed globe injury, visual acuity has prognostic value and may indicate other injuries that is not visible without specialist ophthalmic examination such as retinal injury. If the patient has sickle cell trait, this increases the risk of raised pressure and complicates management.

Retinal Detachment and Dialysis

Retinal detachments occur when a break in the retina allows fluid to pass from the vitreous cavity into the subretinal space. These breaks often occur when the vitreous detaches from the retina and causes tears at points of residual attachment (posterior vitreous detachment, PVD). PVD may occur spontaneously with ageing, is more common in people who are short-sighted and may also be precipitated by an eye injury. Patients with PVD will usually complain of flashing lights, as the vitreous pulls off the retina, and floaters by clumps of degenerate vitreous or blood. Once retinal detachment develops (usually

weeks after the closed globe injury), the patient will be aware of a peripheral shadow in their vision that will gradually progress to affect the central vision.

A retinal dialysis occurs most commonly after trauma when the retina detaches at its anterior base, and PVD may not occur. The patient will still have a shadow that starts peripherally (often superonasal) and progresses to involve the central vision over several days.

When the central vision is not involved (and visual acuity is normal), retinal detachments and dialyses are emergencies, requiring repair before the central vision becomes involved. These are termed macula on retinal detachments (because the macula has not yet detached). The usual timeframe within which macula on detachments should be repaired is 24 hours. Once the macula has detached and central vision is reduced, the repair is less urgent and is usually scheduled within 1–2 weeks.

The other type of retinal detachment that occurs after trauma is tractional retinal detachment, which affects around 50% of military eye injuries after repair. For this reason, open globe injuries should have access to subspecialist vitreoretinal surgery, which is a Role 4 capability, within 2 weeks of repair.

Closed Globe Injuries After Refractive Surgery

Corneal injury after refractive surgery can rarely dislocate the surgical flap after laser-assisted in situ keratomileusis (LASIK) surgery and remains to be a small long-term risk afterwards. A dislocated flap should not be confused with a contact lens or a foreign body.

A corneal abrasion within one year of any type of refractive surgery may cause corneal scarring, and therefore, early ophthalmology consultation should be sought if there is a concern about eye injury in a patient with a history of refractive surgery.

UNDERSTAND HOW TO SAFELY TEMPORISE AND PACKAGE SERIOUS OCULAR PATHOLOGY

All the time-critical eye injuries discussed earlier require specialist ophthalmic assessment and management.

Chemical Injury

The ocular chemical injury requires immediate irrigation.

Irrigation is aided by the application of topical anaesthetic, the use of a Morgan lens and a speculum, and is ideally conducted using sterile balanced buffered solution but should not be delayed for any reason. If tap water is the only fluid available, then it should be used until better equipment becomes available. During irrigation, the ocular surface should be inspected – including the upper and lower fornices under the eyelids – and any debris removed with a cotton-tipped applicator or forceps.

After 2-L irrigation, the pH should be reassessed. If the pH is still abnormal, then this cycle is repeated until pH is normal. If the other eye is uninjured, pH may be compared between the two eyes. Once pH is normal, irrigation may stop, but pH must be rechecked 20–30 minutes later to ensure that it remains normal.

After irrigation, ocular chemical injuries should be thoroughly assessed, including visual acuity, and then given antibiotic ointment (after testing visual acuity, as ointment will reduce visual acuity). The patient should be evacuated for ophthalmology assessment within 24 hours, as further medical and surgical treatment may be required. Severity may be gauged by a reduction in visual acuity and eye appearance. The loss of normal blood vessel pattern on the white of the eye and around the limbus and corneal haziness obscuring iris and pupil details indicates severe injury.

Orbital compartment syndrome

Orbital compartment syndrome should be managed as follows:

- Perform immediate lateral canthotomy and cantholysis (Figure 16.6).
- Evacuate urgently for ophthalmology assessment and possible secondary procedures (including medical management and orbital decompression).
- If performed competently, this is a low-morbidity procedure, and the lateral canthus heals well by secondary intent, with no need for surgical repair. When doubt exists as to whether an orbital compartment syndrome is present, it is, therefore, preferable to perform an unnecessary canthotomy/cantholysis than fail to perform a necessary one.

- Do NOT perform only a lateral canthotomy. This is an ineffective procedure.
- Assess the globe again, as this will be improved once the lateral canthotomy/cantholysis has been performed.

Open Globe Injuries

Open globe injuries should be managed as follows:

- Administer systemic fluoroquinolone antibiotics such as ciprofloxacin 750 mg or moxifloxacin 400 mg orally to reduce the risk of devastating intraocular infection.
- Administer anti-emetics, as these injuries often cause nausea, and vomiting causes extrusion of intraocular contents.
- Administer adequate systemic analgesia because eye pain causes patients to squeeze their eyes, which extrudes ocular contents.
- Avoid topical medications because many contain preservatives which are toxic to ocular contents.
- Apply a hard shield with stand off from the eye and secure with tape or a bandage. Do NOT apply a pad, as pads press on the eye and extrude ocular contents.
- Seek early teleophthalmology consultation.
- Evacuate to allow repair within 12–24 hours of injury. Open globe injuries are not generally a contra-indication to aeromedical evacuation or an indication for ground-level cabin pressure.

Closed Globe Injuries

Closed globe injuries with hyphaemia should be managed as follows:

- Apply preservative-free atropine (or preserved if preservative-free is not available).
- Seek early teleophthalmology consultation.
- Evacuate to allow ophthalmology assessment within 24 hours of injury.

Retinal Detachments

Retinal detachments (without other globe injuries) should be evacuated to allow repair within 24 hours if macula not involved (i.e. with good visual acuity).

(a)

(b)

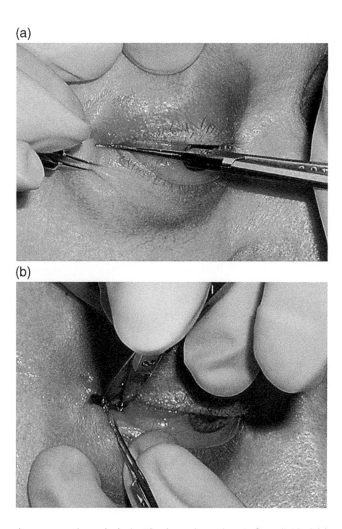

Figure 16.6 Lateral canthotomy and cantholysis. The lateral canthus is first divided (a) and then the lateral canthal tendon cut (b) to detach the lower lid from the lateral orbital margin and allow forward movement (proptosis) of the globe to decompress the orbit. If inferior cantholysis is insufficient, superior cantholysis may also be performed. The lateral canthotomy wound does not require repair and heals well by secondary intent.

If visual acuity is poor, evacuation should occur within one week. Progression may be slowed by applying double eye pads gently to both eyes so that they are unable to see light and dark. In theory, this reduces eye movements and, therefore, reduces vitreous traction on the retina and may allow a detachment to settle.

Closed Globe Injuries After Refractive Surgery

Refractive surgery procedures such as LASIK and photorefractive keratectomy (PRK) have been shown to be safe and effective. Post-operative complications including traumatic LASIK flap dislocations are rare. Never attempt to repair an eye after trauma or remove a LASIK flap. Traumatic corneal abrasions occurring after PRK can lead to corneal haze and loss of uncorrected and corrected visual acuity. In addition to topical antibiotics, an ophthalmologist may recommend topical steroid drops, oral vitamin C, and ultraviolet (UV) light protection, using sunglasses to prevent the development of corneal stromal haze.

UNDERSTAND SOME OF THE ISSUES AROUND PROLONGED CARE OF EYE INJURIES, INCLUDING THE EFFECT OF DELAY AND THE RISK OF SYMPATHETIC OPHTHALMIA

In British operations in Iraq and Afghanistan, the average time to specialist ophthalmic assessment was 1.5–2.6 days, which represents a massive achievement in terms of speed of aeromedical evacuation [14]. The standard of care in Western medical practice is access to specialist assessment to allow primary repair within 24 hours of injury but there is some evidence that this should be shortened to 12 hours to reduce the risk of devastating intraocular infection [10]. The outcomes of British eye injuries in British soldiers in the two published case series from these conflicts was comparable to other reports of military injuries, despite being higher in civilian times to repair, although there was some evidence that increasing time to repair was associated with worse visual outcomes. In civilian series, delayed repair beyond 12–24 hours worsen final visual acuity by approximately one Snellen line per 24 hours and increases the risk of endophthalmitis and post-operative wound leak.

It is therefore clear that primary repair within 12–24 hours is the most desirable treatment. It is also clear, though, that delays to primary repair do not prevent good outcomes, although they may make them less likely on average. Indeed, one series reported primary repairs as long as 1 month after injury, with some good outcomes.

Aside from the detrimental effect on visual outcome in the eye affected, the main risk of very delayed, absent, or incompetent repair is sympathetic ophthalmia. Sympathetic ophthalmia is an autoimmune granulomatous inflammatory disorder that occurs after open globe injury or intraocular surgery and affects the uninjured (as well as the injured or operated) eye. The risk of sympathetic ophthalmia after intraocular surgery is low, at between 1/1,000 and 1/10,000, but is higher after open globe injury. In a large series of 1,392 patients with open globe injury, 1,283 underwent primary repair (889 patients), evisceration (491 patients), or enucleation (3 patients) of whom none developed sympathetic ophthalmia. 109 patients did not have primary surgical management, and of these patients, two developed sympathetic ophthalmia (1.83%), suggesting that this risk is low except when primary repair or eye removal is not performed.

Need 10 Key points:

FURTHER READING

1. Wong TY, BE Klein, and R Klein, *The prevalence and 5-year incidence of ocular trauma. The Beaver Dam Eye Study. Ophthalmology*, 2000;**107(12)**:p. 2196–2202.
2. Blanch RJ and RA Scott, *Military ocular injury: presentation, assessment and management. J R Army Med Corps*, 2009;**155(4)**:p. 279–284.
3. Breeze J, et al., *Skill sets required for the management of military head, face and neck trauma: a multidisciplinary consensus statement. J R Army Med Corps*, 2018;**164(2)**:p. 133–138.
4. Breeze J, et al., *Comparing the management of eye injuries by deployed US and UK military surgeons during the Iraq and Afghanistan conflicts. Ophthalmology*, April 2020;**127(4)**:p. 458–466.
5. Soliz BA, *Saving lives in prolonged care scenarios at role 1 requires changes in leadership, force structure, and training. US Army War College, Carlisle, PA*, 2018.
6. Keenan S, *Deconstructing the definition of prolonged field care. J Spec Oper Med*, 2015;**15(4)**:p. 125.
7. DeSoucy E, et al., *Review of 54 cases of prolonged field care. J Spec Oper Med*, 2017;**17(1)**:p. 121–129.
8. Allied Joint Doctrine for Medical Support. *Ministry of Defence*, 2015, p. 1–280.
9. Gerard M, et al., *Experimental study about intra-ocular penetration of ammonia. J Fr Ophtalmol*, 1999;**22(10)**: p. 1047–1053.
10. Essex RW, et al., *Post-traumatic endophthalmitis. Ophthalmology*, 2004;**111(11)**:p. 2015–2022.
11. Blanch RJ, et al., *Effect of time to primary repair on final visual outcome after open globe injury. Br J Ophthalmol*, 2019.
12. Coles WH, *Traumatic hyphema: an analysis of 235 cases. South Med J*, 1968;**61(8)**:p. 813–816.
13. Fong LP, *Secondary hemorrhage in traumatic hyphema. Predictive factors for selective prophylaxis. Ophthalmology*, 1994;**101(9)**:p. 1583–1588.
14. Blanch RJ, et al., *Ophthalmic injuries in British armed forces in Iraq and Afghanistan. Eye (Lond)*, 2011;**25(2)**:p. 218–223.
15. Cruvinel Isaac DL, et al., *Prognostic factors in open globe injuries. Ophthalmologica*, 2003;**217(6)**:p. 431–435.

16. Kong GY, et al., *Wound-related complications and clinical outcomes following open globe injury repair.* Clin Exp Ophthalmol, 2015;**43(6)**:p. 508–513.

17. Lesniak SPLiX, Bauza A, Soni N, Zarbin MA, Langer P, Bhagat N, *Characteristics and outcomes of delayed open globe repair.* Mathews J Ophthalmol 2017;**2(1)**:p. 1.

18. Kilmartin DJ, AD Dick, and JV Forrester, *Prospective surveillance of sympathetic ophthalmia in the UK and Republic of Ireland.* Brit J Ophthalmol, 2000;**84(3)**:p. 259–263.

19. du Toit N, et al., *The risk of sympathetic ophthalmia following evisceration for penetrating eye injuries at Groote Schuur Hospital.* Br J Ophthalmol, 2008;**92(1)**:p. 61–63.

Resource-Limited Environment Plastic Surgery

17

Johann A. Jeevaratnam, Charles Anton Fries,
Dimitrios Kanakopoulos, Paul J. H. Drake,
and Lorraine Harry

INTRODUCTION

Soft tissue injury due to high or low energy trauma may occur in isolation but is more often associated with concomitant injury to bone and neurovascular structures. Altered soft tissue integrity increases the chances of infection, impairment of function and immobility, and a potential loss of limb or life. The appreciation of the mechanism of injury is paramount to understand how each tissue type is susceptible and enables a full understanding of the 'zone of injury'. This is the concept whereby tissue surrounding the direct or indirect damage is disrupted in variable severity, with potential for irreversible or reversible impairment. This relates to the extent of microvascular compromise and is compounded by wound contamination such as soil and vegetation. Understanding the zone of injury, each individual tissue's response to trauma, and how it can change with time enables appropriate decision making for optimal treatment. This involves adequate debridement (excision of necrotic tissue and removal of contaminants and foreign bodies), assessment of the resulting defect, and reconstruction using well-established, robust plastic surgical techniques.

Tissue Response to Injury

Each tissue is variably susceptible to the mechanism of injury. Skin, the largest organ of the body, is particularly vulnerable to sheer and torsional forces, which disrupt the delicate network of vascular plexi that supply it from the underlying tissue planes. Large areas of skin can effectively be 'degloved' or lifted off the fascial and subfascial vasculature, struggling to survive. However, this may not be evident immediately and can take several days to evolve and declare itself as non-viable. The underlying fat is far more at risk from trauma compared to its durable cover. Fat is easily injured, often beyond the zone of skin injury. Necrosis quickly ensues once blood supply is interrupted, with the potential to form discrete nodules which undergo liquefactive necrosis. Muscle tissue can be bruised, sprained by stretch, or lacerated, with variable degrees of injury severity. It is extremely sensitive to direct trauma, where tearing and subsequent necrosis of the myofibrils creates space for haematoma formation and proliferation of inflammatory cells, as part of the repair process. Finally, nerve injury is well described and can be classified from mild bruising (neuropraxia) to complete disruption of the fascicles (neurotmesis), corresponding to cell death and loss of ability to transmit sensory or motor impulses.

Once resuscitative surgery has been undertaken and physiological restoration achieved, the principles of the management of traumatic wounds are those of wound excision, followed by delayed reconstruction. It is axiomatic that debridement of devitalised tissues is meticulous and comprehensive; however, the placement of fasciotomy, or other wound extending incisions, must be with respect to future reconstructive efforts. For example, the relative positions of neurovascular structures, joints, and skin perforating vessels must be respected.

The debridement itself must also be tailored to the tissues being excised. Where low volumes of normally well-vascularised tissues that have vital functional significance are encountered, a more expectant approach can be effective. The tissues of the head, neck, and hands have been found to be extremely resistant to infection and necrosis; where there is ambiguity of vitality, it is safe to leave these smaller areas to declare themselves. Clearly, this is not the case for large muscular compartments – if left, they can have life-threatening systemic effects.

Debridement

Extensive damage to the soft tissues must be accurately assessed in the intraoperative environment. An initial wash with soapy chlorhexidine once under anaesthetic enables gross contaminants to be removed, prior to formal prep and drape of the affected body part. Often in the extremities, accurate assessment of the wound is better achieved with use of a pneumatic tourniquet (authors' preference), although there is debate regarding its use. Tourniquet inflation after exsanguination allows clear inspection of the tissue planes, without continuing blood staining as well as haemorrhage control. Proponents of non-tourniquet technique will highlight the lack of ability to assess healthy tissues via bleeding. This, however, can be achieved with deflation.

The term 'debridement' comes from the French word 'débrider', meaning 'to unbridle' or release. A more accurate description of the technique would be excision of the wound, removing all contaminants and dead tissue. This must be performed in a systematic fashion so that all areas of the wound are included. This may be preferentially from superficial to deep, peripheral to central, with anterior and posterior structures included. Often, it is helpful to consider the wound a clockface, and systematically go around to ensure complete assessment and removal of all non-viable tissue. It can be difficult to assess the viability of some tissue where there is some potential functional compromise, if excised. Preservation of the neurovascular structures is vital even in the zone of injury.

It may be possible to perform serial debridement to allow the evolution of junctional areas which may or may not recover. However, it has been demonstrated – particularly in the case of open fractures – that repeated debridement and delay to appropriate vascularised soft tissue cover, increases the risk of infected non- or malunion of bones, and is to be avoided.

Extension Lines

When considering the lower limb, debridement of both soft tissue and bone is required, in the same meticulous stepwise manner. However, the delivery of bone ends required may not be permitted through the breached soft tissue envelope. Therefore, the wound must be extended, in a controlled fashion, using the same incisions as would be required in fasciotomies of the lower limb. This enables the bone ends of the tibia to be delivered and debrided back to bleeding bone. The extension also allows inspection of the posterior compartment muscles in case there are contaminants or bone fragments which would be easily missed. Other benefits of these extension lines include the ability to formally decompress the four compartments of the lower limb and finally preserve the perforating branches of the posterior tibial artery on the medial side for potential local flap coverage of small distal defects of the leg.

Revascularisation of limbs in resource-constrained environments will depend on the expertise of the surgeons deployed and optical systems available to them. However, the named vessels of the forearm and lower limb can reliably be re-anastomosed using loupe magnification only, including the interposition of vein grafts.

Once debridement and revascularisation are complete, the protection of vital structures is considered. Simple mobilisation of muscles or fasciocutaneous flaps may be adequate to achieve temporary coverage of neurovascular structures and tendons, preventing desiccation and loss of function, prior to dressing and transfer, or definitive closure.

Definitive reconstruction in a resource-limited environment must consider not only the suitability of the patient and the medical facility but also local rehabilitation and prosthetic services.

Broadly speaking, simple robust solutions are required. That being said, reliable local muscle or fasciocutaneous flaps can be transposed with basic equipment with minimal monitoring.

FASCIOTOMY OF THE EXTREMITIES

Overview

Compartment syndrome of the extremities is a limb-threatening scenario, which may occur when pressure is raised in any closed osseo-fascial compartment. Causes of increased pressure include bleeding, crush injury, ischaemia-reperfusion injury, electrical burns, injection, posture, and iatrogenic causes. A persistent rise in interstitial pressure within the compartment, above that of tissue perfusion pressure, results in infarction of contents of the compartment. The ischaemic damage is irreversible beyond a certain time, leading to loss of function, systemic effects, and even death from reperfusion injury. This may occur in as little as 1 hour in a shocked polytrauma patient.

Surgeons should, therefore, perform fasciotomies without hesitation.

Resource Limitation Concerns

Following fasciotomy patients will require a return to theatre at 24–48 hours for a 'second look' +/- closure.

Equipment

1. Surgical blade No.15
2. Soft tissue retractors (Weitlaner self-retainer, Senn, Langenbeck)
3. Dissecting scissors (McIndoe, Jameson, Stevens)
4. Electrocautery
5. Sterile drapes and gloves
6. Sterile non-adhesive dressings (Jelonet, Adaptic, Atrauman)
7. Dressing gauze
8. Softband
9. Elastic bandage
10. Optional dressing to replace the preceding: VAC at 80 mmHg

Diagnosis

The diagnosis of compartment syndrome is clinical and based on a high index of suspicion.

Pain is the most reliable symptom and is disproportionate to the underlying injury. It is severe, progressive, unrelieved by analgesia (escalating analgesic requirements is a telling sign), and worse on passive stretch of muscles within the compartment. The limb may feel tense and other signs – such as weakness of muscles within the compartment and altered sensation in the distribution of nerves passing through the compartment – may be noted, though these are often late. Examination of the pulse is not useful, as its absence is an extremely late sign, and its presence does not rule out the diagnosis.

Importantly, one should be aware of occult compartment syndrome in the multiply- or head-injured patient and understand that the presence of open wounds does not exclude the diagnosis.

The measurement of compartment pressures is prone to false-positive and -negative error, and for that reason, is not advocated. If any degree of clinical suspicion exists, the relevant compartments should be decompressed urgently, as the implications of missed compartment syndrome are severe. If not therapeutic, a diagnostic decompression will serve as a prophylactic measure. Indeed, prophylactic fasciotomies should be considered in cases of revascularisation of limbs following prolonged ischaemia, for example.

Key Concepts: Fasciotomy

1. Appropriately anaesthetised patient (avoid nerve block regarding post-operative monitoring) with a high tourniquet to enable safe exposure.
2. Bold is beautiful: incisions should be through both skin and fascia and should be full length; aim to avoid exposing nerves/tendons.
3. Minimise damage to cutaneous nerves and preserve longitudinal veins.
4. Once the fascia is released, ensure that the skin is not acting as a constricting band.
5. Systemically examine the viability of each individual muscle belly in each compartment, and if tight, incise overlying epimysium.

   Viable muscle is pink, contracts when stimulated, and bleeds when cut.

6. Frankly, necrotic muscle should be excised while the tourniquet is inflated.

   It will not bleed or twitch but will look dark or extremely pale and will feel soft.

   If doubt exists, deflate the tourniquet, and reassess muscle viability.

7. Be aware of potential reperfusion injury and inform anaesthetist when tourniquet is due to be released.

8. Do not close primarily but temporise with simple dressings, or topical negative pressure, if available.

9. Monitor for symptoms and signs of compartment syndrome and, if in doubt, redo fasciotomies.

10. Relook at 24–48 hours; if healthy, consider closure +/− split-thickness skin graft.

SURGICAL TECHNIQUE

Leg

The leg is the most common site for compartment syndrome. The four compartments of the leg – anterior, lateral, superficial/deep posterior (Figure 17.1) – should be decompressed via two incisions. **Other more minimal, less invasive methods are not appropriate in the trauma setting.**

1. Identify and mark anatomical landmarks: medial tibial border, fibula head to lateral malleolus (the course of the fibula; Figure 17.2).

2. Mark incisions before starting; landmarks will become distorted once an incision is made.

   The lateral incision should be marked one finger breadth *anterior to* the fibula, from the level of the fibula head to the level of the malleolus (Figure 17.2).

   The medial incision should be marked one thumb breadth *posterior* to the palpable medial edge of the tibia, from the level of the tibial tuberosity to the level of the malleolus (Figure 17.2).

3. Lateral incision

   As per markings, the skin and underlying fascia – lying over the anterior compartment – are both incised completely to enter the anterior compartment. Dissecting laterally, one will encounter the intermuscular septum between the anterior and lateral compartments which should be divided to decompress the lateral compartment (Figure 17.1).

   The superficial peroneal nerve, lying posterior to the intermuscular septum in the lateral compartment, should be identified and protected.

   Be mindful of placing the initial incision too far laterally and risking entering the lateral, rather than anterior, compartment with the first incision and potentially injuring the peroneal nerve.

4. Medial incision.

Both posterior compartments (superficial and deep) are released via a single medial incision, as marked. Incise through skin only, before dissecting on top of the fascia to identify the saphenous vein and nerve and retracting both anteriorly.

Protect the saphenous vein and nerve.

Identify the medial border of the tibia and incise fascia to access the superficial compartment, containing gastrocnemius and soleus muscles. Release soleus from the medial border of the tibia, before incising the fascia over flexor digitorum longus and tibialis posterior, to decompress the deep compartment. Identification of the posterior tibial neurovascular bundle confirms that the compartment has been entered (Figure 17.1).

Ensure the deep posterior compartment is released.

Do not be confused by the interval between gastrocnemius and soleus, thinking that you have entered the deep compartment. The Plantaris tendon is a useful landmark in this regard.

Adequate decompression requires the release of soleus from the posterior border of the tibia.

Foot

The nine compartments of the foot fall into four groups – intrinsic, medial, central, and lateral (Figure 17.3) – and should be decompressed via a single medial incision (Figure 17.4).

1. Mark the incision from a point below the medial malleolus (midway between malleolus and sole) to the base of the first metatarsal.

2. Incise through skin and plantar fascia.

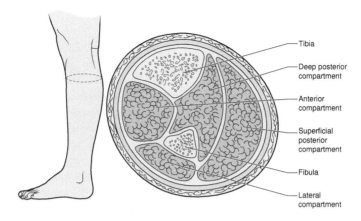

Figure 17.1 Anatomical cross-section of the leg, showing fascia, four compartments of the leg, intermuscular septae, and location of neurovascular structures.

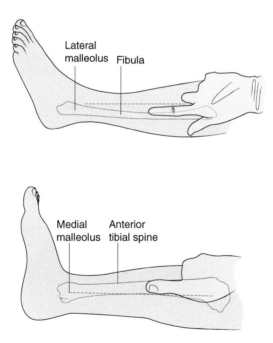

Figure 17.2 To show surface anatomy of leg with key anatomical landmarks: medial tibial border, fibula head to lateral malleolus (the course of the fibula). Highlighting lateral and medial incisions: Lateral marked one finger breadth anterior to the fibula, from the level of the fibula head to the level of the malleolus. Medial incision marked one thumb breadth posterior to the palpable medial edge of the tibia, from the level of the tibial tuberosity to the level of the malleolus.

The neurovascular bundle is identified and retracted.

3. Incise the fascia over abductor hallucis and flexor hallucis brevis to enter the medial compartment.
4. Incise the medial intermuscular septum longitudinally to enter the central compartment.
   Note the lateral plantar neurovascular bundle runs over quadratus plantae.
5. The remaining compartments (lateral and intrinsic) are entered by blunt dissection.

The lateral (abductor) compartment can be identified by retracting flexor digitorum brevis.

Thigh

Compartment syndrome of the thigh is uncommon, both due to its large volume and the possibility for fluid to track beyond the compartment. The three compartments of the thigh – anterior, posterior, and medial –

are usually decompressed via one lateral incision. In severe cases, a medial incision may also be required.

1. The lateral incision is marked one finger breadth anterior to tensor fascia lata, which is identified as a tense band of tissue running from the greater tuberosity to the lateral aspect of the knee (Figure 17.5).
2. Incise through skin only and raise skin flaps above the fascia anteriorly and posteriorly.
3. Make two separate longitudinal incisions in both the anterior compartment fascia and posterior compartment fascia, decompressing both. These two incisions are joined by a transverse incision through fascia lata (leaving an H-shaped incision) to ensure adequate release, which is usually sufficient to decompress the thigh.
4. If further release is required, a separate medial incision can be made posterior to the adductor longus tendon, palpated with the thigh abducted and knee flexed.

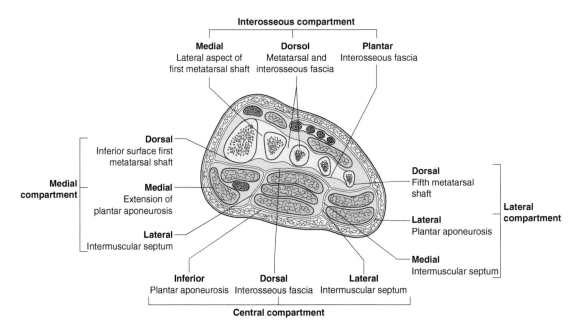

Figure 17.3 Cross section of the foot similar to these diagrams but without the dorsal incisions. Individual muscles do not need to be labelled but rather muscle compartments and intermuscular septae, as per the right diagram.

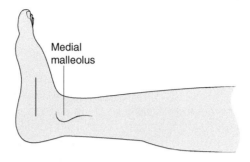

Figure 17.4 Medial view to show surface anatomy of the foot with incision marked from a point below the medial malleolus (midway between malleolus and sole) to the base of the first metatarsal.

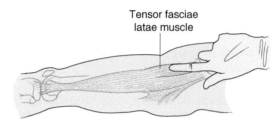

Figure 17.5 The lateral incision is marked one finger breadth anterior to tensor fascia lata, which is identified as a tense band of tissue running from the greater tuberosity to the lateral aspect of the knee.

HAND

The 10 anatomical compartments of the hand – four dorsal (interossei), three palmar (interossei), adductor, thenar, and hypothenar – are decompressed via two dorsal and one palmar incision (Figure 17.6).

DORSAL

To decompress four dorsal interossei, three palmar interossei, and the adductor compartment.

1. Make two skin incisions, one between the second and third metacarpal and another between the fourth and fifth metacarpal (Figure 17.6).

Preserve dorsal veins.

2. Incise the fascia over the second and fourth dorsal interossei; then elevate the skin to enable incision over the first and third dorsal interossei.

   When dissecting over the first dorsal interosseous, look for and preserve branches of the superficial branch of the radial nerve.

3. To decompress the first palmar interosseous and adductor compartment, insert tenotomy scissors in a palmar direction along the ulnar border of the second metacarpal. One should feel the dorsal fascia of the palmar/adductor compartment give way as the scissors pass through, at which point they can be spread to fully decompress the compartment.

4. In a similar fashion to step three, the second and third palmar interossei are decompressed by inserting scissors along the radial aspect of the fourth and fifth metacarpal.

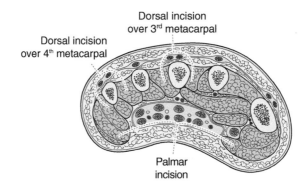

Figure 17.6 Above diagram to be adjusted, placing incisions between second or third and fourth or fifth metacarpals. Palmar incision remains the same.

PALMAR

To decompress the thenar and hypothenar compartment and median and ulnar nerves (Figure 17.6).

1. A step incision is made across the distal wrist crease, continuing as a longitudinal incision between the thenar and hypothenar eminences up to at least the proximal palmar crease (Figure 17.7).
2. The flexor retinaculum is divided to release the carpal tunnel and median nerve, which lies immediately underneath.

    The motor branch of the median nerve passes radially into the thenar muscles, at the distal end of the carpal tunnel, and should be preserved.
3. The thenar compartment is decompressed by incising the overlying fascia.
4. Guyon's canal, through which the ulnar nerve and artery run, is decompressed by deepening the incision in an ulnar direction, superficial to the flexor retinaculum.
5. Continuing in an ulnar direction allows decompression of the hypothenar compartment.

During dissection, preserve deep motor branches of the ulnar nerve running into the hypothenar wad and, additionally, the ulnar artery as it branches.

DIGITAL

If required.

1. Mid-axial incisions, which are dorsal to the neurovascular bundles, can be made to decompress the digits. These should be sited on the non-dependant side of each digit (radial aspect of thumb and little finger, ulnar aspect of index, middle, and ring).
2. Decompression is achieved by dissecting dorsal to neurovascular bundles (NVBs), volar to the flexor sheath, then dorsal to the NVB as the other side of the digit is reached.

Forearm

Four compartments – superficial flexor, deep flexor, and two extensors (dorsal and mobile wad) – should be decompressed via one or two incisions.

1. From the proximal end of the above palm incision, drop the incision towards the ulnar aspect of the wrist and then continue proximally along the ulnar border of the forearm for around 5 cm, before curving the incision toward the radial aspect of the antecubital fossa (ACF) and continuing in the flexion crease of the ACF towards the ulnar aspect of the elbow (Figure 17.7).

2. It may be possible to reach the extensor compartments via the volar incision. If not, a separate midline longitudinal incision is made over the dorsal aspect of the pronated forearm, starting 2 cm medial and distal to the lateral epicondyle (Figure 17.8).

3. All muscles and both median and ulnar nerves should be systemically examined and decompressed. Care must be taken to decompress the deep flexor compartment (including pronator quadratus), which can be found deep to and on retraction of the long flexors.

   Identify and protect the palmar cutaneous branch of the median nerve, arising from the radial aspect of the median nerve 5 cm proximal to the wrist crease, and the dorsal branch of the ulnar nerve, which arises from the ulnar aspect of the ulnar nerve, 5 cm proximal to the pisiform, and passes dorsally.

4. The median nerve should be released in the antecubital fossa, which requires division of the lacertus fibrosis and proximal edges of pronator teres and flexor digitorum superficialis.

Arm

1. The proximal extent of the forearm fasciotomy incision is continued proximally along the medial aspect of the arm, over the posteromedial aspect of biceps (Figure 17.9).

2. Both anterior and posterior compartments are decompressed through one incision.

Avoid damage to the radial nerve as the posterior compartment is decompressed.

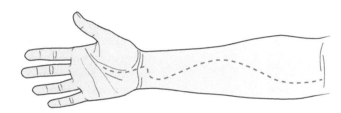

Figure 17.7 Surface anatomy of the volar aspect of the hand and forearm, showing a step incision across the distal wrist crease, continuing as a longitudinal incision between the thenar and hypothenar eminences up to the proximal palmar crease. Extending proximally, from the proximal end of the above-palm incision, the incision drops towards the ulnar aspect of the wrist and then continues proximally along the ulnar border of the forearm for around 5 cm before curving toward the radial aspect of the antecubital fossa (ACF) and continuing in the flexion crease of the ACF towards to the ulnar aspect of the elbow.

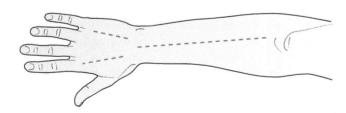

Figure 17.8 Surface anatomy of the dorsal aspect of the pronated forearm, showing a midline longitudinal incision starting 2 cm medial and distal to the lateral epicondyle.

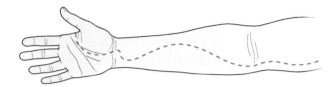

Figure 17.9 Surface anatomy of the medial aspect of the arm, showing a continuation of the proximal extent of the forearm fasciotomy incision along the medial aspect of the arm, over the posteromedial aspect of biceps.

BURNS

Overview

Burn injuries may be obvious or concealed. Around one-third of conflict burns have other, potentially life-threatening, injuries, which may be missed due to the more obvious burn injury. Therefore, all patients should be assessed with a full primary and secondary surgery, in line with Advanced Trauma Life Support (ATLS) and Emergency Management of Severe Burns (EMSB) principles.

Resource Limitation Concerns

The management of burns is resource-heavy, therefore, in a limited resource environment, the aim should be to stabilise the casualty by accurately assessing the injury, adequately resuscitating the casualty, addressing any life or limb-threatening sequelae, and transferring on to a definitive care facility as soon as possible. In the military context, eligibility matrices should be in place relating to the care of local national burns casualties, which carry a considerable logistical burden.

Considerations of futility in the management of major burns in the resource-limited environment are a particular challenge and exert a psychological effect on all staff members. Paediatric patients are particularly at risk to burn injuries, and this scenario is even more difficult. Senior medical and executive commanders should liaise with facility burn care providers ahead of time to establish what may be realistically achieved in a given environment. When faced with such patients, discussion can be informed, but not dictated, by this prior planning.

Regardless of the situation, the goal of burn treatment should be early wound closure and the avoidance of sepsis – based on an accurate assessment of the burn injury and appropriate, adequate resuscitation. The methods, sequence, and timing of interventions may be different from those we are accustomed to in modern specialist burn centres, and some ingenuity may be required to adapt the facilities and equipment at our disposal. These principles should be used to guide particular adaptations that will be dictated by the context of the environment. It is important to recognise that normal practice may not be possible in constrained situations and insistence on this may overstretch not only available physical resources, but the capability of available personnel and can, in fact, also be dangerous. Mature and pragmatic judgement is required to define appropriate and realistic expectations:

- Early complete excision may not be possible and may be dangerous.
- Limited temporising cover with allograft and the like will not be available/sustainable.
- Utilising all required donor sites increases the wound burden and may be life-threatening outside of a properly equipped burn centre.
- Excision, therefore, has to be staged while managing the remaining eschar appropriately.
- Priority to be given to tracheostomy site, line sites, and hands.
- Special considerations for delayed presentations and presentations with established burn wound sepsis (techniques such as antibiotic clysis become useful).

- Adrenaline infiltration of all sites during excision and skin graft harvest to minimise blood loss.
- Potential to favour fascial excision over tangential excision to allow greater surface area debridement and lower blood loss.

Acute Management

STOP THE BURNING PROCESS

Remove any remaining thermal or chemical source (foreign body, clothes) and cool, or neutralise in case of chemical burn, by irrigating with tepid water (so as not to excessively cool the casualty).

Acute management should then proceed in an ABC fashion.

AIRWAY

Apply high-flow oxygen.

The potential for airway injury may not be apparent and should be anticipated based on history, clinical signs, and symptoms.

Seek urgent anaesthetic review if any concern exists regarding the airway.

Do not watch and wait as any deterioration in the airway is likely to be harder to address.

The emergency management of all inhalational injury (above the larynx, below the larynx, and systemic intoxication) involves securing the airway and providing respiratory support by way of high flow oxygen.

BREATHING

Examine chest movement.

If any deep circumferential chest burns cause restriction of chest movement to perform an emergency escharotomy.

Emergency escharotomy

Escharotomies are painful and should ideally be performed under general anaesthetic. In time-critical cases, they may need to be performed in the Emergency Department.

The aim is to release tight constriction of burnt tissue. Cutting diathermy is used to divide through the necrotic layer of unyielding skin. The end point should be determined by reaching unburnt tissue and achieving the desired release (Figure 17.10).

Chest escharotomy

Not all sides of the 'breastplate' need to be completed. Start by performing both sides of the subcostal incision,

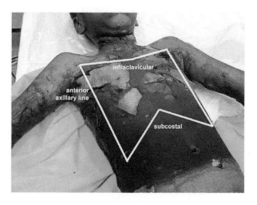

Figure 17.10 Markings for chest escharotomy.

then seek feedback from the anaesthetist to assess any potential ease in ventilation. If restriction persists, proceed to both anterior axillary line incisions. Finally, if required, the infraclavicular incision can be performed.

Limb escharotomy

Incisions are made as per Figures 17.11 and 17.12 (dotted lines), avoiding important marked structures. To achieve full release, incisions should be extended into adjacent non-burnt tissue, though in extensive burns this may not practically be possible. On release of the eschar, be prepared for potential limb hyper-perfusion and associated blood loss. If any suspicion exists regarding underlying compartment syndrome, then fasciotomies should be performed.

Ensure haemostasis is achieved, after which, the wounds can be dressed in the same manner as the burnt surrounding tissue.

CIRCULATION

Acute burns do not cause profound hypovolaemia; therefore, assess for potential occult injuries.

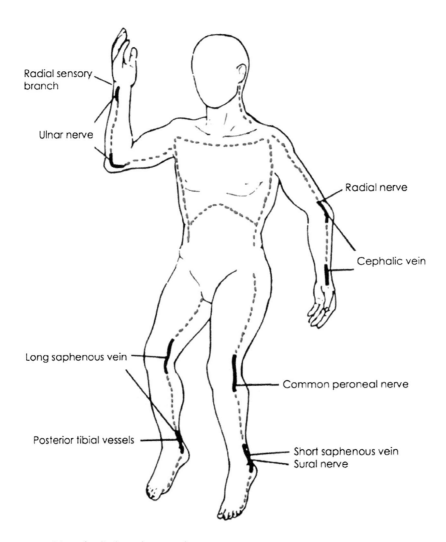

Figure 17.11 Markings for limb escharotomies.
http://acuclinic.com.au/pocit/Escharotomy.htm

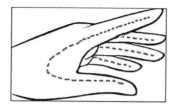

Figure 17.12 Markings for digital escharotomies.
http://acuclinic.com.au/pocit/Escharotomy.htm

Establish vascular access and commence crystalloid resuscitation fluids (rate adjusted later).

Assess for circumferential limb burns, which may be compromising limb perfusion. If any concern exists regarding either venous return – which would likely occur first – or arterial inflow, perform emergency escharotomy.

DISABILITY

Patients with an altered state of consciousness, confusion, or restlessness after sustaining a burn injury have carbon monoxide poisoning until proved otherwise.

However, do not forget other potential contributing injuries.

EXPOSURE

Ensure patient is kept warm during this phase.

Uncover one limb at a time and, if possible, maintain a warm environment. Remove any potentially constricting clothing or jewellery.

Assess and document total body surface area (TBSA) of burn and depth (Table 17.1) – this is more relevant than transfer and ongoing, rather than acute, management.

Photographs are helpful both for documentation and in seeking third-party advice.

Estimation of burn extent

Assessment of the extent of the burn (%TBSA) is important to guide fluid resuscitation and to provide prognostic information with regard to mortality (the greater the area of burn, the greater the mortality).

Blisters should be de-roofed, and any debris or soot should be removed to enable an accurate assessment. Areas of simple erythema should not be included in the calculation.

Small or non-confluent areas can be assessed using the patient's own palm, which equates to approximately 1% TBSA.

The Rule of Nines lends itself to larger confluent areas and breaks the body regions into multiples of nine (Figure 17.13).

Table 17.1 Examination of burn depth

Depth	Colour	Blisters	Capillary Refill	Sensation	Healing
Epidermal	Red	No	Present	Present	Yes
Superficial dermal	Pale pink	Small	Present	Painful	Yes
Mid dermal	Dark pink	Present	Sluggish	+/–	Usual
Deep dermal	Blotchy red	+/–	Absent	Absent	No
Full-thickness	White	No	Absent	Absent	No

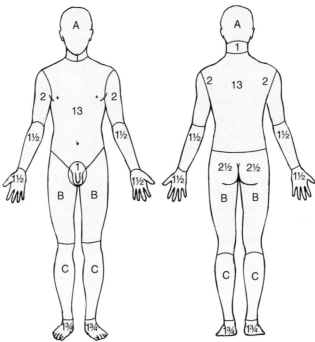

Relative percentage of area affected by growth

Age in years	0	1	5	10	15	Adult
A Head	9	8	6	5	4	3
B Thigh	2	3	4	4	4	4
C Leg	2	2	3	3	3	3

Figure 17.13 The Lund and Browder chart. (From Williams, N. et al. (eds). *Bailey & Love's Short Practice of Surgery, 27th Ed.,* ch. 41, p. 621. Taylor & Francis Group, 2018.)

This is less accurate in children, due to differing body proportions, so the Paediatric Rule of Nines should be used (right side of Figure 17.12, for a child aged 1 year). For every year over one, the head decreases in size by 1% and each leg increases by 0.5%, reaching adult proportions by 10 years of age.

The Lund-Browder chart provides the most accurate estimation of TBSA (Figure 17.13).

FLUIDS

Initiate resuscitation fluids if the burn is >15% TBSA in adults or >10% TBSA in children.

Calculate fluid requirements according to the Parkland formula:

2 − 4mL × bodyweight (kg) × % TBSA of burn

= total volume of crystalloid to be given in the

first 24 hours

Half of the total 24-hour fluid volume should be given within 8 hours of the burn and the remaining half over the next 16 hours.

The formula only provides a guide; therefore, the rate of infusion should be titrated against urine output (catheterise patient) aiming for $0.5–1 \text{ mL kg}^{-1} \text{ hour}^{-1}$.

ADJUNCTIVE MEASURES

Analgesia: intravenous opioid titrated to response and respiratory rate.

Investigations: consider baseline arterial blood gas, full blood count, and renal function.

Note persistent metabolic acidosis despite adequate fluid resuscitation may be due to cyanide toxicity – consider administration of hydroxocobalamin.

Nasogastric tube: consider in burns over 20% TBSA for gastric decompression and to initiate early feeding as soon as feasible.

Tetanus status: burns are tetanus-prone.

DRESSINGS

Loose, non-adherent dressings, such as paraffin gauze, should be applied, followed by wrung-out betadine-soaked gauze and outer dressings to manage likely high exudate. The outer dressings can be changed when soiled, leaving the non-adherent base layer intact to avoid undue pain associated with dressing changes. Limbs should be elevated, and splinting, considered.

BURN EXCISION

Formal burn excision, in the case of deep or slow-to-heal burns, should be undertaken at a definitive care facility.

ELECTRICAL BURNS

Low-voltage (<1000 V) injuries are likely to present with a contact wound and may cause cardiac arrest but are unlikely to cause deep tissue damage.

High-voltage (>1000 V) injuries may cause flash burns +/– deep injury via transmission of current. In addition to potentially innocuous-looking entry and exit wounds, deep tissue damage may be extensive.

Once the power source has been cleared, management is as discussed earlier with a few areas warranting additional focus:

Fluids: haemochromogen pigmentation of the urine is to be expected in the presence of deep tissue damage; therefore, aim for a urine output of 1.0–1.5 mL/kg^{-1}/hour^{-1} to prevent acute kidney injury.

Dysrhythmia: all patients should have an electrocardiogram and those who have had a cardiac arrest or passage of current through the thorax will require continuous monitoring.

Fasciotomy: significant deep tissue damage to an extremity may lead to compartment syndrome, requiring fasciotomy.

CHEMICAL BURNS

Constant flow of water, until a neutral pH is reached, is the key acute management of chemical burns.

Alkali burns require irrigation longer than acid burns.

If eyes are affected, apply topical chloramphenicol following irrigation to prevent secondary infection.

Certain chemical agents require specific management:

Hydrofluoric (HF) acid:

A seemingly trivial cutaneous HF burn can be fatal. Systemic hypocalcaemia and hypomagnesaemia can lead to arrhythmias.

> *Irrigate copiously.*
> *Apply topical 10% calcium gluconate gel to inactivate fluoride ions, titrated to relief of pain and reapply when pain returns.*
> *Subcutaneously infiltrate burn wounds refractory to topical therapy with 0.5 mL of 10% calcium gluconate per cm^2.*
> *Intravenous calcium gluconate should be considered if extensive subcutaneous infiltration is not possible.*
> *If pain persists, consider early excision to halt systemic absorption.*

Phosphorous

Though extinguished by water, embedded phosphorous particles will continue to burn.

> *Visible particles should be removed.*
> *Apply 0.5% copper sulphate solution, which turns the particles black, facilitating their removal.*
> *Note that systemic absorption may lead to hypotension and renal injury.*

It is in non-surgical burn treatment that we might benefit most from the often-forgotten heirlooms of early burns management such as the following:

- Stabilisation of burn eschar
- Antibiotic clysis
- Topical Mafenide (Sulfamylon)
- Flamazine
- Flammacerium
- Silver
- Hypochlorite (Dakin's Solution)

These can all be discussed with advantages/disadvantages, antibiotic spectrum, and so on. These techniques have been largely superseded in modern specialist burn care but provide potentially valuable tools in austere environments and mass-casualty events. Mafenide, in particular, has been valuable in the field, especially in Afghanistan and the Iraq wars.

Key Concepts: Burns

1. **Stop the burning process by removing the source and irrigating.**
2. Perform primary survey and rule out coexisting injury.
3. Have a low threshold for seeking anaesthetic review of the airway.
4. Consider escharotomy if deep burns are comprising chest movement or limb perfusion.
5. Estimate burn extent and initiate appropriate fluid resuscitation, titrated to urine output.
6. Administer appropriate analgesia and review tetanus status.
7. Keep the patient warm.
8. Dress with loose, non-adherent dressings, betadine-soaked gauze, and an absorbent outer layer.
9. Be aware of the potentially severe implications or relatively innocuous-looking electrical or chemical injuries.
10. Burn management is resource-heavy; therefore, transfer as soon as possible.
11. Consider the definition of treatment futility with respect to your facility ahead of time.

PERIPHERAL COLD INJURY

Overview

The highest proportion of frostbite injuries recorded in the Western world are secondary to prolonged exposure to cold within the military population. Prolonged application of cooling therapy in cases of musculoskeletal injuries can also lead to significant frostbite injury.

The management of these injuries differs from that of thermal injuries.

Cold injuries may be general (hypothermia) or local (freezing cold injury [FCI] and non-freezing cold injury [NFCI]). Irreversible FCI is termed frostbite, reversible FCI is termed frostnip, the latter may still have long-term sequelae including dysesthesias. The severity of injury, and the degree of irreversible tissue necrosis, is directly proportional to both the temperature and duration of exposure, and is influenced by the area of tissue exposed. Poorer outcomes are seen in lower extremity involvement, concomitant infection, and delayed injury presentation. NFCI, or 'trench-foot' is due to prolonged exposure to sub-physiological temperatures that do not lead to tissues freezing.

Resource Limitation Concerns

The majority of these injuries are small and innocuous, but widespread, life-threatening areas of tissue necrosis, as with burns, will require significant resources to manage.

After rewarming, every attempt should be made to avoid potential re-exposure. For this reason, rewarming must not be initiated until in an environment that can prevent refreezing.

Early transfer is advocated.

Clinical Presentation

The extremities are usually affected first, with digits, ears, nose, and penis most frequently affected. Presentation may range from mild tingling of a digit to a moribund patient with extensive tissue loss.

Patients report the affected area to be cold to touch and numb. It usually appears pale, with mottling at the interface of affected and unaffected tissue, and may feel woody, due to oedema. As the injury evolves, blistering of the dermis may be noted. Ultimately, the tissue will either deteriorate further or recover, which is very much dependant on initial management.

The gross appearance of the tissue at the time of presentation will indicate the severity of injury (Table 17.1).

This is not an equivalent measure to classification of burn depth.

Frostbite should be considered in all trauma patients in cold environments.

Nearly one-quarter of patients with frostbite injuries have been reported to have significant coexisting traumatic injuries. It is also important to be aware of the potential for hypothermia (core temperature below 35 °C) in patients presenting with frostbite.

Assessment

Life-threatening or associated pathology, including compartment syndrome, should be ruled out by ATLS assessment.

Affected areas and severity of injury, as per Table 17.2, should be documented. Photographs are helpful both for documentation and in seeking third-party advice.

Routine radiology is not helpful.

Management

Management is primarily non-operative.

The patient should first be stabilised, associated injuries managed, and any hypothermia corrected (to above 35 °C).

The mainstay of treatment is local rewarming; however, this should only occur if there is no further risk of refreezing, as thawing and refreezing will result in more extensive tissue injury.

Rewarming should only be commenced in the field if there is no further chance of freezing. Rubbing the affected area to stimulate warmth should similarly be

avoided. Even walking on the affected limb to an appropriate facility would be better than the risk of rewarming and refreezing. One should also bear in mind the availability of appropriate analgesia prior to commencing rewarming, as it is often associated with significant pain, which may be long-lasting and, in severe cases, progress to complex regional pain syndrome.

Once the above criteria are met, rewarming should be initiated using a hot bath of water mixed with antiseptic solution, such as chlorhexidine, at a temperature of 37–39 °C. Higher temperatures lead to more significant pain. The water temperature should be monitored and regulated. Foot spa–type baths greatly increase the ease of rewarming. This should be undertaken for a minimum of 30 minutes, aiming for the clinical end point of soft, pliable tissue with a reddish-purple hue.

Post-thaw reperfusion injury may lead to compartment syndrome, which in limb injuries should be specifically assessed following rewarming.

A low threshold should be maintained for urgent escharotomy or fasciotomy in cases of escalating analgesia requirements.

Prostaglandin F2-alpha and thromboxane A2 cause platelet aggregation and vasoconstriction. As long as there are no contraindications, a systemic prostaglandin inhibitor should be administered, such as oral ibuprofen, at a dose of 12 mg/kg^{-1} twice daily (up to a maximum of 2400 mg day^{-1}), or aspirin at 300 mg once a day.

In a pre-hospital environment, it may be prudent to leave intact simple areas of non-tense clear blistering to reduce the risk of infection. Aspiration can be considered to reduce the exudate rich in prostaglandin F2-alpha and thromboxane A2. When in an appropriate facility, where asepsis may be

Table 17.2 Severity of cold injury				
	Depth of freezing	Tissue colour	Oedema	Skin compromise
1st degree	Partial skin thickness	Hyperaemic	Minor	None
2nd degree	Full skin thickness	Erythematous	Substantial	Clear blistering
3rd degree	Subcutaneous tissues	Dark blue/black	Substantial	Haemorrhagic blistering +/− necrosis
4th degree	Muscle/tendon/bone	Black with mummification	Minor or none	Major necrosis

managed, blisters should be debrided to aid with wound care and accurate assessment of the depth of injury. In more severe cases, this debridement may require a general anaesthetic.

A topical thromboxane inhibitor, such as *aloe vera,* should be applied, followed by simple, loose, non-adherent dressings. Affected limbs should be elevated to reduce dependant oedema and the potential for progression of necrosis in watershed areas. A splint should be considered and patients with lower limb injuries should remain non-weight-bearing.

Patients should be strongly advised to stop smoking. As with thermal burn injuries, prophylactic antibiotics are not routinely required and should be reserved for cases of infection/contamination. Appropriate tetanus cover should be ensured, as frostbite injuries are tetanus-prone.

Management is almost universally non-operative, aside from those required for compartment syndrome or infection. As the depth of injury is difficult to ascertain, tissues should be allowed to demarcate and the extent of injury reassessed. Tissues frequently, though initially appearing unsalvageable, recover and severe cases rarely require surgery even down the line. Late debridement may be indicated once clearly demarcated necrotic tissue remains, as this may pose an infection risk.

Thrombolysis has been shown to reduce the rate of late amputation in severe cases of frostbite; therefore, Tissue Plasminogen Activator should be considered in severe cases, presenting within 24 hours of injury. It should be administered within a high-care environment, following careful consideration of absolute contraindications, such as associated trauma, and the associated risks of haemorrhage, reperfusion injury, and compartment syndrome.

Key Concepts: Cold Injury

1. Rule out coexisting traumatic injury.
2. ***Correct hypothermia and ensure no chance of refreezing before rewarming with water at 37–39 °C for at least 30 minutes.***
3. Analgesia including NSAID (unless contraindicated) and review tetanus status.
4. Escharotomy +/− fasciotomy in cases of compartment syndrome.

5. Consider thrombolytic therapy in severe extremity injuries.
6. Debride blisters (may require general anaesthetic).
7. Apply topical *aloe vera* (or other anti-thromboxane gel) and loose, non-adherent dressings, splinting, and elevation.
8. Administer antibiotics if concerned with infection.
9. Abstain from smoking.
10. Debridement should only be undertaken when clear demarcation of tissues has occurred following appropriate initial management.

Plastic Surgery Reconstructive Elevator

PRINCIPLES

The concept of reconstruction of the soft tissues is straightforward as we consider the plastic surgery ladder. This is the stepwise progression of reconstructive options and underlies the basic principles of reconstruction. When a wound is created, the first option to close this is by primary intention or direct suture. If the wound is left to heal, it will progress through secondary intention with the phases of inflammation, reparation, and final maturity, with the definitive scar formed once re-epithelialisation has occurred. This can take several months and leads to a significant hypertrophic scar. A wound can be freshened and closed by delayed primary intention.

Once the defect is too large even for undermining the edges to allow apposition and closure, techniques such as skin graft and flap reconstruction must be considered.

The idea of a ladder is simple, although it can be misleading; therefore, consideration of the plastic surgery elevator will allow for correct decision making. A ladder is suggestive of climbing through each rung until the suitable reconstructive option is reached which will be successful. An elevator takes you to the most appropriate technique for the defect straight away.

SKIN GRAFTS

Skin grafting is a surgical procedure that involves removing skin from one area of the body and moving

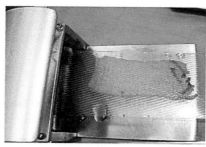 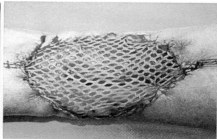

Figure 17.14 STSG.

it – or transplanting it – to a different area of the body. It is completely detached from its vascular supply and relies on the blood supply of the recipient wound bed to survive.

Skin grafts have been widely used to cover superficial defects.

It provides a barrier to infection, alleviates pain, and may act as a permanent or a temporary wound cover.

Classification

- *Autograft* (most common) is a graft taken from one part of an individual's body that is transferred to a different part of the body of that same individual.
- *Isograft* is a graft from the genetically identical donor and recipient individuals, such as identical human twins.
- *Allograft* is taken from another individual of the same species (can be cadaveric).
- *Xenograft* is a graft taken from an individual of one species that is grafted onto an individual of a different species.

Types

Split-thickness skin graft (STSG; Figure 17.14)

- It contains epidermis and a variable amount of dermis.
- It does not carry epithelial appendages.
- Instruments required to harvest an STSG may include a pneumatic or electric dermatome, or freehand blades such as a 'Watson' knife, a 'Goulian', or a 'Silvers' knife.
- The thinner the STSG (0.005–0.01 in.), usually the better the 'take', as the faster the perfusion is re-created.
- It usually requires 5 days to 'take'.
- Aesthetically and functionally, it is inferior to FTSGs as it tends to contract pigments to look like a patch and is more vulnerable to injury.
- Donor site is usually dressed and allowed to heal by secondary intention over a period of 2–3 weeks.

Full-thickness skin graft (FTSG; Figure 17.15)

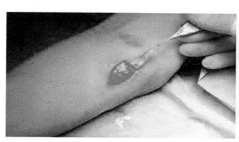 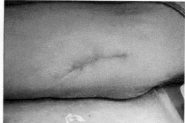

Figure 17.15 FTSG.

- It includes all of the dermis as well as the epidermis.
- It contains epithelial appendages (hair follicles, sebaceous glands, sweat glands).
- A surgical scalpel is necessary to harvest a full-thickness skin graft. Any fat remaining on the dermis must be removed completely to allow unrestricted ingrowth of blood vessels essential for skin graft survival.
- A well-vascularised wound bed is required, usually demanding 7 days to 'take'.
- FTSGs look more natural compared to STSGs, they are more elastic and resistant to traumatic forces.
- Donor site is usually sutured primarily and may be alternatively closed by an STSG.

Reverdin or 'pinch' grafts (Figure 17.16)

- It is a cone of skin where the peripheral margins of the graft are quite thin, gradually increasing in thickness towards the centre, to include a variable thickness of the dermis.
- It may contain epithelial appendages depending on dermal thickness.
- A fine hypodermic needle is inserted horizontally to the skin or forceps is used to elevate a cone of skin, followed by transverse tangential shaving of the pinch graft using a scalpel.
- The grafts are implanted into the wound bed as spread-out islands of skin to serve as centres of epithelialization and growth.
- Useful in medium-to-large superficial defects, such as burns, ulcers, etc.
- It usually requires 7–10 days to 'take'.
- They do contract comparably to STSG, are not very resistant to stress forces, and aesthetically may be substandard.

- If the pinch grafts have been taken in a linear fashion, the donor site can be sutured primarily. If not, then donor site can heal by secondary intention or resurfaced by an STSG.

LOCAL FLAPS

A flap is a unit of tissue transferred from a donor site to a recipient site while maintaining its own blood supply. In environments with limited resources, simple defects could be reconstructed with the use of skin grafts or local flaps. Complex defects, though, would require either regional or distant flaps. Flaps raised in the immediate vicinity of defects are called *local flaps* and provide excellent texture and colour match to the defect. Tissue transferred from an anatomic site not in the immediate vicinity to the defect is known as a *distant* flap. Distant flaps may transfer still attached to their original blood supply, known as *pedicled* flaps, or may be completely disconnected from their blood supply and then re-anastomosed to vessels at the recipient site, known as *free* flaps. Local flaps and pedicled flaps are much quicker and easier to raise and transfer, representing an excellent choice in patients requiring reconstruction of defects in a surgically challenging setting. Free flaps require microsurgical expertise, special instruments such as a microscope, and they entail lengthy operating times and special post-operative monitoring – all of which may not be available in austere conditions. For this reason, free flap reconstruction will not be discussed in this chapter.

Flaps are usually required to/for

- cover wounds with poor vascularity;
- cover vital structures;
- pad body prominences;
- provide temporary cover that may be necessary to

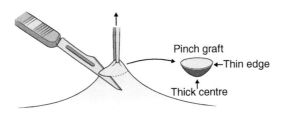

Figure 17.16 Pinch grafts.

operate through the wound at a later date to repair underlying structures;

- provide a functional motor unit;
- control infection in the recipient area; and
- for aesthetic reasons.

They range in composition – from simple skin and subcutaneous tissue flaps, to composite flaps more commonly including skin, fat, fascia, muscle and bone – and can potentially bare tendon, nerve, lymph nodes, or even a joint.

Can be classified according to

- the *vascularity* of the transferred tissue;
- tissue *composition* of the flap; and
- the *method of movement* to transfer the tissue.

Vascularity

- *Random* flaps – no named blood supply. Circulation is random via subdermal plexus, which in turn is supplied by direct or indirect cutaneous perforator vessels.

  o Can only be local flaps/
  o Most flaps in dermatologic surgery on the face but can be raised anywhere in the body.
  o Length-to-width ratio may be 1:1 in lower limb (poor blood supply) or up to 6:1 on the face (rich blood supply).
  o Length-to-width ratio limitations restrict their reliability to reconstruct moderate to large defects.

- *Axial* flaps – supplied by distinct and named blood

vessel(s) within the longitudinal axis of the flap. Their reliable blood supply makes them preferable in the reconstruction of moderate to large or compound defects.

  o Can be local, regional, or distant (including free) flaps.

Composition

- Cutaneous – skin and fat only
- Fasciocutaneous – skin, fat, **and** fascia
- Fascial – fascia **only**
- Musculocutaneous – skin, fat, fascia, **and** muscle
- Muscle only
- Osseocutaneous – skin, fat, **and** bone (may or may not contain fascia and muscle depending on donor area)
- Osseous – bone **only**
- Visceral – colon, small intestine, and omentum flap

Method of Movement

Flaps that can transfer to the defect from an adjacent area are known as local flaps and are of two types:

1. Ones that rotate about a pivot point – transposition, rotation, interpolation flaps.

- *Transposition* flap – tissue moved into adjacent defect, leaving a secondary defect that needs closing directly (i.e. rhomboid, Figure 17.17) or by other methods, such as an STSG (i.e. scalp

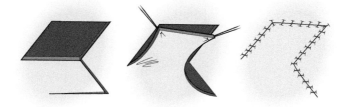

Figure 17.17 Rhomboid flap. Defect may have 60° and 120° angles as in a rhombus or can be more circular in clinical practice. Commonly used in head and neck area but can be used anywhere in the body. Can be single, bilateral, or triple-limbed. In its simplest form, the defect is measured, and an identical adjacent skin flap is marked and raised including a cuff of fat matching the defect's depth. Flap is pivoted and inset into the defect, while the donor site is sutured directly.

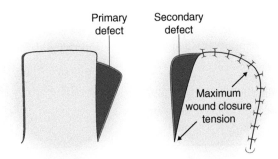

Figure 17.18 Transposition flap requiring closure of 2° defect. The flap must be designed slightly larger than the defect, so it doesn't fall short after transfer. Raising the flap can be chosen to reconstruct small to moderate defects almost anywhere in the body, but if performed in the scalp, the galea aponeurotica should be included. The flap is raised and transferred over a pivot point, leaving 2° defect needing closure with other methods (i.e. STSG).

transposition flap, Figure 17.18). The bilobed flap (Figure 17.19) is an example of two transposition flaps on a common pedicle, where the secondary defect of the first lobe is closed by another local flap (the second lobe), and the tertiary defect of the second lobe is closed directly.

- *Rotation* flap (Figure 17.20) – tissue rotated into adjacent defect, i.e. scalp rotation flap. The flap circumference should be 5–8 times the size of the defect to permit direct closure at the donor site. If the donor site cannot be closed directly, then a back cut at the flap's base or a Burrow's triangle may facilitate closure or another method may be needed to close if it's too large (another flap, skin graft, secondary intention, etc.).

- *Interpolation* flap – tissue moved into defect near – but not adjacent to – the donor site, over or

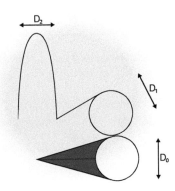

Figure 17.19 The bilobed flap. A versatile flap that can be used to reconstruct small to moderate superficial defects anywhere in the body. The first lobe of the flap should match the size of the defect. The second lobe should be narrower at its base but a bit longer compared to the first lobe. The horizontal axis across the midpoint of the defect and the vertical axis across the midpoint of the second lobe are the pivot points of each transposition flap lobe, respectively. This produces a total transposition arc of 90–100°, with each transposition flap having an arc of 45–50°. Usually, a triangle of skin needs to be excised at the base of the defect (shaded area on the figure) adjacent to the first lobe to avoid a standing cutaneous deformity on closure.

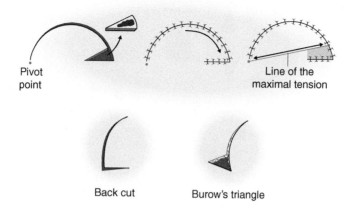

Figure 17.20 Rotation flap. A semicircular flap consisting of skin and fat, rotated about a pivot point, to close a defect. It should be designed with the arc directed towards an area of tissue redundancy. The circumference should be 5–8 times the size of the defect. Extensive undermining may have to be performed while maintaining the broad attachment of the flap to preserve blood supply. A back cut or a Burrow's triangle at the pivot point may facilitate closure or another method may be needed to close if too large (another flap, skin graft, secondary intention, etc.).

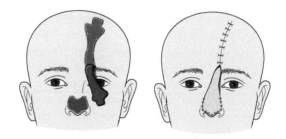

Figure 17.21 Paramedian forehead flap is an example of interpolated flap of the axial category, as it is based on the supratrochlear vessels. It is commonly used for reconstruction of the nose but can also be used in paranasal and forehead areas and usually carried out in two stages, sometimes three. A template of the defect is taken, and the forehead is marked accordingly. The path of the supratrochlear artery is marked at the medial aspect of the eyebrow, superolateral to the root of the nose and the base of the flap is designed 1.5 cm wide to include the pedicle. Elevation of the flap begins from the superior most end of the forehead markings at the subcutaneous plane for the first 2 cm to create a thin, pliable flap tip. As the elevation proceeds inferiorly, it is extended to the subperiosteal layer about 2 cm superior to the brow region, careful not to injure the pedicle. The medial portion of the pedicle should be extended in a curvilinear fashion towards the medial canthus to aid pivoting the flap medially at a point below the level of the eyebrow. The flap lies over an area of intact skin over the root of the nose and glabellar region to reach the more distal nasal defect, what makes it an interpolated flap. Inset follows thinning of the tip of the flap to the level of the dermis. Donor site may be possible to close directly to its entirety with a few deep dermal absorbable monofilament sutures and a layer of nylon skin sutures on top. If this is not feasible, then the area that cannot be closed directly can be left to heal by 2° intention using simple dressings. The raw part of the flap overlying the intact skin over the root of the nose can also be dressed with simple non-adherent dressings. The second stage can be performed as soon as 10–14 days later, but it is safer to wait 3–4 weeks to allow maximal vascularity and reduced oedema. Pedicle overlying the intact skin over the root of the nose is divided and discarded. The distal flap is elevated and further thinned as required and contoured, with sutures removed 7 days later.

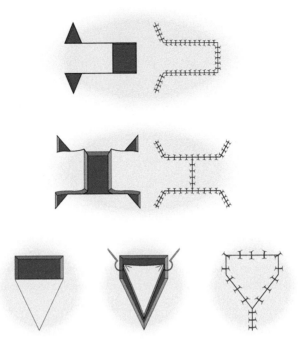

Figure 17.22 One of the commonest advancement flaps is the V-Y advancement flap. Can be performed almost anywhere in the body. For smaller defects, it can be unilateral or bilateral, while for moderate defects it is usually bilateral. Procedure requires a triangular incision down to subcutaneous tissue, with the base of the triangle adjacent to the d. The height of the triangle is usually 1.5–2times the length of the base. The flap is undermined laterally, sometimes undermining of the tip of the triangle, and the base may be required to facilitate mobility but not under the actual pedicle to avoid blood supply compromise of the flap. Once mobilised, the flap is brought into position using a skin hook, and an anchor nylon suture is placed between the middle of the V base and the opposite wall of the defect to hold flap in place. Another two similar sutures are placed to the angles of the base of the triangular V flap. The donor site can now be closed, directly creating a vertical limb, transforming V to a Y. This also releases the tension to the anchored V flap and allows tension-free closure of the triangular flap with nylon stitches.

under adjacent intervening tissue (i.e. paramedian forehead flap (Figure 17.21), Littler's neurovascular island flap).

2. Ones that advance into the defect – advancement flaps (i.e. V-Y, keystone, etc.).

- *Advancement* flap – relies on skin elasticity and is moved by sliding (advancing) directly into the adjacent defect. If skin elasticity alone is not enough to advance the flap adequately, then a counter incision or a Burrow's triangle or a Z-plasty at the base of the flap will increase it. Examples (Figure 17.22) are a simple or modified advancement flap, V-Y, keystone, bipedicled, and so on.

Procedure and Equipment Details for Local Skin Flaps

All procedures can be carried out under LA, and/or sedation, or GA. A minor operations surgical set and bipolar diathermy is more commonly necessary to perform these procedures. This includes the following:

- 1 × Mosquito artery forceps 5″ straight
- 1 × Gillies toothed dissecting forceps 6″
- 1 × Kilner needle holder 5.25″

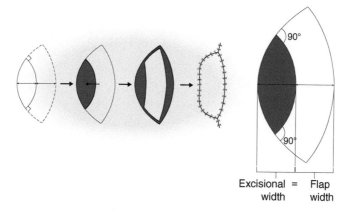

Figure 17.23 Keystone flap.

- 1 × Iris scissors 4.5″ curved
- 1 × Martins splinter forceps 4.5″
- 1 × Mayo scissors 6.5″ straight
- 1 × Gillies skin hook
- 1 × Stitch scissors 5″ sharp/sharp
- 1 × Allis tissue forceps 6″
- 1 × Scalpel handle No.3 (to take blades 10–5)
- 1 × Spencer Wells artery forceps 5″ straight
- 1 × McIndoe plain dissecting forceps 6″
- 1 × Volkmann spoon

Keystone flap is another interesting advancement flap which can be recruited to reconstruct from small to large defects anywhere in the body. It employs immediately adjacent skin and soft tissue that provide a good colour match in addition to reconstructing the contour of the defect. The defect is converted to elliptical shape to favour proper closure with outstanding cutaneous deformity. The side of the defect with greater tissue laxity is chosen as the flap donor area. If a single flap is not sufficient to cover the defect, then another flap from the opposite side of the ellipse can be raised to make it a bilateral keystone flap. The width of the Keystone flap must be equal to the width of the defect. The flap length depends upon the length of the elliptical defect. An incision at 90° at either end of the ellipse meets the curvilinear line of the flap outer

margin. The incision is made along the markings, as described earlier, down to the deep fascia, which is divided along the outer border of the flap. This will allow mobilisation without any undermining that may compromise the blood supply to the flap. An anchor nylon suture is placed between the middle portion of the flap and the middle of the opposite wall of the defect. The rest of the flap can then be sutured with a number of monofilament absorbable deep dermal sutures, followed by nylon sutures or staples to skin. If the Keystone is bilateral due to a large defect, then placement of a drain is recommended for a few days (Figure 17.23).

Single and bilateral advancement flaps with Burrow's triangles excision. V-Y advancement flap.

SUGGESTED READING

- Advanced Trauma Life Support Student Course Manual.
- Emergency Management of Severe Burns Candidate Manual.
- Joint Service Publication 539 Heat illness and cold injury: prevention and management.
- Trauma: Code Red Companion to the RCSEng Definitive Surgical Trauma Skills Course.

Acute Acoustic Trauma and Blast-Related Hearing Loss

18

Jameel Muzaffar, Christopher Coulson, Jonathan D. E. Lee, and Linda E. Orr

Acute hearing injuries may occur alone or as part of multisystem trauma, and acute acoustic trauma (AAT) should be suspected in any patient exposed to blast or who have sustained a blast injury to any part of their body. The severity of the hearing injury experienced may vary widely from a conductive hearing loss caused by tympanic membrane rupture or middle ear disruption, to sensorineural loss due to acoustic overexposure, temporal bone fracture, or any combination of these.

Until recently, acute hearing injuries have been treated by removal from further potential hearing insults. Prevention has rightly been the mainstay of protection, with the use of hearing protective devices (HPDs); however, AAT in the military setting can be unpredictable, and the use of HPDs has been beset by the belief that it may compromise situational awareness. Recent work has highlighted the potential for steroid therapy delivered orally, intravenously (IV) or via intratympanic injection (ITSI) as salvage following AAT. Prompt recognition and early intervention are associated with improved outcomes and such treatment may allow injured personnel to return to active duty following a period of recuperation.

A trade-off exists between oral administration – which is relatively easy to deliver but achieves lower intra-cochlear drug levels and risks systemic side effects – and intratympanic administration which requires expertise to deliver and carries some procedural risks but achieves higher intra-cochlea levels without systemic side effects. The risk – benefit judgement may be influenced by other injuries, particularly head injury, polytrauma, and burns; the treatment of which may be compromised by systemic administration of high dose oral or IV steroids. Wider occupational consideration may also come into play (e.g., a fast jet pilot or diver may have a different opinion as to the relative risk–benefit analysis of oral versus trans tympanic injection of steroid).

Resource constraints may make both diagnosis and treatment more challenging. This is a rapidly evolving field with technological developments, such as boothless audiometry and endoscopic imaging, allowing accurate testing near the point of injury. Whilst hearing injuries are an emergency, there is almost always time to seek specialist advice with interventions undertaken over a period of hours to days.

RESOURCE LIMITATION CONCERNS

Limitations of Diagnosis

Diagnosis of hearing injuries can be challenging even in resource-rich environments. Other injuries – fear of letting colleagues down – and potential occupational consequences may prevent patients from reporting subjective reduction in their hearing. Examination may be difficult due to blood and debris in the ear canal, the lack of access to microsuction, and the contraindication of water-based syringing without knowledge of the status of the tympanic membrane (TM), or even the lateral skull base. Such canal obstruction may contribute up to 30 dB of conductive hearing loss – roughly the same as putting your fingers in your ears. If the ear canals are clear and assessment confirms the presence of a perforation, there are concomitant risks; development of infection and a probable cause of hearing loss not amenable to repair in the operational environment.

With most blast-related injuries presenting as a sensorineural or mixed loss, the biggest challenge in the deployed area or in a mass casualty situation is often obtaining a reliable hearing threshold test in a timely way. Until recently, this required testing in a soundproofed audiometric booth; however, boothless audiometry headsets now combine an audiometer and acoustic shielding, allowing testing away from the traditional setting. These devices generally look like ruggedised over-ear headphones, typically connected to a small tablet or laptop computer which can electronically transmit audiology results and images to a central location positioned remotely for expert review and formulation of an individual management plan. Such devices, combined with endoscopic imaging of the tympanic membrane, have already been used successfully in carefully controlled situations, but given the frequency of AAT and the difficulty of conventional hearing testing, it is almost inevitable that their adoption will become widespread. Caution must be exercised if pure self-report will be used as an initial screening for AAT, as experience has shown that in the deployed setting, this often poorly correlates with objective testing, and it is recommended that all members of a team with a significant exposure are assessed with boothless audiometry downrange, if the equipment is available. Much less satisfactory is the use of tuning forks, which may provide some information to help differentiate types of hearing loss and identify the worse-hearing ear but are inadequate for decision-making if serious suspicion of hearing injury exists.

Limitations of Treatment

The best mitigation of noise-induced hearing injury is avoidance of exposure. If this is not possible, then appropriate use of personal protective equipment is the next most effective option. Several potential prophylactic and treatment options have been mooted, including a variety of vitamins, antioxidants, and, more recently, near-infrared light. None of these yet have convincing evidence to support their routine use; glucocorticoid steroids have the strongest evidence base for post-exposure treatment of AAT. Some of the

rationale for this originated from the treatment of other conditions, such as Idiopathic Sudden Onset Sensorineural Hearing Loss (ISSHL). Current evidence for the treatment of ISSHL suggests intratympanic injection is superior to oral administration of steroid as salvage and as first-line treatment. The authors' own case series has shown very promising initial results for the treatment of AAT, with more than 80% of patients treated showing significant recovery following early ITSI +/- oral steroid treatment.

Options include the following:

Oral Steroids – Typically given as Prednisolone 1 mg/kg^{-1} up to a maximum of 60 mg once a day with a Proton Pump Inhibitor (PPI) cover to prevent gastric side effects.

- **Advantages:** Readily accessible, does not require specialist equipment or skills to administer, and can be commenced soon after injury.
- **Disadvantages:** The main concerns are lower levels of steroid in the inner ear compared to other routes of administration and the risk of systemic side effects. Whilst PPI cover may mitigate gastric side effects, the risks of sleep disturbance (common), steroid psychosis (uncommon), and avascular necrosis of the hip (uncommon) are particularly concerning in a military population. The risk of sleep disturbance and steroid psychosis necessitate the possible removal of access to weapons, avoidance of driving, and machine operation. In the presence of other injuries, particularly head injury, polytrauma and burns systemic steroid administration may be contraindicated.

Intratympanic Steroids – Typically given as Methylprednisolone 125 mg dissolved in water for injection (instructions for the procedure below); variable total dose dependant on volume of the middle ear. Dexamethasone is less irritant to middle ear mucosa and is reported to be less painful, but controversy exists as to which medication produces higher intracochlear steroid concentrations. ITSIs can be repeated, and the efficacy of this is an area where further research is needed. Typical protocols involve audiometry prior to ITSI, 1 week and 1, 6, and 12 months post-steroid administration.

- **Advantages:** High intracochlear steroid levels and much lower systemic concentration. Hence, the lower risk of potentially career-ending systemic side effects.
- **Disadvantage:** Requires specialist skills and equipment that may not be available near the point of injury. Small procedure associated risks if done by an otologist or ENT surgeon.

Intravenous Steroids – Can be administered without the equipment or expertise for intratympanic administration.

- **Advantages:** Intravenous administration allows high systemic levels in rapid time. Does not require specialist skills or equipment.
- **Disadvantages:** High systemic steroid levels are accompanied by increased associated risks. Some expertise required to administer, and the patient will require 'bedding down' with monitoring whilst the treatment is given.

Combination Approach (Oral and Intratympanic Administration) - As the evidence base for steroid treatment is still evolving, a lack of certainty exists as to the optimum agent, dose, and route of administration. A combination approach, where oral steroids start as close to the point of injury as possible once a hearing injury is objectively recorded and evacuation to a location where intratympanic treatment may be given, has much appeal.

- **Advantages:** Allows prompt treatment by oral administration and subsequently high intracochlear concentrations via intratympanic route.
- **Disadvantages:** Likely to require removal from an operational environment for intratympanic treatment.

Bone Conducting Hearing Systems

Conductive losses, such as those caused by blast-induced perforation, may benefit from the use of bone conductive hearing aids. Recent devices, such as the ADHEAR™ (MED-EL) or via a headband, may avoid the need for skin-penetrating osseo-integrated components, though they are limited to patients with well-preserved bone conduction thresholds.

Such devices are used immediately after injury to overcome the conductive element of an AAT may allow consents to be taken, and reduce anxiety resultant from a sense isolation a victim may have after a blast exposure.

Knowledge Update (Brief Review of Material)

The interaction between occupational noise exposure and hearing loss in the military was first documented in the 1500s by Amboise Paré, a French war surgeon, who noted that his patients suffered hearing loss as a result of weapon firing. Three hundred years later, John Fosbroke described both acute and chronic noise-induced hearing injuries. Despite these observations, combat deployment is still associated with high rates of hearing injury. Currently, hearing injuries account for approximately 4% of medical discharges across all three services in the UK.

Hearing impairment has been shown to impact service personnel performance in several environments including tank combat, dismounted close combat, and ship-to-ship communications. In close combat scenarios, even a relatively modest simulated hearing impairment has been associated with reduced situational awareness, lethality, reduced willingness to operate aggressively (i.e. reluctance to go forward), and a significant increase of in the risk of a 'blue on blue' incident. There may be operational considerations which take priority and necessitate acutely hearing injured personnel continuing in the fight, but this must be weighed against the increased risk to the person themselves and to their colleagues because of their potentially impaired performance.

In blast-exposed military patients, approximately 10–50% will have tympanic membrane rupture. Amongst this group, approximately 75% report hearing loss and 50% tinnitus. Spontaneous healing occurs in approximately 50%, with the other 50% requiring surgical closure.

In the past, the established understanding of the mechanism by which noise-induced hearing loss occurs was that acoustic overexposure caused impairment of outer hair cell function within the cochlea, worsening hearing. If the exposure were moderate and for a brief period, the effects would reverse in what was termed a 'Temporary Threshold Shift

(TTS).' If the hearing impairment did not improve, it was termed a 'Permanent Threshold Shift (PTS).' Recent improvements in understanding have shown more clearly other major influences such as the frequency of exposure and individual susceptibility.

Some consider a TTS of up to 50 dB may recover completely, though this opinion is far from universal and controversy exists as to the length of time at which a change should be classified as a PTS. Most TTS recovery is expected within 16–24 hours, but animal studies have shown improvement up to three weeks post-exposure. More recent animal studies (mice, rats, chinchillas, and non-human primates) have shown that even in animals, following noise exposure where complete recovery of hearing thresholds has been noted, histological examination of the cochlear demonstrates the loss of up to 90% of the synapses between the inner hair cell and the spiral ganglion neurone (the first part of the auditory nerve). This suggests that the idea that a TTS is harmless may not be true and, if this is correct, current health and safety guidelines regarding safe levels and durations of exposure are based on a misconception. Second, whilst outer hair cells are responsible for amplification within the cochlea, it is the inner hair cell/spiral ganglion area that is responsible for the encoding of complex signals, such as speech in background noise. Poor-quality encoding due to injury at this synapse could explain the

tinnitus and hyperacusis often associated with blast injury – as a result of increased central gain – as a compensatory mechanism for impaired encoding. Human studies looking for 'Hidden Hearing Loss' – Cochlear Synaptopathy, as it is more accurately termed – have not yet provided any firm evidence and studies, including that of Armed Forces personnel are ongoing. It may be that humans are more resistant to this phenomenon than animals, but it is more likely that either current test measures are not sensitive enough to detect synaptopathy without histological analysis of the temporal bone or that the civilian populations studied so far have not had sufficient noise exposure to induce it. Improved understanding of the site of lesion within the auditory pathway is an essential stepping stone to the validation of novel therapeutics that are currently in animal and early phase human trials for the regeneration of inner ear structures, or for pharmacological protection of structures prior to noise exposure.

Step-by-step procedure

Description of technique for intratympanic steroid injection – This procedure should currently only be undertaken by a consultant otologist/ENT surgeon (Figures 18.1–18.6):

1. Prior to the procedure, the patient should be warned about the risks of bleeding, infection,

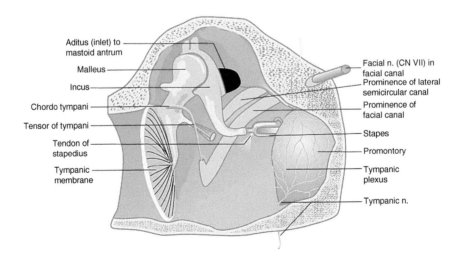

Figure 18.1 Middle ear anatomy. (Reproduced with permission from Tysome, J. and Kanegaonkar, R. *ENT: An Introduction and Practical Guide*. Taylor & Francis Group, 2018.)

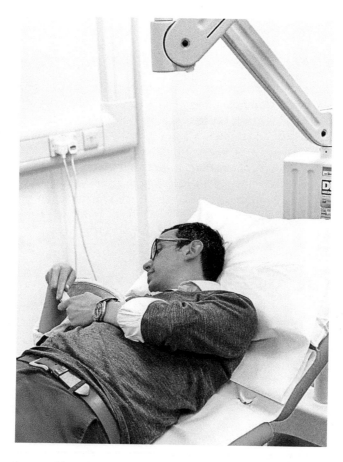

Figure 18.2 Step 2: patient positioned with vomit bowl for saliva to avoid swallowing.

pain, persistent perforation, failure to improve, worse hearing/tinnitus, transient dizziness, sleep disturbance; the very rare risks of ossicular disruption, steroid psychosis, avascular necrosis of the hip; and the unknown effect of steroid on the ossicles long term.

2. The patient should be warned that after injection, they should remain with the injected ear upwards and avoid swallowing or speaking, as such movements cause the opening of the Eustachian Tube and drainage of the steroid away from the middle ear and into the nose. A vomit bowl or similar should be provided for the patient to spit into rather than swallowing their own saliva.

3. The patient should be positioned supine with the otologist sitting on the side of their injured ear.

4. The patient's head is gently positioned away from the otologist, so the injured ear is upwards and there is a clear view down the ear canal with either a microscope or endoscope.

5. Options for local anaesthetic include Xylocaine (Lidocaine/Lignocaine) spray, typically at 5% or 10% – the latter is the authors' preference. Other options include injection of 2% Lignocaine with 1:80,000 Adrenaline. Some clinicians suggest that local anaesthetic is not required if a sufficiently small spinal needle is used; however, this is not the authors' usual practice.

6. Using a 25G spinal needle attached to a 2-mL syringe, gently inject steroid (typically 125 mg Methylprednisolone but Dexamethasone can be used as an alternative), at body temperature

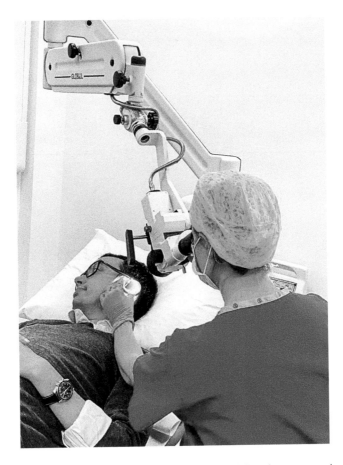

Figure 18.3 Steps 3 and 4: otologist positioned with the patient's injured ear upwards.

through an anterio-superior puncture. A fluid level rising behind the tympanic membrane should be visible. Fill the middle ear to capacity. The tympanic cavity varies in size from approximately 0.5–1 cm^3, though due to potential drainage into the mastoid cavity or via the Eustachian Tube, injecting until capacity is reasonable.

7. Methylprednisolone irritates the middle ear mucosa so patients often report a burning sensation following injection, which may last until the next day. Some clinicians reduce this by mixing the steroid with a local anaesthetic, the disadvantage is that this reduces the volume of steroid instilled and local anaesthetics are emetogenic and vestibulotoxic may increase the risk of post-procedure dizziness, so the solution is not recommended by the authors. To help reduce discomfort, simple analgesia is given prior to the procedure.

8. After the procedure, the patient should remain injected ear up, not speaking or swallowing for 30 minutes.

9. Given the small iatrogenic perforation caused by the injection, the patient should be encouraged to keep their ears dry to reduce the risk of infection until the hole has been observed to have healed. This includes using cotton wool rubbed in Vaseline placed in the conchal bowl when they shower. They should also be advised to avoid Valsalva, blowing their nose, or sneezing without their mouth open.

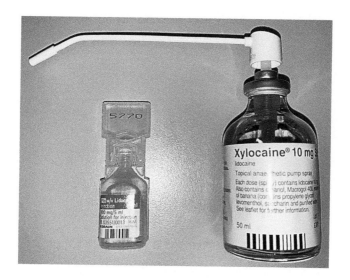

Figure 18.4 Step 5: local anaesthetic – shown here 10% Xylocaine spray and 2% Lignocaine.

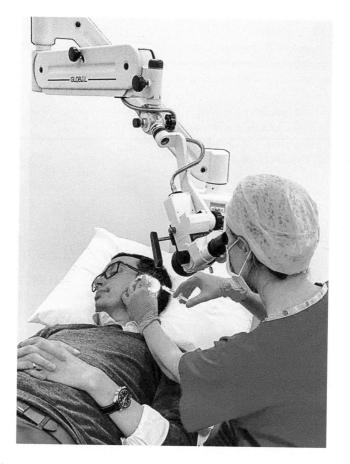

Figure 18.5 Step 6: (We've got two pictures showing this stage. I'm not sure if you want to keep both or rename one). First picture: Methylprednisolone, 25G spinal needle and syringe.

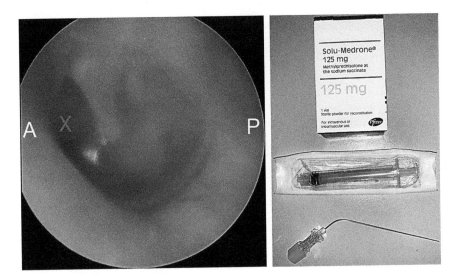

Figure 18.6 Step 7: Second picture: Injection of steroid. Left TM with red X is the location for TM puncture marked with red X. A, Anterior; P, Posterior.

10. Currently, post-AAT patients are reviewed with audiometric testing at one week, but this may change if evidence shows more frequent ITSIs are more efficacious. Subsequent follow up is at 1, 3, 6, and 12 months if no second injection is administered.
11. Post-treatment advice, in collaboration with Occupation Health, is given to the patient for the degree to which they should or should not be exposed to noise. This is currently a challenging area as the degree of risk to the remaining hearing after a person has had a hearing injury +/− successfully rescued, who then sustains another injury, acute, or chronic, is poorly understood.

KEY CONCEPTS

1 – Acute hearing injury should be suspected in any person in the vicinity of a blast or exposure to significant noise when hearing is unprotected.

2 – Treatment of acute hearing loss involves removal from further noise exposure, objective testing of hearing, and may require the administration of steroids – the efficacy of treatment can be significantly affected by delays in its' administration.

3 – The evidence base is rapidly evolving so all cases should be discussed with a Role 4 ENT surgeon to plan a treatment regime and MEDEVAC if required.

Key Points

1. Hearing injuries due to blast and acoustic trauma are common and should be suspected when reported by the patient or in the presence of other blast injuries to the patient or others injured close by.
2. In the military hearing, injury may severely impair the patient's warfighting performance including reluctance to go forward, misinterpretation of instructions, and significantly increasing the risk of 'blue on blue' casualties.

3. Injuries may be conductive, sensorineural, or mixed in nature, and appropriate examination involves an examination of the ears to ensure they are not occluded with debris and the drum is intact through an appropriate hearing assessment.

4. The use of boothless audiometry equipment may allow quantitative assessment of hearing but typically require at least a quiet room (i.e. less noise than typical conversation).

5. Emerging evidence supports the use of steroid treatment as rescue following acute hearing injury.

6. A trade-off exists between the ease and efficacy of oral steroid administration when compared to intratympanic injection. Oral steroids are easier and require no specialist equipment or expertise. Intratympanic steroids allow higher concentrations of medication to reach the inner ear without elevated levels of systemic absorption but require equipment and expertise that may not be available close to the point of injury if the incident occurs outside the UK.

7. There is increasing evidence that an earlier hearing injury predisposes the individual to worse outcomes with a subsequent hearing injury. As such, all those affected should receive an Occupational Health consultant review and, at the very least, have maximum hearing protection and minimal noise in their role.

8. Blast and impulse noise exposure—significant enough to cause a Temporary Threshold Shift—are associated with higher levels of reported hearing difficulties in the future. This may be due to injury further along the hearing pathway which may not be reflected in the patient's Pure Tone Audiogram.

9. Owing to the potential career and long-term quality of life implications, meticulous documentation and counselling are required.

10. Due to the potential risks and benefits involved, all military cases should be discussed with a Role 4 ENT surgeon to formulate the most appropriate management plan and expedite evacuation for intratympanic treatment, if required.

FURTHER READING

Keller MD, Ziriax JM, Barns W, Sheffield B, Brungart D, Thomas T, Jaeger B, Yankaskas K. Performance in noise: impact of reduced speech intelligibility on Sailor performance in a Navy command and control environment. *Hearing Res.* 2017 Jun 1;**349**:55–66.

McIlwain DS, Gates K, Ciliax D. Heritage of army audiology and the road ahead: the Army Hearing Program. *Am J Public Health.* 2008;**98(12)**:2167–2172. doi:10.2105/AJPH.2007.128504.

Peters LJ, Garinther GR. *The effects of speech intelligibility on crew performance in an M1A1 tank simulator.* Human Engineering Lab Aberdeen Proving Ground MD; 1990 Oct.

Phalguni A, Bayliss S, Moore D & Dretzke J. *Existing evidence on noise-induced hearing loss and tinnitus in the military and other occupational groups.* University of Birmingham. 2017. Available from http://epapers.bham.ac.uk/3036/1/Existing_evidence_on_NIHL_and_tinnitus_in_the_military_and_other_occupational_groups.pdf.

Ritenour AE, Wickley A, Ritenour JS, Kriete BR, Blackbourne LH, Holcomb JB, Wade CE. Tympanic membrane perforation and hearing loss from blast overpressure in Operation Enduring Freedom and Operation Iraqi Freedom wounded. *J Trauma Acute Care Surg.* 2008 Feb 1;**64(2)**:S174–8.

Ryan AF, Kujawa SG, Hammill T, Le Prell C, Kil J. Temporary and permanent noise-induced threshold shifts: a review of basic and clinical observations. *Otol Neurotol.* 2016 Sep;**37(8)**:e271.

Sheffield B, Brungart D, Tufts J, Ness J. The effects of elevated hearing thresholds on performance in a paintball simulation of individual dismounted combat. *Int J Audiol.* 2017 Jan 23;**56(sup1)**:34–40.

Taylor IG, Markides A. *Disorders of auditory function*: Volume III. Elsevier 2014. P17 US DoD Hearing Center of Excellence Website. Available from https://hearing.health.mil/.

Wells TS, Seelig AD, Ryan MA, Jones JM, Hooper TI, Jacobson IG, Boyko EJ. Hearing loss associated with US military combat deployment. *Noise Health.* 2015 Jan; **17(74)**:34.

Obstetrics in Limited-Resource Settings 19

Carlos Pilasi Menichetti and Rebekka Troller

INTRODUCTION

The reproductive health risks that all women face are greatly exacerbated when healthcare facilities are inadequate, equipment and medications are in short supply, and well-trained medical staff are few and far away. This is unfortunately the reality of many women living in resource-limited environments (RLE). Human resources present, or sent to collaborate in a humanitarian mission, are reduced in number; therefore, they are required to be flexible and cover areas that may be out of the surgeons' comfort zone. This is certainly what happens to a general surgeon sent to assist in a natural disaster or an armed conflict when exposed to obstetric emergencies. It must be mentioned that assisting in a humanitarian capacity or military operations may cover a spectrum of resources and environmental constraints when delivering emergency surgical care.

As published by the Lancet commission, there is a high proportion of the world's population without access to safe surgical and anaesthetic care. Moreover, if you also consider the density of surgeons, anaesthetists, and obstetricians, we can see that the same geographical regions around the world have less access to safe surgery; these regions are also the highest in maternal mortality related to childbirth and caesarean sections worldwide.

A peak in maternal mortality occurs during the intrapartum period around childbirth and the first day post-partum. Women are at risk of dying because of obstetric problems, and these are unfortunately prevalent in RLE; it is very likely that these women will present at a medical facility even though it has not been defined as a maternity.

Regarding armed conflicts, there is growing evidence to show the profound negative impact of conflict on maternal mortality: populations that have experienced armed conflict have among the highest rates. For these reasons, whenever an emergency response team is deployed to a limited resource area where a sudden onset disaster (SOD) has occurred or to medically assist victims in an armed conflict emergency obstetric skills must be ensured.

The five main causes of direct maternal death are the following:

1. Haemorrhage
2. Hypertensive disorders
3. Sepsis
4. Obstructed labour
5. Abortion

What are effective interventions to reduce maternal mortality?

There have been many strategies to reduce maternal mortality; however, the only proven approach to save the lives of the 75% of women who die in pregnancy and giving birth, and the 25% who die after birth, is the provision of emergency obstetric and newborn care. This can either be basic (BEmONC) or comprehensive (CEmONC). CEmONC interventions include safe blood transfusion, capacity to perform caesarean sections, manual removal of the placenta, assisted vaginal delivery, abortion, and resuscitation of the newborn; BEmONCs do not provide blood transfusion nor caesarean sections.

What can be done for each problem?

HAEMORRHAGE

Obstetric haemorrhage remains the leading cause of maternal mortality worldwide. In 2012, the World Health Organization (WHO) published new guidelines for the prevention and treatment of postpartum haemorrhage.

The management must cover adequate resuscitation, including the use of tranexamic acid, and identification of the cause for adequate treatment.

The antifibrinolytic therapy in post-partum haemorrhage has shown to be effective in reducing maternal mortality by 31% (reduction in death from bleeding when given to women for treatment of postpartum haemorrhage (PPH) within 1–3 hours after delivery).

> **The treatment, as with other life-threatening Haemorrhage, is to resuscitate the patient and identify the cause.**

Causes of PPH: (remember the 4Ts)

Postpartum haemorrhage, the loss of more than 500 mL of blood after delivery, is the most common maternal morbidity in developed countries. It may be caused by uterine atony after delivery, partial or complete placenta separation disorder, laceration of the genital tract, or uterine rupture.

The 4Ts for the common cause of bleeding (Figure 19.1):

Tone – Atonic uterus
Tissue – Retained placenta
Tears – Perineum/Cervix
Thrombin – Clotting abnormalities

Management

Rapid assessment, resuscitation, and observations (HR, BP, RR) should be undertaken. The patient should lie flat. Uterine atony is treated by bimanual uterine compression and massage, followed by drugs

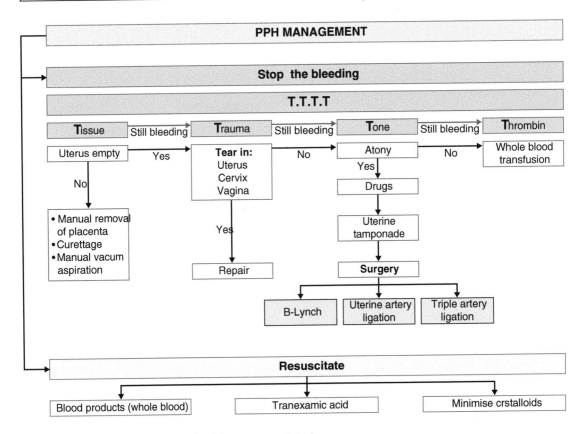

Figure 19.1 PPH management algorithm rest annotated.

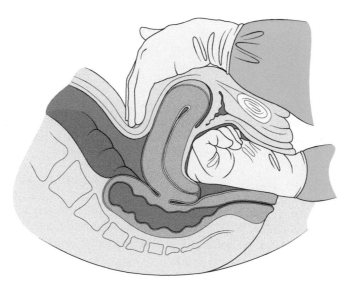

Figure 19.2 Technique of bimanual massage.

(Oxytocin 20 IU L^{-1} of normal saline, Carboprost 0.25 mg IM, Misoprostol (Cytotec) 1000 mcg rectally, Methylergonovine 0.2 mg IM). Two large-bore cannulas and blood test should be sent; then the bladder must be catheterised.

Diagnose the cause of the bleeding (4Ts) and stop the bleeding.

Bimanual compression of the uterus (Figure 19.2): one hand is introduced into the vagina, the fist compressing the cervix, while the external hand presses the fundus against the internal hand (Hamilton manoeuvre). The compression is maintained until the bleeding is controlled and the uterus contracted.

Examination under anaesthetic for persistent uterine atony often caused by retained placenta or clots. Ensure the uterine cavity is empty and suture tears if necessary.

Internal uterine tamponade:

A **Foley catheter** with a 30-mL balloon is easy to acquire (Figure 19.3). Insert the catheter inside a condom and tie the condom to the catheter with a vicryl suture without closing the catheter channel. Insert some water to ensure it is not leaking or too loose.

The condom can be inserted into the vagina and

uterus and the catheter filled with water. Make sure the catheter is spigoted; otherwise, the water will pour out.

The balloon will take 200–500 mL, depending on the type.

Leave the balloon in place for 6–24 hours with antibiotic cover.

A sterile glove can also be used in place of a condom.

B-Lynch Suture:

The most common and effective technique is the B-Lynch suture (Figure 19.4). The aim of this suture is to reduce the volume of the uterus. The

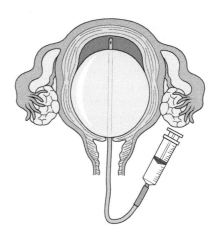

Figure 19.3 Foley catheter.

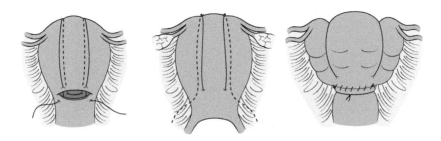

Figure 19.4 B-Lynch suture.

technique is described later. It can be done after normal delivery or caesarean section.

Packing the uterus with gauze soaked in antiseptic. The pack should be removed after 12 hours. Major haemorrhage needs compression of the aorta, ligation of the internal iliac arteries, or a hysterectomy (Figure 19.1).

HYPERTENSIVE DISORDERS

Pre-eclampsia and eclampsia are still estimated to cause approximately 30,000 maternal deaths annually worldwide, mostly in low- and middle-income countries.[11]

The first line of treatment is resuscitation with antihypertensive drugs; magnesium sulphate for severe preeclampsia and eclampsia.

The definitive treatment of eclampsia and pre-eclampsia is the termination of the pregnancy. This can be achieved by inducing labour, conducting a spontaneous labour, or via caesarean section. It is very important to highlight that in RLE, it is not possible to ensure that the patient will have access to a medical facility in her next pregnancy. This is relevant as the risk of leaving a uterine scar can be life-threatening for the mother following pregnancy. Having said that, if it is indicated, every effort should be made to provide caesarean section for the woman in need.

SEPSIS

The WHO published a statement on maternal sepsis in 2017: 'Maternal sepsis is a life-threatening condition defined as organ dysfunction resulting from infection during pregnancy, childbirth, post-abortion, or post-partum period'. Undetected or poorly managed maternal infections can lead to sepsis, death, or disability for the mother and increased likelihood of early neonatal infection and other adverse outcomes.

ABORTION

Unsafe abortion is a persistent, preventable pandemic. The WHO defines unsafe abortion as a procedure to terminate an unintended pregnancy either by individuals without the necessary skills, an environment that does not conform to minimum medical standards, or both. The main causes of death from unsafe abortion are haemorrhage, infection, sepsis, genital trauma, and bowel injuries. There are fewer data on nonfatal long-term health complications, but they include poor wound healing, infertility, consequences of organ injury (urinary and stool incontinence from vesicovaginal or rectovaginal fistulas), and bowel resections.

> **Provision of safe abortion (medical and surgical options) is a proven strategy to reduce maternal mortality.**

OBSTRUCTED LABOUR

Another important source of mortality is obstructed labour. Despite some indications and conditions for instrumental deliveries (vacuum or forceps), caesarean section is probably the most frequent technique. When medically justified, a caesarean section can effectively prevent maternal and perinatal mortality and morbidity. However, there is no evidence showing the benefits of caesarean delivery for women or infants who do not require the procedure. As with any surgery, caesarean sections are associated with short- and long-term risk which can extend years beyond the current delivery and affect the health of the woman, her child, and future pregnancies. These risks are higher in women with limited access to comprehensive obstetric care.

- It must be remembered that leaving a woman with a uterine scar increases her risks in future pregnancies (higher risks of uterine rupture and abnormal placentation), and therefore, the decision deserves a thoughtful analysis.
- Even though there are different options for management, there is also a role for surgery in all five main causes of maternal death.
- Providing safe caesarean section and managing the bleeding related to pregnancy, especially post-partum haemorrhage (PPH), can reduce up to 70% of direct maternal deaths.
- Caesarean section provision and PPH management are two skills that a surgeon deployed to assist in a humanitarian projects must be familiar with.
- It is not expected that an emergency hospital dealing with different pathologies will transform into a maternity; however, women with obstetric complications will present if there is no other facility. Having the availability to perform emergency caesarean section as well as blood transfusion and management of post-partum haemorrhage must be part of the services provided.
- Training on caesarean sections as well as management of post-partum haemorrhage are skills a general surgeon must acquire *before* deployment to humanitarian missions in low resource settings.

CAESAREAN SECTION

Indications

In austere environment, emergency indications for caesarean section (CS) are predominant – there is rarely an elective operation, dictated by rudimental infra-structure. Severe pre-eclampsia or eclampsia are the most important indication due to maternal condition. More frequent indications are when the foetus is at risk such as cord prolapse, strangulation, protracted or obstructed labour, placental insufficiency, infection, or prematurity causing fetal distress.

Obstructed labour, amnion infection, and placental abruption are the most important ones.

If the foetus has already died, caesarean section should be avoided in cases with placental abruption.

Techniques

Preoperative:

> Check fetal heart.
> Blood test (group and safe, Hb), electrolytes, coagulatory test.
> Consent and examine the patient prior to caesarean section.
> Epidural anaesthesia and IV line with infusion. Premedication with Ranitidine or Magnesium trisilicate 300 mg.
> 2 units of blood ready, if available.
> Urinary catheter, WHO safety checklist, skin disinfection, and patient covered with sterile sheets.
> Tilt the operating table to reduce aorto-caval compression.

Operation technique:

Ensure adequate analgesia by testing the area below umbilicus with forceps.

Right-handed surgeons stand on the right side of the patient. A Pfannenstiel incision (Figure 19.5) is performed: 10–12-cm straight incision 2 cm above the symphysis pubis. Alternatively, a lower abdominal midline incision (between umbilicus and symphysis) provides fast opening of the abdomen and it's easier to perform. The subcutaneous tissues are incised and brought down to the fascia at the centre of the incision.

The fascia is incised transversely with the scalpel (2 cm) and extended laterally with heavy curved Mayo scissors, or blunt with fingers. The superior edge of the fascia is grasped and elevated, and the fascia gently pulled cranially and caudally. Slowly stretch the muscle and subcutaneous tissue by bimanual bilateral traction and separate the rectus muscles with fingers. Use a Doyen's retractor to handle the lower segment and pull the bladder down (Figure 19.6).

The peritoneum is opened sharply transversely and extended bluntly with both index fingers, aiming high

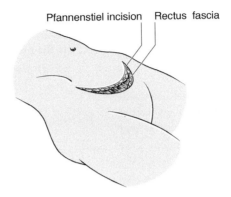

Figure 19.5 Pfannensteil incision.

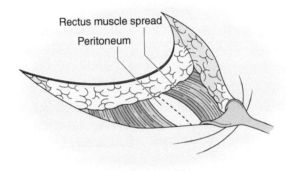

Figure 19.6 Doyen's retractor to handle the lower segment and pull the bladder down.

up the peritoneum (Figure 19.7). The gravid uterus will now be under direct vision. After the peritoneum is opened, the serosa at the site of the plica vesico-uterina has to be cut transversely; push the bladder downwards.

Replace the bladder retractor under the opened peritoneum.

> **Make sure the bladder is reflected down, exposing the uterus. You do not want to enter the uterus via the bladder!**

A 3-cm transverse incision is made with a scalpel in the lower uterine segment; approximately 1 cm below the upper margin of the peritoneal reflection in the midline is the incision of choice until the membranes bulge (Figure 19.8). Insert fingers and open the uterus by stretching laterally.

> *Be careful not to injure the foetus, particularly in cases where the fluid is reduced or has already drained by premature rupture of the membranes.*

The operator's right hand is passed into the uterine cavity between the foetal head and symphysis pubis. The head is carefully flexed and elevated

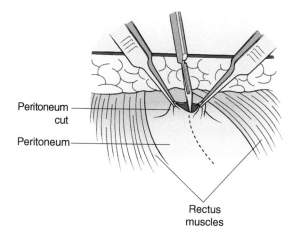

Figure 19.7 Sharp dissection of the peritoneum.

upwards into the uterine opening, and only then will the assistant provide mild fundal uterine pressure (Figure 19.9).

After the head, both shoulders are delivered with gentle traction. Two clamps are placed on the umbilical cord at least 10 cm from the abdomen and cut between the clamps with scissors. Hand the baby to the midwife.

Asked the anaesthetist to give Syntometrine or Oxytocin and antibiotic prophylaxis.

Now, the placenta is removed manually by a constant but controlled traction on the cord. Massaging the uterus with one hand can be helpful.

The placenta should be inspected for completeness and the womb should be checked for retained tissue or membranes using fingers or sterile swab.

Grab inferior and posterior edge of uterine incision and suture the uterus with a running-lock suture about 1 cm apart for haemostasis using Vicryl O suture. Start a second layer of suture just lateral to the lateral angle sutures. If necessary, additional cross-stitches can be placed wherever significant bleeding is still prevalent. Large blood clots are removed in the paracolic gutters with a swab on a stick. Haemostasis should be checked at each layer. Fascial closure is done by running suture using Vicryl or PDS; skin closure with Monocryl or clips. A vaginal examination is performed to spot ongoing bleeding. Clots of blood from the vagina can be removed with a swab on a stick.

Postoperative Care

Assess the patient for vaginal bleeding prior to transfer to the ward. Do regular observations; consider 24 hours of antibiotics in cases of sepsis or prolonged rupture of membranes.

CAESARIAN SECTION FOR BREECH DELIVERY

Good exposure is essential. The abdominal and uterine incision should be of sufficient size. If the head is stuck in the pelvis, pulling the head from below could be necessary to deliver the baby.

Female genital mutilation (FGM)

This problem is not considered as a main source of mortality worldwide; however, it is prevalent in certain countries. More than 200 million girls and women alive today have been cut in 30 countries in Africa, the Middle East, and Asia, where FGM is concentrated.

Surgeons who will be deployed to high-prevalence FGM regions require a more in-depth preparation and information on this matter.

Some facts about FGM:

- FGM includes procedures that intentionally alter or cause injury to the female genital organs for non-medical reasons.

(a)

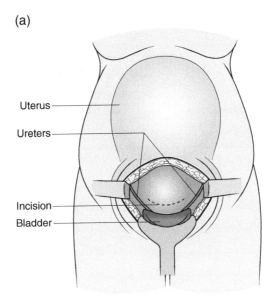

(b)

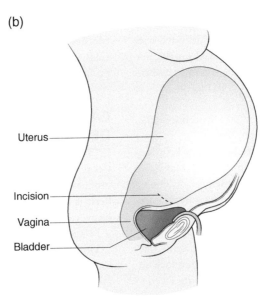

Figure 19.8 Uterine incision location.

- The procedure has no health benefits for girls and women.
- Procedures can cause severe bleeding, infection, and – in the longer run – urinating problems as well as complications in childbirth and increased risk of newborn deaths.
- FGM is mostly carried out on young girls between infancy and age 15.

- FGM is a violation of the human rights of girls and women.

TYPES AND DEFINITIONS

Female genital mutilation is classified into four major types by the WHO. These procedures are

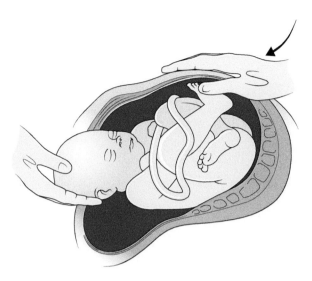

Figure 19.9 Delivery of foetus.

almost always done by traditional circumcisers who often play other central roles in communities, such as attending to childbirths. The poor hygiene conditions contribute to the already massive harm done to these girls. However, surgeons as any other health care providers, must not perform it based on the erroneous belief that the procedure is safer when medicalised.[16] The WHO clearly and strongly call on health professionals not to perform such procedures because there is no medical indication for it and there are not health benefits. On the contrary, it violates a person's rights to health, security and physical integrity, their right to be free from torture and cruel, inhuman or degrading treatment, and the right to life when the procedure results in death. It is nearly always carried out in minors and, therefore, is a violation of the rights of children.

- **Type 1:** Often referred to as **clitoridectomy**, this is the partial or total removal of the clitoris or, in very rare cases, only the prepuce.
- **Type 2:** Often referred to as **excision**, this is the partial or total removal of the clitoris and the labia minora, with or without excision of the labia majora.
- **Type 3:** Often referred to as **infibulation**, this is the narrowing of the vaginal opening through the creation of a covering seal. The seal is formed by cutting and repositioning the labia minora, or labia majora, sometimes through stitching, with or without removal of the clitoris.
- **Type 4:** This includes all other harmful procedures to the female genitalia for non-medical purposes (e.g., pricking, piercing, incising, scraping, and cauterising the genital area).

It is unlikely for an expatriated surgeon to face acute complications because of the hidden nature and cultural beliefs where this procedure is performed. It is more frequent to face late complications that will become more evident during childbirth. Because of scarring and alteration of normal anatomy, FGM can be a cause of obstructed labour that will require some specific management.

Deinfibulation. This term refers to the practice of cutting open the sealed vaginal opening in a woman who has been infibulated, which is often necessary to improve health and well-being and to allow intercourse or facilitate childbirth. If the scarring tissue allows then deinfibulation as shown in Figure 19.10 can be undertaken. In case the introitus is exposed and there is scarring, an episiotomy (even bilaterally) may be needed during delivery.

As a medical professional, it is not accepted to re-infundibulise (cannot be sutured back to the way it was prior to deinfibulation) because it would counter the principle of 'do not harm' that all doctors subscribe to.

(a)

(b)

(c)

(d)

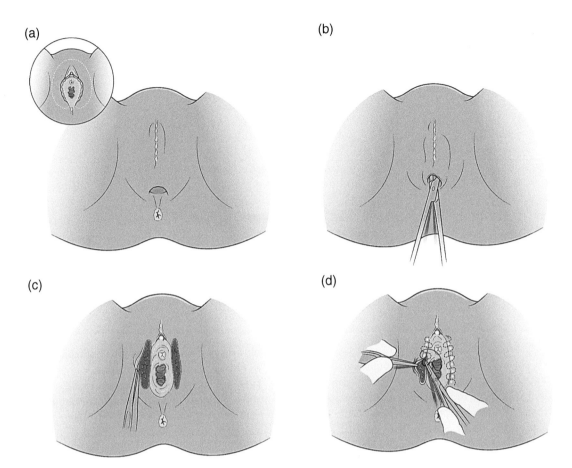

Figure 19.10 Deinfibulation

KEY POINTS:

The five main causes of direct maternal death are the following:

1. Haemorrhage
2. Hypertensive disorders
3. Sepsis
4. Obstructed labour
5. Abortion

The **4Ts** for the common cause of bleeding:

1. **Tone** – Atonic uterus
2. **Tissue** – Retained placenta
3. **Tears** – Perineum/Cervix
4. **Thrombin** – Clotting abnormalities

Resuscitate and address reversible causes.

FURTHER READING

1. World Health Organization. *WHO recommendations for the prevention and treatment of postpartum haemorrhage.* WHO; 2012.
2. Dildy GA, Belfort MA, Adair CD, et al. Initial experience with a dual-balloon catheter for the management of postpartum haemorrhage. *Am J Obstet Gynecol.* 2014;**210**:136.e1–136.e6.
3. Waves of burden of disease during a disaster graphed as hospital resources required over me. (*von Schreeb J, Riddez L, Samnegård H, Rosling H. Foreign eld hospitals in the recent sudden-onset disasters in Iran, Hai, Indonesia, and Pakistan. Prehospital and disaster medicine* 2008;**23(02)**:144–51.
4. Campbell OMR, Graham WJ. Strategies for reducing maternal mortality: getting on with what works. *Lancet.* 2006;**368(9543)**:1284–1299.

5. Filippi V, Ronsmans C, Campbell OMR, Graham WJ, Mills A, Borghi J, Koblinsky M, Osrin D. Maternal health in poor countries: the broader context and a call for action. *Lancet.* 2006;**368**(**9546**):1535–1541.

6. O'Hare BAM, Southall DP. First do no harm: the impact of recent armed conflict on maternal and child health in sub-Saharan Africa. *JRSM.* 2007; **100**(**12**):564–570.

7. Shakur-Still, H. et al. The WOMAN Trial (World Maternal Antifibrinolytic Trial): Tranexamic acid for the treatment of postpartum haemorrhage: An international randomised, double blind placebo controlled trial. *Trials.* **11**. 40. doi:10.1186/1745-6215-11-40.

8. B-Lynch C, Coker A, Lawal AH, Abu J, Cowen MJ. The B-Lynch surgical technique for the control of massive postpartum haemorrhage: an alternative to hysterectomy? Five cases reported. *Brit J Obstet Gynaecol* 1997;**104**(**3**):372-375.

9. World Health Organization. *The prevention and management of unsafe abortion. Report of a Technical Working Group.* http://whqlibdoc.who.int/hq/1992/WHO_MSM_92.5.pdf (accessed July 6, 2006)

10. World Health Organization. *Unsafe abortion, authors. Global and Regional Estimates of the Incidence of Unsafe Abortion and Associated Mortality in 2003.* 5th ed. Geneva: World Health Organization; 2007.

11. Hannah ME, Hannah WJ, Hewson SA, Hodnett ED, Saigal S, Willan AR. Planned caesarean section versus planned vaginal birth for breech presentation at term: a randomised multicentre trial. Term Breech Trial Collaborative Group. *Lancet.* 2000;**356**(**9239**):1375–1383.

12. Lumbiganon P, Laopaiboon M, Gulmezoglu AM, Souza JP, Taneepanichskul S, Ruyan P, et al. Method of delivery and pregnancy outcomes in Asia: the WHO global survey on maternal and perinatal health 2007–08. *Lancet.* 2010;**375**:490–499.

13. Villar J, Carroli G, Zavaleta N, Donner A, Wojdyla D, Faundes A, et al. Maternal and neonatal individual risks and benefits associated with caesarean delivery: multicentre prospective study. *BMJ.* 2007;**335**(**7628**): 1025.

14. Souza JP, Gulmezoglu A, Lumbiganon P, Laopaiboon M, Carroli G, Fawole B, et al. Caesarean section without medical indications is associated with an increased risk of adverse short-term maternal outcomes: the 2004-2008 WHO Global Survey on Maternal and Perinatal Health. *BMC Med.* 2010;**8**:71.

15. https://www.who.int/news-room/fact-sheets/detail/female-genital-mutilation.

16. https://www.unicef.org/media/files/FGMC_2016_brochure_final_UNICEF_SPREAD.pdf

17. Johnson, C. et al. Surgical techniques: surgical techniques: defibulation of type III female genital cutting. *J Sex Med.* Volume **4**, Issue **6**; 1544–1547

18. http://nationalfgmcentre.org.uk/fgm/fgm-medical-examination/.

Index

Note: *Italicized* page numbers refer to figures, **bold** page numbers refer to tables